Meet LifeSmart...

LifeSmart was designed with YOU in mind. Through real-world examples, career applications, and online interactivities, *LifeSmart* offers a dynamic learning experience designed for today's students.

What's Inside?

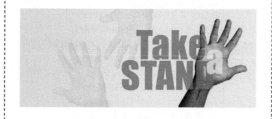

"Take a Stand" asks you to take an informed position on a controversial issue.

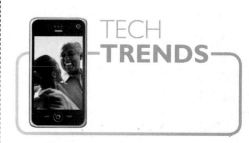

"Tech Trends" show how technology can aid in understanding human development.

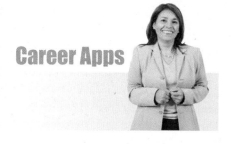

Career Apps

"Career Apps" apply the concepts of human development to real-life careers.

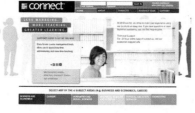

"Connect Psychology" is a response to the learning preferences of today's student. The groundbreaking adaptive diagnostic tool helps students "know what they know" while guiding them to experience and learn what they don't know through engaging interactivities, exercises, and readings.

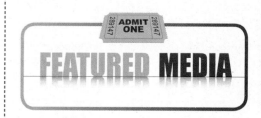

"Featured Media" connects popular movies and television shows to topics in the chapter, helping to bring key concepts to life.

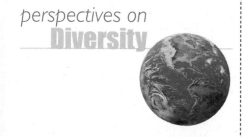

perspectives on **Diversity**

"Perspectives on Diversity" discuss human develpment in the context of race, ethnicity, and cross-cultural issues.

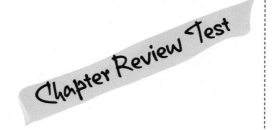

Chapter Review Test

"Chapter Review Test" allows you to check your mastery of core concepts.

My friend has a **baby.** *I'm* recording *all the* **noises** *he makes so later I can* ask *him* **what he meant.**

STEPHEN WRIGHT

"Short quotations" help make the content memorable.

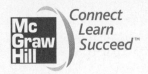
LifeSmart

VICE PRESIDENT, EDITORIAL **Michael Ryan**
EDITORIAL DIRECTOR **Beth Ann Mejia**
PUBLISHER **Michael Sugarman**
DIRECTOR OF DEVELOPMENT **Dawn Groundwater**
EXECUTIVE EDITOR **Krista Bettino**
DEVELOPMENT EDITOR **Joanne Fraser**
EDITORIAL COORDINATOR **Megan Stotts**
EXECUTIVE MARKETING MANAGER **Julia Larkin Flohr**
MARKETING MANAGER **Yasuko Okada**
PRODUCTION EDITOR **Regina Ernst**
MANUSCRIPT EDITOR **Margaret Moore**
DESIGN MANAGER AND COVER **Cassandra Chu**
INTERIOR DESIGN **Maureen McCutcheon**
LEAD PHOTO RESEARCH COORDINATOR **Alexandra Ambrose**
PHOTO RESEARCHER **Judy Mason**
ART MANAGER **Robin Mouat**
ILLUSTRATORS **Bill Graham, John and Judy Waller, and Lachina Publishing**
MEDIA PROJECT MANAGERS **Thomas Brierly and David Blatty**
SENIOR PRODUCTION SUPERVISOR **Louis Swaim**
COMPOSITION **10/12 Times by Lachina Publishing Services**
PRINTING **45# Influence Gloss, Quad/Graphics**
COVER IMAGES FRONT COVER: BLINK/CORBIS; BACK COVER: PURESTOCK/GETTY IMAGES; INSIDE COVER (TOP TO BOTTOM): BALLYSCANLON/GETTY IMAGES,
AMOS MORGAN/GETTY IMAGES, RUBBERBALL PRODUCTIONS, RYAN MCVAY/GETTY IMAGES, AMOS MORGAN/GETTY IMAGES, CORBIS/PUNCHSTOCK,
RUBBERBALL PRODUCTIONS, RYAN MCVAY/GETTY IMAGES, RYAN MCVAY/GETTY IMAGES

Library of Congress Cataloging-in-Publication Data

Fiore, Lisa B., 1970-

Lifesmart / Lisa Fiore.
p. cm.
ISBN-13: 978-0-07-803524-1 (alk. paper)
ISBN-10: 0-07-803524-4 (alk. paper)
1. Longevity. 2. Life spans (Biology) I. Title.
QH528.5.F56 2010
155—dc22

2010034721

Meet LIFESMART from McGraw-Hill.

LifeSmart is the newest member of the McGraw-Hill M Series, the series that started with YOUR students.

WE LISTENED TO STUDENTS.

Based on extensive student research, we have created a complete learning resource to meet the needs and maximize the workflow of today's college students. Students told us they wanted a briefer text with more visual appeal . . . and a lower price.

WE ALSO LISTENED TO INSTRUCTORS.

We learned about the challenges that they faced in their classrooms every day and what their ideal course materials would look like. They told us they needed an engaging solution for their course needs—but without sacrificing quality and content.

WE RESPONDED.

LifeSmart blends core content and research with a wealth of real-world examples, career applications, and online interactivities to create a dynamic and engaging learning solution for today's students.

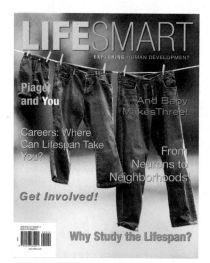

Meet the Author

Name: Lisa Beth Fiore

Occupations: Mom (24/7); developmental and educational psychology professor and director of Early Childhood Education

Family: husband Steve, son Matthew (8), and daughter Talia (6)

Hobbies: theater, "making art" (as Talia says), walking

Childhood ambition: to solve mysteries with the Hardy Boys

Last book read: Norton Juster's The Phantom Tollbooth and Rachel Vail's Just in Case

Favorite film: Shakespeare in Love

Favorite tune to beat the blues: Beautiful by Christina Aguilera (and almost anything by James Taylor)

Latest accomplishment: learning to feel less guilty about saying "no"

Future feat: to run the Boston Marathon

Quote: "At some point in life the world's beauty becomes enough. You don't need to photograph, paint, or even remember it. It is enough."   —Toni Morrison, from Tar Baby

LifeSmart

BRIEF CONTENTS

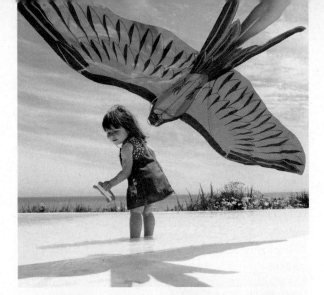

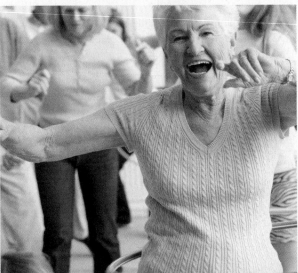

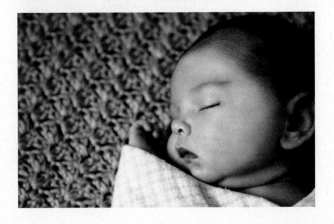

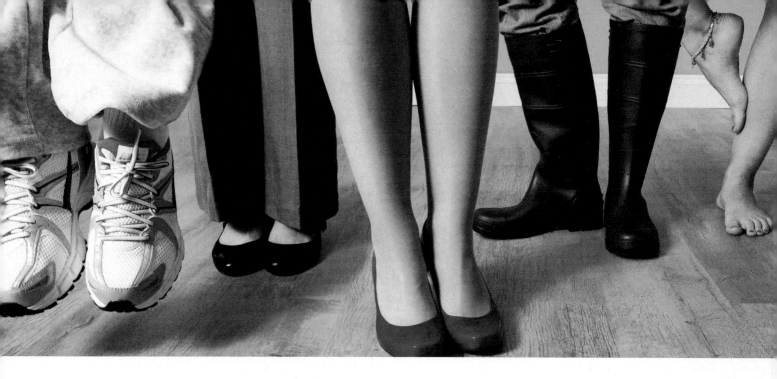

1 > Lifespan Development: An Introduction

2 > Theories of Development: Interpreting the Lifespan

Table of Contents

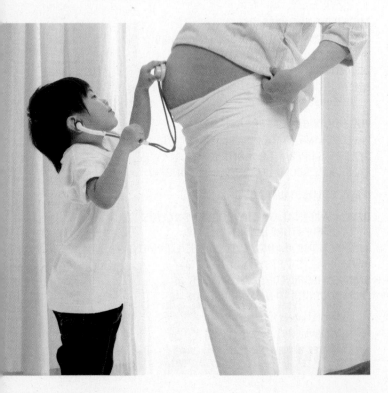

5 > Infancy

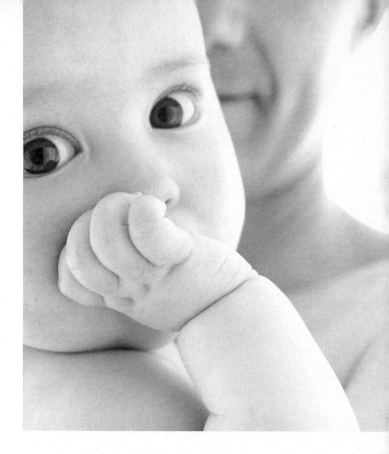

6 > Early Childhood

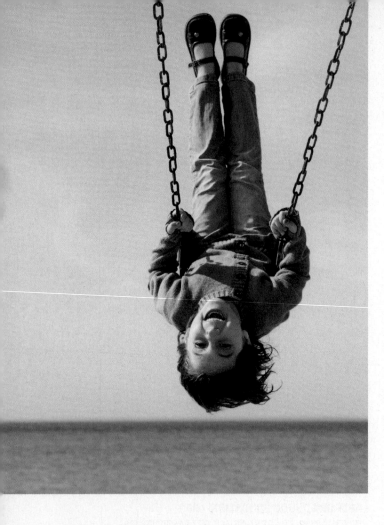

8 > Adolescence

7 > Middle Childhood

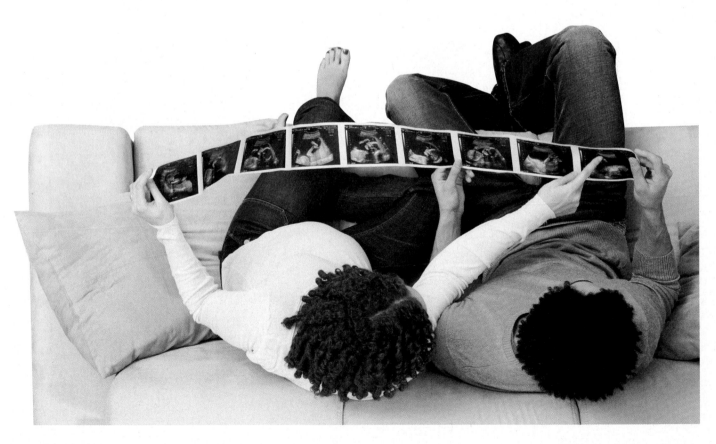

11 > Late Adulthood

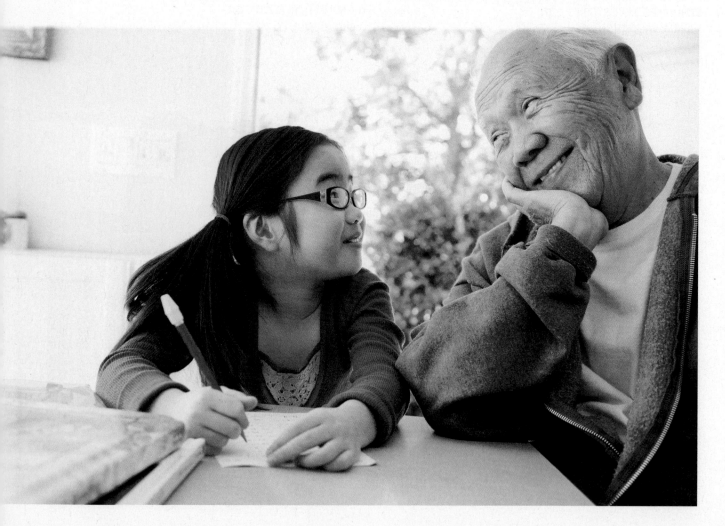

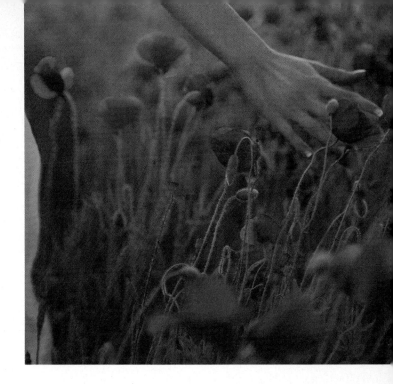

12 > Dying and Spirituality

13 > Putting It All Together: Lifespan Development in Action

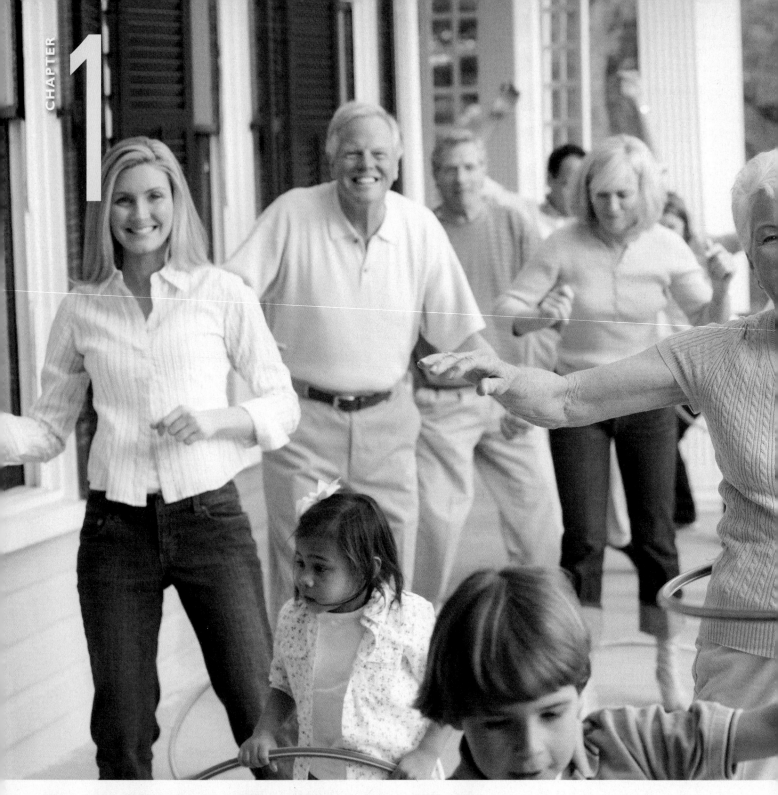

LIFESPAN DEVELOPMENT:

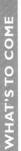

As You READ

After reading this chapter, you should be able to answer the following questions:

- How would you define and describe lifespan development?

- What are the different views of lifespan development?

- What role do biopsychosocial interactions play in lifespan development?

- What are the major issues in lifespan development?

- What is the role of research in studying lifespan development?

AN INTRODUCTION

re you curious?

A One of the traits that sets humans apart from other living creatures is the innate desire to find out the answer to the biggest, most commonly asked question since the dawn of time: "Why?" Over the course of a person's life this question takes different forms. For example:

- **Why** is the sky blue?

- **Why** do I need to go to bed so early?

- **Why** can't I find work to inspire me?

- **Why** do I have to pee *again*? (I just went 15 minutes ago!)

If you try to pinpoint which age is the one during which one of the sample "why" questions is most typically asked, you would have a difficult time. A 2-year-old might ask why the sky is blue, as might a graduate student in environmental studies. Similarly, an elderly man might wonder why he has to urinate so frequently, just as a pregnant woman in her mid-20s ponders the same phenomenon. It is precisely this questioning spirit and the desire to search for answers that propels the researcher in all of us to study human development. The material you will read as you work through this book will reveal much new information and some information that you, as a living and breathing individual on Earth, already understand by virtue of being—human being.

The process of following our questions, also called hypotheses, and generalizing our findings to a larger population is the foundation of scientific research. Scientific research is the work on which the field of lifespan development was built, as you will learn in the chapters that follow. The assumptions and biases that are part of the scientific method may or may not be stated explicitly, either in the original research articles or in the pages of this text. It is for this reason that you should keep the big questions in your mind as you read on. Never be afraid to ask, "Why?" . . . it is the beginning of a journey that leads you to some answers and, ultimately, more questions.

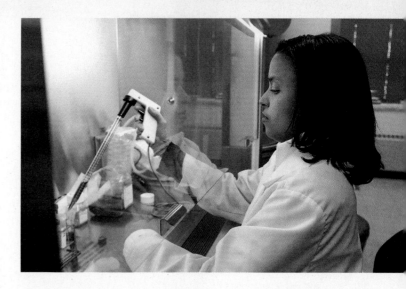

The highly popular youth fiction series Choose Your Own Adventure remains popular with young readers because the books are designed to let the reader have some control over the outcome of the stories. What a concept—control over one's (or a fictional character's) destiny! This concept of having control over our own lives is one that researchers have investigated for centuries and one that businesses take advantage of as they sell products that promise us that ability. As researchers have studied human development, certain factors have been identified as "risk" factors—things that seem to influence our lives in negative ways. The more risk factors a person is faced with in her life, the harder it will be for her to be happy and successful throughout her life. Other factors have been identified as protective factors that allow someone to succeed—or even survive—great challenges. The following study underscores the idea that a host of factors, positive and negative, work together in an extremely complex way to influence human development over time.

During the year 1955, psychologists Emmy Werner and Ruth Smith (1992, 1995, 2001) began to collect data on every child born on the Hawaiian island of Kauai. That year, a total of 837 children were born. Amazingly, Werner and Smith studied 505 of these children from their prenatal days until they were in their early 30s. (The drop in the

From time to time ... you will be asked to **make a choice.** *Your choice may lead to* **success or disaster!** .... *The adventures you take are a result of your choice. You are responsible because you choose!* .... **Remember**—*you cannot go back!* **Think carefully** *before you make a move! One mistake can be your last ... or it may lead you to fame and fortune!*—**WARNING!!!**

—DISCLAIMER FROM *THE CAVE OF TIME*, THE FIRST BOOK IN THE CHOOSE YOUR OWN ADVENTURE SERIES, BY EDWARD PACKARD (1979)

number of children studied was due to some of the children dying, some moving to other islands, and some moving to the U.S. mainland.)

Of the 505 children in the group, one in three was born with the threat of serious developmental difficulties, such as the effects of a difficult birth or an environment that triggered tough challenges. Some faced the prospect of a life of grinding poverty. Throughout their lives, others experienced divorce, desertion, alcoholism, or mental illness. Two out of three people in this so-designated vulnerable group were born exposed to four or more daunting risk factors—factors that scientists had determined to predict negative life outcomes. And yet, one in three of these high-risk children developed into a confident, competent adult.

Why do some individuals beat the odds? What developmental forces enable some people to overcome dramatically difficult obstacles and yet permit others to succumb? In a sense, the children of Kauai provide us with a window through which we can view the events that shape the lifespan—the biological, psychological, and environmental interactions that contribute to what we are. These brief glimpses of human development in one study lead us to ask even more questions: What combinations of these forces interact at what levels to produce differences in human development? What are the processes at work that *explain* what happened? Why?

With these ideas in mind, then, let's first explore the meaning of lifespan development and follow the developmental path of one well-known individual. **Lifespan development** refers to an examination of the biological, cognitive/psychological, and social changes that occur over the course of a human life. As the field of psychology has evolved as a discipline, lifespan development has emerged as one lens through which researchers look for explanations for many phenomena.

Looking closely at one example of lifespan development illustrates how peaks and valleys come into all our lives. Although we all chart an individual course, there remain many similarities in our lives. We walk, we talk, we learn, and we search for satisfying occupations. Yet within this sameness, we all have and choose different experiences that shine a unique light on our journey through the lifespan. To aid in this analysis of lifespan development, throughout this book we'll explore the notion of **biopsychosocial interac-tions,** those biological, psychological, and social/environmental forces that act together to shape the path of development.

Such biopsychosocial interaction in turn leads to a consideration of several issues that must be addressed in any scrutiny of lifespan development. Finally, this introductory chapter concludes with an explanation and analysis of relevant research techniques used in studies of human development.

An Example of Development Through the Lifespan

If you think about the course of your own life—events you've experienced and those you hope or fear you might experience—you begin to appreciate the complexity of development. Because it's usually difficult to look at ourselves objectively, let's examine the life of one individual—Barack Obama—whose rise to fame and power with all its accompanying triumphs and tragedies offers some insight into concepts of lifespan development.

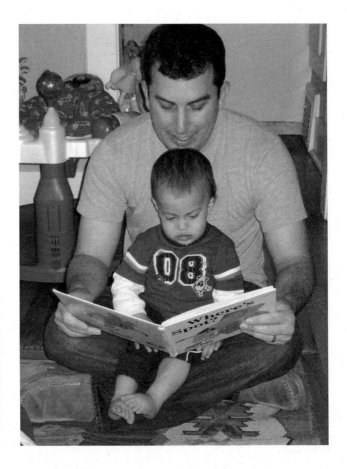

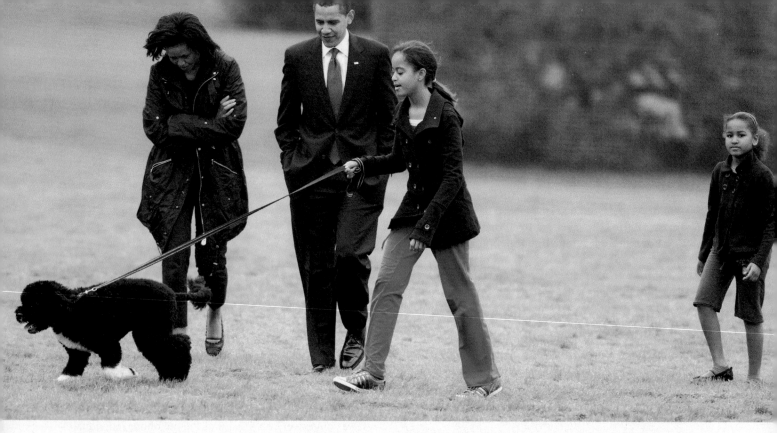

Tonight is a particular honor for me because—let's face it—my presence on this stage is pretty unlikely. My father was a foreign student, born and raised in a small village in Kenya. He grew up herding goats, went to school in a tin-roof shack. His father—my grandfather—was a cook, a domestic servant to the British.

I stand here today, grateful for the diversity of my heritage, aware that my parents' dreams live on in my two precious daughters. I stand here knowing that my story is part of the larger American story, that I owe a debt to all of those who came before me, and that in no other country on earth is my story even possible.

These words, spoken on July 27, 2004, to a tumultuous gathering at Boston Garden were part of Barack Obama's keynote address at the Democratic National Convention. At the time, he was a junior U.S. senator from Illinois. His remarkable story is a great example of the potential inherent in human development. Tracing the path that Obama followed in his lifespan dramatically illustrates the trials and tribulations and the successes and joys of human development.

Born in 1961 in Honolulu, Hawaii, Obama is the son of Barack Obama Sr. and Ann Dunham of Wichita, Kansas. At the time of his birth, Obama's parents were both students at the East-West Center of the University of Hawaii. Following the divorce of his parents, his mother later married Lolo Soetoro from Indonesia, where the family then lived for several years. Obama returned to Hawaii to live with his maternal grandparents and finish his early education. He later graduated from Columbia University. After several years as a community organizer in Chicago, Obama

attended Harvard Law School, received his law degree, and returned to Chicago, where he joined a corporate law firm. He met and married Michelle Robinson, a lawyer from the same firm. Obama became active in community affairs and joined a Chicago civil rights law firm. He also lectured on constitutional law at the University of Chicago.

In 1996, Obama took the first step in a political career when he was elected to the Illinois state senate. After an unsuccessful campaign for Congress in 2000, an overwhelming majority elected Obama to the U.S. Senate in 2004. In 2006, he led a congressional delegation to several African countries and made international headlines as he traced his family's origins in Kenya. As one prominent Kenyan noted, "He's a role model for all of Africa." In 2005, *Time* magazine selected Obama as one of the "100 most influential people in the world." Two years later, on February 11, 2007, he announced his candidacy for the presidency, and ran a long and ultimately successful campaign. On January 20, 2009, Barack Obama was sworn in as the 44th president of the United States and the first African American to serve in this position. His inauguration was celebrated around the world.

If you don't know **where** *you are going, any road will get you* **there.**

LEWIS CARROLL

How did this individual from a modest background achieve such a lofty position? One path leads to the conclusion that Obama's family—parents, wife, children—are of paramount importance to him. Another path identifies those personal concerns that shaped his thinking. His decision to follow a political career provided opportunities for him to influence legislation affecting education, the poor, minorities, and international affairs. Barack Obama is an example of an individual proceeding through his lifespan by remaining faithful to his values, recognizing opportunities, and making the most of his unique abilities. Considered separately, the components of Obama's life may be common or familiar to millions of individuals, and could be the result of choice, luck, or destiny. But woven together, the pieces form the unique fabric of one man's life as viewed through the lens of our particular moment in time. Barack Obama's biography is a remarkable story of human development.

Thinking About Lifespan Development

Lifespan development studies human development from conception to death. This text presents a *normative* approach to development, that is, studying the typical or average developmental path that people follow, but also casts a spotlight on individual variations throughout the chapters, accordingly.

WHY STUDY THE LIFESPAN?

As a discipline, **lifespan psychology** gained momentum when developmental psychologists began to agree that development didn't cease when human beings passed from adolescence to adulthood. A lifespan perspective took psychologists into a wider field. A range of influences, including brain research, analysis of the development of the mind, and research into the ways developmental levels influence individuals' responses to their experiences (Rutter, 2006), prompted the acceptance of development as a lifelong process. Each age or stage (infancy, adolescence, and so on) has its own developmental agenda and contributes to the entire lifespan.

The following are several objectives of lifespan development:

• To offer an organized account of development across the lifespan

• To identify the interconnections between earlier and later events

• To account for the mechanisms responsible for lifespan development

• To specify the biological, psychological, and social factors that shape an individual's development

Once these objectives are identified, developmental psychologists attempt to trace the range of individual development, encourage individuals to live their lives as positively as possible, and help them avoid negative outcomes (Baltes, Lindenberger, & Staudinger, 2006).

WHAT IS DEVELOPMENT?

Few readers would argue with the notion that individuals respond to the events of their lives in a manner consistent with their age at that time. Our lives are not static and unchanging, and **development** reflects this underlying assumption of change.

Age alone cannot account for varied responses to life events. Age, as Rutter (2006, p. 314) points out, is an inadequate explanation for behavior because

• age tells us about biological maturity and little else,

• different elements of biological growth proceed at different rates,

• age reflects past experiences that may influence current behavior,

• age reflects current social situations, and

• age tells us little about the underlying causal mechanisms.

Two 5-year-olds, Talia and Sora, are sitting on a blanket at a park. Talia pulls a peanut butter and jelly sandwich out of her backpack, and Sora starts to whine, "I'm hungry!" Talia'a mom comes over and breaks the sandwich into two pieces, giving each girl one piece. Sora gleefully exclaims, "Now I have a sandwich, too!" and Talia starts to whine, "Now I only have a haaaalf." Age alone doesn't inform us of the psychological mechanism at work here. What seems to happen is that in some contexts, dividing one larger object into two smaller objects does not cause upset, whereas in other situations, the act of dividing implies something negative despite the result of the social act of sharing or mathematical process of making more. You can see that what may appear on the surface to be solely age-related changes is due to factors such as social relationships and cognitive development.

Development indeed implies change, but the two terms are not equal. For change to be used in a developmental sense, it must possess a systematic, organized structure that contains a successive theme; that is, it should be clear that the changes that occurred at a later time were influenced by earlier changes. Thus the concept of development signifies systematic and successive changes over time (Lerner, 2002). (Keep in mind, though, that even this definition may vary according to the orientation of the psychologists involved—biological, philosophical, and so on.) Our focus will therefore be on *what* changes

lifespan psychology Study of human development from conception to death.

development The process of changing and the changes that occur through the lifespan.

TABLE 1.1

Developmental Periods of the Lifespan

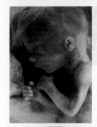
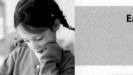
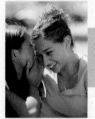
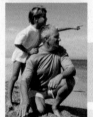
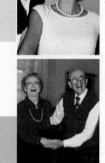

Period	Characteristics
Prenatal (conception to birth)	Nine months of rapid growth in which organs and systems appear; extreme sensitivity to environmental influences.
Infancy (birth to 2 years)	Continued rapid growth; brain development provides the basis for the emergence of motor, cognitive, and physiological accomplishments.
Early childhood (3 to 6 years)	Physical growth slows somewhat; substantial gains in cognitive and language development; the interplay between socialization and individualization shapes personality and influences adjustment.
Middle childhood (7 to 11 years)	School becomes a major force in development; physical cognitive, and psychosocial abilities become apparent.
Adolescence (12 to 18 years)	Puberty affect all aspects of development; thought becomes more abstract, academic achievement begins to shape the future; the search for identity continues unabated.
Early adulthood (19 to 34 years)	Higher education or the beginning of work beckons; relationships are a major focus of these years; marriage and children become central concerns of the lifespan.
Middle adulthood (35 to 64 years)	Heightened responsibility; may include care of children and aging parents; growing community involvement; peak period for leadership and influence; a time of physical change (for example, menopause).
Late adulthood (65+)	Retirement; eventual declining health and strength; adjusting to death of loved ones; facing one's own mortality; changing lifestyle to enhance "successful aging"; enjoying greater wisdom.

> *What a distressing* **contrast** *there is between the radiant intelligence of the* **child** *and the feeble mentality of the average* **adult.**
>
> **SIGMUND FREUD**

come about, *whether* they are maintained or lost, and *how* the course of development varies from individual to individual (Rutter & Rutter, 1993). In other words, "Why?" For example, "Why does change occur?" or "Why do individuals change?"

For purposes of research and analysis, the human lifespan is typically divided into developmental stages or periods. It's important to remember that each particular period is part of a greater whole, and these distinct periods will be discussed in detail in this text. The most widely acknowledged sequence of developmental periods includes the following categories: prenatal period, infancy, early childhood, middle childhood, adolescence, early adulthood, middle adulthood, and late adulthood (see Table 1.1). Let's take a look at the varied interpretations that society has embraced regarding lifespan development over hundreds of years.

Changing Views of the Lifespan

If we agree that development indeed implies change, then interpretations of the lifespan over the years should also reflect the notion of change. And, not surprisingly, they do. As the different, evolving images of children, adolescents, and adults are presented in this book, keep in mind that these developmental snapshots were influenced by cultural forces reflecting the dominant ideas and values of a particular era. The power dynamic that exists within a society, culture, or the world cannot be ignored or underestimated.

CHANGING VIEWS OF CHILDHOOD

Although written decades ago, Freud's words strike a familiar chord and highlight a major assumption about lifespan development: along the path from childhood to adulthood something vital changes. But is it the child who changes, or does the way the individual is viewed by society change? Children encapsulate innocence, a joie de vivre, that gets diluted as life becomes more complicated and children either take on increasing responsibilities or have responsibility thrust upon them as demanded by society. The assumption thus creates a challenge in any attempt to understand children: Without understanding a specific context, how can we interpret children's growth, development, and behavior more generally? How does any society define what a "child" is? Are children seen as miniature adults or as competent, curious youths? What is appropriate for children, and who are the stakeholders in any outcomes?

If historians wish to understand children of the past, they must first discover how adults have viewed the young (Heywood, 2001). The concept of childhood has changed from period to period, place to place, and culture to culture. Viewing children as miniature adults (and treating them this way) is quite different from recognizing the significance of the interactions of heredity and environment in a child's development.

The manner in which societies viewed children has differed throughout history according to culture and prevailing values of the historical period. Greek and Roman scholars believed that ideal human development involved disciplined

FEATURED MEDIA

Perspectives on Childhood

***Big* (1988)** – A film in which a 12-year-old makes a wish to be "big" and wakes up the next day as a 30-year-old. He encounters grown-up responsibilities and relationships and faces the ultimate decision of whether or not to return to childhood.

***The Crepes of Wrath* (1990)** – In the 11th episode of the first season of *The Simpsons,* Bart travels to France as an exchange student and must work like a slave for two winemakers while his own family falls for the student they've taken in, Adil, who is really an Albanian spy. This episode speaks to the competence and resilience of young children and the power of adults' perceptions of children and their place in society.

***Freaky Friday* (1976, 2003)** – A mother and daughter each wish that they could trade places with the other to experience the "easy" life of the other. The result forces the mother to understand her daughter's perspective and remember what it's like to be a young girl.

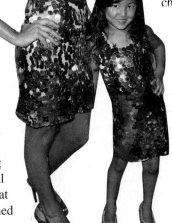

cultivation of body and mind, and children (mostly male children of wealthy families) were brought up according to specific values and expectations for their life practices. With the gradual spread of Christianity and the belief that humans are inherently evil and need to be shaped to allow optimal moral growth, formal classrooms and schools began to appear. The playful, cheerful spirit of children was considered a hindrance to living a moral life. But great changes in the world's technological capabilities, such as the invention of the printing press and the industrial age and subsequent child labor laws, prompted changing concepts of childhood, and children entered the symbolic world of the written word. Children were slowly becoming objects of concern on a grand scale.

Throughout history, philosophers such as John Locke and Jean-Jacques Rousseau presented challenging, often contradictory, ideas of child rearing. Locke proposed that children were like a *tabula rasa,* or blank slate. Therefore, the role of the parents was to instruct children's minds. Locke believed that by carefully observing children's natural inclinations, parents could use them to motivate children toward the best paths. Rousseau, on the other hand, believed that children develop naturally and learn behaviors and freedom through the natural course of their everyday being. Verbal learning or forced instruction was not something Rousseau supported. Both Locke and Rousseau agreed, however, that childhood should be joyful and celebrated and that the success of nations depends on it. As the concept of childhood became more accepted and subject to various interpretations, an important work by the biologist Charles Darwin, titled *Biographical Sketch of an Infant* (1877), heralded a new and innovative analysis of childhood. The book, which consisted of Darwin's careful observations of his infant son's early development, provided a scientific basis for studying children.

When Darwin's book was followed in 1882 by William Preyer's *The Mind*

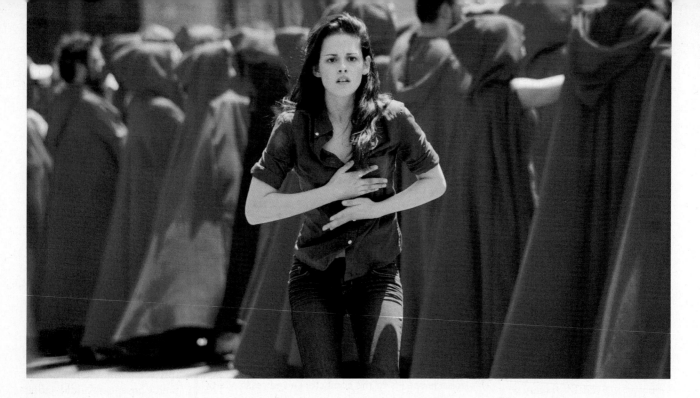

When I came here as a child, he would always **remove** the bullets as soon as he walked in the door. I guess he considered me **old enough** now not to shoot myself by accident, and not depressed enough to shoot myself on **purpose.**

BELLA SWAN, IN STEPHENIE MEYER'S *TWILIGHT*

of the Child, a rich, scholarly account of children's competencies based on careful observation, childhood was firmly entrenched as a separate subject deserving of study to answer growing questions about human development. The 19th century yielded remarkable studies of child development, particularly Alfred Binet's study of intelligence and G. Stanley Hall's writings on childhood and adolescence. As the notion of childhood acquired more credence, one of the most powerful interpreters of childhood was Sigmund Freud. In Freud's view, much of adults' behavior could be linked to experiences in the early years of life. Careful psychoanalysis would reveal these connections and shed light on resulting behaviors. Today, children are viewed as the product of genetic, biological, behavioral, and contextual forces constantly interacting. We see the same level of sophistication applied to the adolescent years.

CHANGING VIEWS OF ADOLESCENCE

In *Twilight,* the 2005 novel by Stephenie Meyer, Bella Swan—a literary figure synonymous with adolescent turbulence—provides a taste of adolescent thought. In her words we read some evidence of the turbulence and uncertainty of adolescence. But she also offers a thoughtful analysis of her own development. Perhaps the best way of thinking

about adolescence is to consider that it begins in biology and ends in culture (Petersen, 1988).

As is true for all periods of the lifespan, the physical maturation of human development initiates the process, but social and emotional adolescent experiences strongly shape the nature and direction of behavior. Lerner and Galambos (1998) summarize the nuances of adolescence when they state that adolescence is that time when a person's biological, cognitive, psychological, and social characteristics are changing from what is considered childlike to what is considered adultlike. A key word is "considered"—considered by *whom*? That is at the heart of the tension that exists for adolescents, who straddle the two distinct realms of childhood and adulthood. What biology deems possible in terms of physical capacity, cognitively and/or emotionally a teenager may not be ready to accept in terms of responsibility or consequences.

As with childhood, the concept of adolescence has changed remarkably through the years. For centuries adolescents were simply viewed as younger adults who were subject to strict rules and harsh discipline. Not until the industrial revolution in Western societies was the need for better education seen, and with the passage of child labor laws and a demand for universal school attendance came a separation of adolescents from children and adults (Grote-

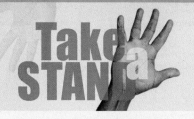
vant, 1998). With the advent of the 20th century, adolescence as a separate phase of development was popularized by the writings and teachings of G. Stanley Hall. In his two-volume text *Adolescence* (1904), he popularized a label of adolescence that is still with us today—a time of "storm and stress." At the beginning of the 21st century, continued speculation and research has changed the picture of adolescence again. Today most psychologists agree that the majority of adolescents have accepted the values and standards of their parents and the greater society, and that friction between the generations is only slightly higher than that of childhood (Dacey, Kenny, & Margolis, 2002).

In spite of numerous risk factors that concern most parents and adults in general, most young adults face the challenges of their environment, adjust to the demands made on them, and, with adult patience and understanding, achieve their goals.

CHANGING VIEWS OF ADULTHOOD

Today we realize that lifespan development involves change throughout the lifespan, adulthood as well as infancy. Development is not complete at adulthood (maturity). Rather, development reaches across the entire life course, and developmental changes involve lifelong adaptive processes unique for each phase of the life course, including adulthood. Compared to childhood and adolescence, adulthood is a relatively complex, long, ever-increasing stretch of time due to the advances of medical and other technologies.

CHANGING PERSPECTIVES ON AGING

As an example of the complexities of aging, consider the results of the Seattle Longitudinal Study of Adult Intelligence (Schaie, 1994). Research suggests that as people age, their physical stamina, memory, and cognitive processing do not decline as much as previously thought. In fact, development continues in significant ways. Although some aspects of cognitive functioning lose a degree of efficiency (for example, speed of processing), such losses in a healthy 60-, 70-, or 80-year-old are more than offset by gains in knowledge and skill due to experience.

Analyzing the cause of an apparent decline in intelligence (as measured by intelligence tests) leads to several conclusions:

- When *physical health* remains good, cognitive performance suffers only a slight decline. Sight, hearing, and motor coordination play key roles in maintaining the link between health and intellectual performance.

- *Speed of response* is the time taken to perform any task that involves the central nervous system such as perception, memory, reasoning, and motor movement. It is the basis for efficient cognitive functioning, especially memory. Much of the decline in memory performance in the later years can be attributed to a decline in verbal speed. If the nervous system involvement is slowed, cognitive performance declines because information may be lost during the required cognitive processing (Birren & Fisher, 1992).

Adult development is neither a footrace *nor a moral* imperative. *It is a road map to help us make sense of where we and where our neighbors might be* located.

GEORGE VAILLANT (2002)

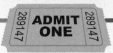

FEATURED MEDIA

Films about Adolescence

***Dead Poets Society* (1989)** – This is the story of several boys at an elite prep school and their teacher, Mr. Keating, who encourages them to "seize the day" and dare to experience life with all of its complications and challenges.

***Hairspray* (1988, 2007)** – Both versions of the film—nonmusical and musical—feature "pleasantly plump" teenager Tracy Turnblad, whose dream is to become a dancer on her favorite television program. She experiences some serious dilemmas, ranging from her weight to racial integration and bigotry.

***Kids* (1995)** – This film features Telly, a skateboarding teen unaware that he is HIV-positive, whose goal is to have sex with as many virgins as possible. One of his previous sex partners, who tests positive for HIV and knows it was Telly who infected her, tries to find him and stop him from passing on the disease to others.

- *Attitude,* especially in a testing situation, affects cognitive performance. Test anxiety lowers test scores when older adults find themselves in strange settings. They may fear that their memory will fail them; they may be uncomfortable with the test's problems; they may simply have an expectation of failure because of all they've heard and read about the declining mental abilities of older adults.

These and similar reasons, either singly or in combination, have often led to an underestimation of older people's intelligence. For example, reasoning, problem solving, and wisdom hold up well, and may even improve, with age. The Seattle study showed that people with higher intelligence test scores tended to be healthier and better educated, have higher incomes and stable marriages, and still be leading active, stimulating lives than those with lower intelligence test scores (Papalia & Olds, 2004). Any standardized test of intelligence, or other area, must be held up to close scrutiny as an accurate measure of assessment for a host of reasons, some of which include cultural bias, contextual factors, and validity.

CHART YOUR OWN LIFESPAN

Endeavoring to illustrate how important knowledge of the lifespan is to each of us, Sugarman (1986) has devised a simple exercise that you can do quickly. Using a blank sheet of paper, assume that the left edge of the page represents the beginning of your life and the right edge where you are today. Now draw a line across the page that indicates the peaks and valleys you have experienced so far.

A sample chart is shown in Figure 1.1.

In this chart, the first valley was a financial reversal for the person's parents. The first peak represents happy and productive high school years, followed by entry into teaching and then marriage. The deep valley was a serious accident followed by years of recuperation and then the birth of children and the publication of a book. You can see that it looks like a temperature chart. Try it for yourself.

When you finish, ask yourself these questions:

Are there more peaks than valleys?

Is there a definite shape to my chart?

Would I identify my peaks and valleys as major or minor?

What caused the peaks and valleys?

Could I have done anything to make the peaks higher and the valleys shallower?

What happened during the plateaus?

What's my view of these highs and lows in my life?

You have drawn a picture of your lifespan, and the questions that you have just answered are the subject matter of lifespan development.

FIGURE 1.1
Milestone Events Across the Lifespan

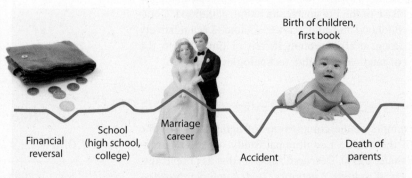

Financial reversal

School (high school, college)

Marriage career

Accident

Birth of children, first book

Death of parents

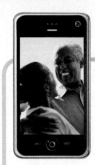
FIGURE 1.2

The Biopsychosocial Model

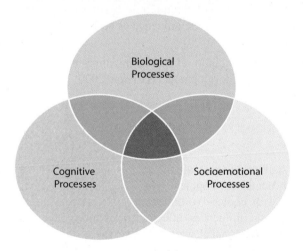

We end this section as we began it: Different eras have conceived different views of the various developmental periods. Any study of lifespan development must recognize that numerous factors account for observable devel-

opmental changes. These differences clearly call for us to appraise the meaning of development more closely.

epigenetic view View of lifespan development that stresses the ongoing interaction between heredity and the environment.

culture The customs, values, and traditions inherent in one's environment.

The Importance of Biopsychosocial Interactions

This book proposes that lifespan development is the product of biopsychosocial interactions—the influence of genetic, biological, psychological, and social/environmental forces on development. This differs from the **epigenetic view** of development, which focuses on the ongoing interaction between heredity and the environment during development. In the biopsychosocial model, development results from the interaction of biological, psychological, and social/environmental factors and processes (see Figure 1.2).

Biological processes range from the role of genes to adult health concerns; psychological processes include all aspects of cognitive and personality development; and social processes refer to the role of family, school/work, peers, and the media. These processes are so tightly intertwined that it is impossible to determine which plays more of a role in development. In many cases, the processes operate in a bidirectional manner. For example, biological forces affect cognitive forces (skipping breakfast can impact students' performance in schools), and it works in the other direction, too (positive thinking and strong friendships can impact elderly people's health). The goal of lifespan psychology is therefore to probe the multiple and integrated layers (genetic, physical, behavioral, and environmental) that drive human development.

UNDERSTANDING THE ROLE OF CULTURE

It's critically important to recognize the contributions that a particular culture makes to the development of individuals and the larger society. **Culture** can be defined as the customs, values, and traditions inherent in one's environment—the features that define values and styles of life (Rutter & Nikapota, 2006). Different cultures have different developmental expectations for their children. Asian children, for example, are encouraged to avoid emotional displays, a characteristic that does not necessarily apply to Asian-American children. This example is simply stated, but to truly understand the previous sentence, you must consider the political and social histories of the countries that are implicitly and explicitly named in the generalization, and the emphasis on keeping harmony among a group of individuals as opposed to striving to be the best individual one can be. We also urge you to remember that the equation *biology + psychology + environment = development* plays out differently within the confines of a particular culture.

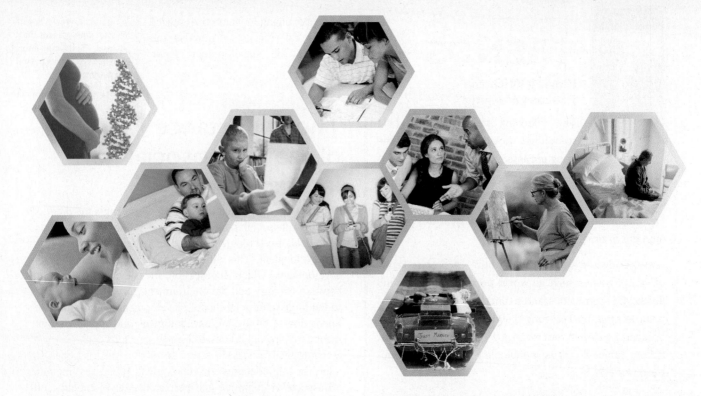

To help you grasp the significance of culture in development, remember that there are three answers to the question "How well do you understand the cultures of your friends, coworkers, and neighbors?"

1. You may understand at a *superficial* level; that is, you know only the facts that make up a person's cultural history.

2. You may understand at an *intermediate* level; that is, you understand the central behaviors that are at the core of a person's social life. Language usage is a good example here: Does a person's culture tolerate, even encourage, calling out in class? Calling out could be a major problem for teachers not familiar with the acceptable behaviors of this person's culture because it goes against acceptable behaviors in traditional classroom culture.

3. You may understand at a *significant* level; that is, you grasp the values, beliefs, and norms that structure a person's view of the world and how to behave in that world. In other words, you change psychologically as a result of your interactions with a different culture (Casas & Pytluk, 1995).

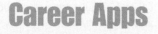

Career Apps

As a developmental psychologist, how might you examine the role that a sense of humor plays in late adolescence?

As you continue studying lifespan development, you therefore need to be aware that different does not mean deficient. Examples of the cultural influence on development are visible in this book in two ways: through Perspectives on Diversity features and by age-specific examples. The following objectives relating to culture specifically are at the core of the biopsychosocial model:

- To understand the relationship between culture and development

- To identify values and attitudes that promote and sustain healthy development

- To trace the impact of cultural transmission, such as parenting practices and the influence of peers, schools, and media

- To assess current cultural change initiatives that encourage successful development (Harrison, 2000)

CONTRIBUTORS TO BIOPSYCHOSOCIAL INTERACTIONS

If you start to imagine all the factors that contribute to biopsychosocial development, you'll see that it's a daunting task with endless combinations of factors. Multiple developmental influences affect growth during the lifespan. More importantly, we would like you to think about the interactions that occur among biology, psychology, and social factors, and how these interactions affect development. By recognizing the significance of biopsychosocial interactions, you'll be able to understand and remember the material of any given chapter. This perspective also helps to emphasize all of the features that so powerfully influence development through the lifespan.

The Impact of Cultural Climate

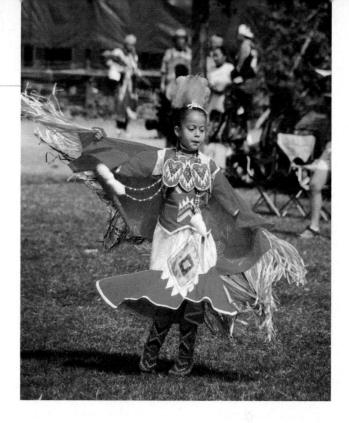

"We are a country of Muslims, atheists, Jews, Christians, Hindus, and devout spiritualists without a specific religious affiliation. We celebrate the winter solstice, Hanukkah, Christmas, Kwanza, and Ramadan. We brought longstanding cultural traditions and rites of passage from Haiti, Laos, Ghana, El Salvador, France, Germany, England, and Samoa, among countless others. Many of our children are taken through rites of passage that include bar and bat mitzvahs, Quinceañeras, debutante balls, and gang initiation." (Muse, 1997, p. 285)

Perhaps nowhere are these words brought to life more dramatically than in the American classroom. A good example of this kind of endeavor can be seen in Kim's (1990) description of Hawaiian children's school experiences. Many Hawaiian children achieve at the lowest academic level and are labeled as lazy and disruptive by their teachers. Yet these same children are remarkably responsible at home—cooking, cleaning, and taking care of their brothers and sisters. They demonstrate considerable initiative and a high performance level. When something needs to be done, they get together and make a group effort to do whatever is necessary. When they find themselves in an individualistic, competitive classroom, however, their performance suffers.

In a series of experiments, teachers were encouraged to model desired behaviors and not assign specific tasks to students. By the end of the academic year, the students would begin the day by examining the schedules of their learning centers and then divide themselves into groups that assigned tasks to individual members, obtained materials, and used worksheets. Although their achievement scores improved significantly, once the students returned to regular classrooms for the fourth grade, a familiar pattern of problems appeared (Kim, 1990).

The classroom is not the only location in which cultures merge. In the business world, people of various cultures and backgrounds work side by side; those designated as minorities may have leadership positions in which members of the dominant culture report to them. As companies become more global and as the number of international markets increases steadily, the workplace begins to resemble the classroom as a meeting place of cultures.

One goal in encouraging you to develop a culturally sensitive perspective is to help you reach a level of significant understanding of people who seem different. If you adopt this perspective, you will come to realize that different people have different worldviews that decisively influence their thinking. Recognizing how diverse people are in their thinking and behavior will help you to identify and comprehend variations in people's backgrounds and how they become functioning members of their culture. In this way, you will work, play, and study more congenially with others, thus fostering more positive relations in our society.

Finally, cultural awareness should also make us aware that we are all alike in important ways. It's mainly in our behavior, the way we deal with the demands of our environment, that we differ.

Issues in Lifespan Development

In lifespan psychology, as in any field, several issues or themes warrant special attention. The following two issues have been the subject of much controversy and great debate, and an awareness of them will increase your understanding of development as you progress through the book.

CONTINUITY VERSUS DISCONTINUITY

In 1980, Orville Brim and Jerome Kagan published *Constancy and Change in Human Development,* which highlighted a long-standing controversy among developmental psychologists. Arguing that humans have a capacity for change across the lifespan, Brim and Kagan brought new life to the question "*How* do these changes occur?" Does each new stage of development contain most of the structures that appeared in an earlier stage (Kagan, 1998)? Do you think you are basically the same person you were when you were 3 years old? 10 years old? 18 years old? Or do you feel quite different? Why? These questions introduce the issue of continuity versus discontinuity. In other words, do developmental changes appear as the result of a slow but steady progression (**continuity**) or as the result of abrupt changes (**discontinuity**)?

To illustrate the distinction between continuity and discontinuity, let's examine the phenomenon known as *attachment* in infancy. Sometime after 6 months of age, babies begin to show a decided preference for a particular caregiver, usually the mother. This is usually described by noting that the infant has attached to the mother. During any time of stress—anxiety, illness, appearance of strangers—the baby will move to the preferred caregiver. With regard to continuity or discontinuity, does attachment develop slowly as the caregiver and infant interact and exchange subtle and more obvious cues, or does it appear suddenly, as a completely new and different behavior?

Continuities and discontinuities appear in each of our lives because the term *development* implies change. Puberty, leaving home, marriage, and career all serve to shape psychological functioning. Continuities occur, however, because our initial experiences, our early learning, and our temperaments remain with us. The form of the behavior may change over the years, but the underlying processes remain the same. For example, the conduct disorders of childhood (such as stealing, fighting, or truancy) may become the violence of adulthood (theft, spousal abuse, child abuse, or murder). Differences or dissimilarities may be evident in types of behavior, but the underlying processes that cause specific behaviors may be identical, thus arguing for continuity in development (Rutter & Rutter, 1993).

Other behaviors in our lives, however, seem to be quite different from those that preceded them—for example, walking and talking. We also negotiate transitions at appropriate times in our lives, such as leaving home, beginning a career, getting married, and adjusting to the birth of children. Events such as these have led some developmental psychologists to highlight the role of accidents, wars, famines, disease, and chance encounters in human experience. Lewis therefore believes that the study of developmental change is actually the study of predictable as well as complex, often random, and certainly unpredictable conditions.

continuity The lasting quality of experiences; development proceeds steadily and sequentially.

discontinuity Behaviors that are apparently unrelated to earlier aspects of development.

Most developmental psychologists now believe that both continuity and discontinuity characterize development. As Lerner notes (2002), any developmental change may be characterized as being either continuous or discontinuous and either stable or unstable. Depending on the particular lens through which behavior is viewed, the interpretations vary.

NATURE VERSUS NURTURE

Another enduring issue in developmental psychology has been the question of which exercises a greater influence on development: our inborn tendencies (nature) or our surrounding world (nurture). Again, most developmental psychologists lean toward an interaction between these two forces in shaping development. Such interaction between genes and the environment explains the individual developmental path each of us follows throughout our lifespan. Lerner (2002) has summarized this argument as follows:

1. Nature and nurture are both involved in the production of behavior.

2. They cannot function in isolation from each other but must interact.

3. The resulting interaction implies that both nature and nurture are completely intertwined.

Perhaps Bjorklund (2005) summarized this issue as well as anyone can when he stated that, for developmental psychologists, there is no nature–nurture controversy because biological factors are inseparable from experiential factors, with the two constantly interacting. It is *how* they interact that produces a particular pattern of development.

These issues help to identify lifespan psychology as a dynamic discipline—one with great theoretical and practical implications. Fascinating though these issues may be, the integrated nature of development is critical to remember. With these ideas in mind to use as we interpret developmental data, let's examine the research techniques that developmental psychologists use while seeking to answer questions about the lifespan.

Research in Lifespan Development

After we identify several key developmental issues and theoretical viewpoints, the question becomes "How can we obtain reliable data about these topics so that we may better understand them?" Today there are many approaches to understanding human behavior, all rooted in a spirit of inquiry, wanting to know "why?" Each has its strengths and weaknesses, and none is completely reliable. Because human beings conduct research, we must accept that humans have conscious or unconscious biases and may make mistakes, and that sometimes pure chance influences the outcomes of an investigation.

Most developmental psychologists employ one of three data collection techniques: (1) descriptive stud-

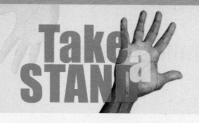

Do Vitamins Increase Life Expectancy?

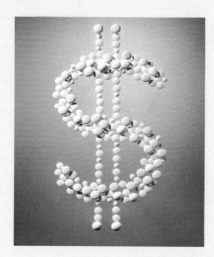

Much research exists on the benefits of nutrition for overall health. Recent findings by experts argue that taking vitamin supplements has no impact on overall health or mortality and that they can actually increase the risk of early death. Despite this, Americans reportedly spend over $20 billion a year on dietary supplements. Consumers are encouraged to buy dietary supplements to increase some functions and decrease other functions, and physicians, pharmacists, and fitness instructors frequently recommend supplements.

Some evidence supports the use of vitamin supplements to improve health, and common knowledge argues that luck plays a major role in how long we live and how healthy we are throughout our lives. The tension between heredity and environmental factors is well exemplified by the desire to supplement what nature/heredity deals us.

Is our destiny determined by genetics/fate (nature) or is it something we can control with environmental input (nurture)?

ies, (2) manipulative experiments, and (3) naturalistic experiments. They also use one of four time-variable designs: one-time, one-group studies; longitudinal studies; cross-sectional studies; and a combination of the last two, called sequential studies. Each type of study varies according to the goal of the research and the effect of time on the results.

DATA COLLECTION TECHNIQUES

At the heart of the study of human development is the **scientific method**—an approach to seeking answers through empirical research, data collection, and testing. When researchers follow the steps of this approach, their work is regarded accordingly in the field as a scientific study. The steps include

1. generating a single research question or a set of guiding questions;

2. developing a **hypothesis**—a prediction about something that can be tested and subsequently supported or rejected;

3. testing the hypothesis through research to collect data;

4. drawing conclusions based on the data and supporting arguments with evidence from the research.

Figure 1.3 shows the steps in the scientific method.

When researchers are curious about a particular question, they choose a specific type of study that best suits their investigation. One of the key aspects of any study is systematic, thoughtful observation. Observations can occur in a laboratory or clinical setting as well as a natural, realistic setting. Careful watching, listening, and recording convey respect for the field and contribute to the effectiveness of the overall study, regardless of which form the study takes.

Descriptive Studies

In **descriptive studies,** information is gathered on participants without manipulating them in any way. Some studies (called *survey* or *self-report studies*) ask people their opinions about themselves or other people. These studies may involve the use of interviews or questionnaires. How happy or unhappy is the average 66-year-old man with his sex life? Other studies (called *observational studies*) describe people simply by counting the number and the types of their behaviors. How many 12-year-olds versus 17-year-olds think the government is doing a good job? How much money does the average 40-year-old woman spend per week? How many pregnant teenage girls were or were not using birth control at the time they became pregnant?

scientific method An approach to investigation that includes empirical research, data collection, and testing.

hypothesis A prediction that can be tested through research and subsequently supported or rejected.

descriptive studies Studies that gather information on subjects without manipulating them in any way.

FIGURE 1.3
The Scientific Method

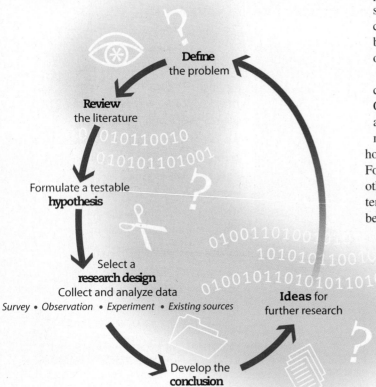

Define the problem

Review the literature

Formulate a testable **hypothesis**

Select a **research design**
Collect and analyze data
Survey • Observation • Experiment • Existing sources

Develop the **conclusion**

Ideas for further research

The scientific method allows researchers to objectively and logically evaluate the data they collect. Their findings can suggest ideas for further research.

Sigmund Freud, Virginia Woolf, and Mahatma Gandhi. From these four cases, he built a new theory about creative innovation.

Descriptive studies have a certain appeal because people can generate a lot of data. However, because the sequence of events is not under a researcher's control, causes and effects cannot be determined; that is, just because two variables are associated does not mean that one causes the other.

The assumption that correlation means causation is a common mistake made in interpreting results of research. Correlation refers to the association between factors, and can be established through a specific statistical technique. This technique provides a number that represents how strong the association is between any two variables. For instance, height and weight are associated with each other, but not perfectly. The taller people are, the more they tend to weigh, but this is not always true; the correlation between height and weight for a typical sample of people is moderately high. Although there is a definite association, we know that height does not cause weight, or vice versa—they are simply correlated. Researchers examine the correlation between variables to find the strength in similar relationships. If high, researchers may want to set up experiments to further examine the relationships.

A third type of study, the *case study,* presents data on an individual or individuals in great detail, in order to make generalizations relating to a research question. An example of this approach was reflected in headlines about the "pregnancy pact" in Gloucester, Massachusetts. In 2008, this town found itself home to an extraordinarily high number of pregnant high school girls. Parents and school officials started to investigate the occurrence, and questions emerged about whether the girls purposely got pregnant and if so, their reasons. Relatives, friends, and teachers were interviewed to shed light on the thinking of the 17 pregnant teenagers, who were also questioned. Although the findings may explain the behavior of only this particular set of girls, researchers hoped to learn more about adolescent psychology and other factors that could have contributed to the unique situation and could be generalized to a wider population.

Another case-study approach involves the study of individual lives from a biographical perspective. For example, Gardner (1997) closely examined the biographies of four eminent persons: Wolfgang Mozart,

manipulative experiments Experiments in which the researcher attempts to keep all variables (all the factors that can affect a particular outcome) constant except one, which is carefully manipulated.

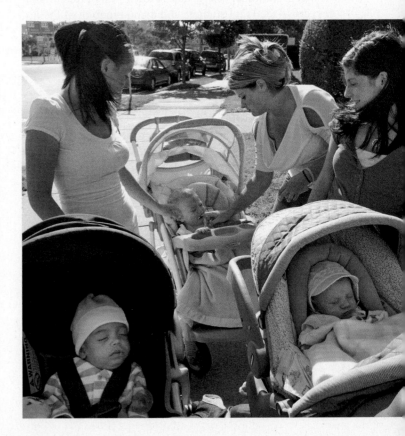

Manipulative Experiments

In an attempt to better learn about the causes of behavior, psychologists design **manipulative experiments.** In these, the investigators attempt to keep all variables (all the factors that can affect a particular outcome) constant except one, which they carefully manipulate. The variables are known as independent or dependent: *independent variables* are those that the researchers specifically manipulate, while *dependent variables* change as a result of the *manipulation,* also called the *treatment*. If differences occur as a result of the experiment, they can be attributed to the variable that was manipulated in the treatment. For example, if researchers are curious about the effect of a book on students' learning of a specific subject, they can assign half a class Book A, and the other half Book B (book = independent variable). The whole class could then take a test to determine which book had a greater influence on students' test scores (score = dependent variable).

Though manipulative experiments often can lead us to discover some causes and related effects, they are open to critique. How can we know if the results are reliable? Was the treatment similar to normal conditions? Do subjects see themselves as special because we picked them and thus react a certain way? For these reasons, researchers may turn to naturalistic experiments.

Naturalistic Experiments

In **naturalistic experiments,** the researcher acts solely as an observer and does as little as possible to disturb the environment. "Nature" performs the experiment, and the researcher acts as a recorder of the results. An example is the study of the effects of the Northeast blizzard of 1978 by Nuttall and Nuttall (1980). These researchers compared the reactions of people whose homes were destroyed with the reactions of people whose homes suffered only minor damage.

Only with a naturalistic experiment do we have any chance of discovering causes and effects in real-life settings. The main challenges with this technique are that it requires great patience and objectivity, and it is impossible to meet the strict requirements of a true scientific *experiment*. True scientific experiments are deemed such due to certain assumptions and expectations about the scientific process. Depending on the field of study, specific biases and assumptions are more or less present, and researchers must be vigilant about accounting for such biases when reporting the results of their investigations.

TIME-VARIABLE DESIGNS

In studies of the human lifespan, researchers often focus on individuals who fall into a specific age group or else people of different ages for comparison within a study. Several **time-variable designs** afford different understandings, depending on the intentions of the investigators and their questions.

One-Time, One-Group Studies

As the name implies, **one-time, one-group studies** are those that are carried out only once with one group of participants. It is almost impossible to investigate cause and effect in such studies because a sequence of events or influence of various factors cannot be known on the basis of a one-time occurrence with one group of people.

Longitudinal Studies

Longitudinal studies, which track the same individuals over a period of time, can answer important questions. The study conducted by Werner and Smith on the island of Kauai, introduced at the beginning of this chapter, is a well-known example of a longitudinal study.

Another engaging example of a longitudinal study is that conducted by filmmaker Michael Apted (2007), represented in the *7 Up* documentary series. Apted has been interviewing and filming the same group of British individuals at 7-year intervals since 1964, when they were 7 years old. Every 7 years, he has returned to ask the participants questions about their lives, and the resulting films capture information about lifespan development that is shown in the personal accounts of each of the individuals and their families.

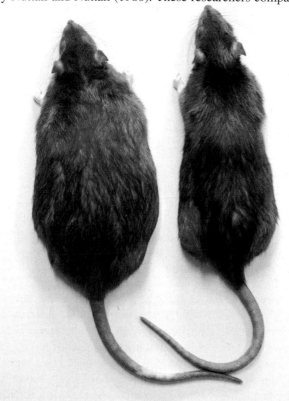

naturalistic experiments Experiments in which the researcher acts solely as an observer and does as little as possible to disturb the environment. "Nature" performs the experiment, and the researcher acts as a recorder of the results.

time-variable designs A specific amount of time (duration) is allowed for a given study, or there is a specific number of times a measure is used in a given study.

one-time, one-group studies Studies carried out only once with one group of participants.

longitudinal studies Studies in which the researcher makes several observations of the same individuals at two or more times in their lives. Examples are determining the long-term effects of learning on behavior; the stability of habits and intelligence; and the factors involved in memory.

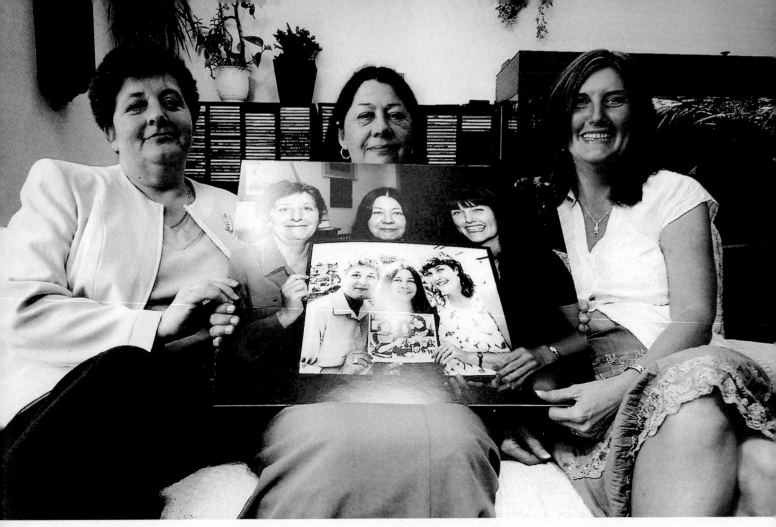

> *There aren't many pieces of work, especially in* film, *that have the patience or longevity or the time to honor the drama of ordinary life; and after all, the* drama *of what we all have to go through—children, jobs, marriage, the things that touch us—is the big* drama *of life, far more so than the drama of movies and television.*

MICHAEL APTED

The amazingly complex array of life issues, including challenges, triumphs, and losses, sheds light on developmental patterns and inconsistencies.

The chief advantage of the longitudinal method is that it permits such discovery of lasting habits and of the periods in which they appear. A second advantage is the possibility of tracing those adult behaviors that have changed since early childhood. Longitudinal research, however, has many challenges. It is expensive and often hard to maintain because of changes in availability of researchers and subjects. Changes in the environment can also distort the results. For example, if a study began in 1960, looking at changes in political attitudes of youths from 10 to 20 years of age, conclusions would likely report that adolescents become more radical as

they grow older. But the war in Vietnam would surely have had much to do with this finding. The results of the same study done between 1970 and 1980 would probably not show this trend, and today the data would show something different and unique to this moment in time.

In a study that began in 1937, researchers have followed a group of Harvard students for more that 70 years as they experience and reflect upon the course of their lives. In *The Atlantic,* author Joshua Wolf Shenk (2009) interviewed primary investigator George Vaillant (whose work has spanned 42 years on this study) and revealed some important messages that Vaillant has come to understand regarding human happiness. To view a short video about the study and learn some of Vaillant's insights gained from the

FIGURE 1.4

Sequential (Longitudinal/Cross-Sectional) Study

Cross-sectional design: people of varying ages studied simultaneously

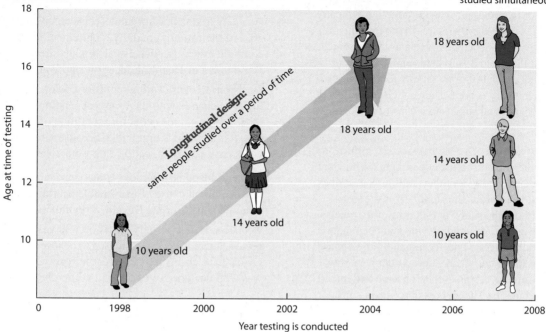

Longitudinal design: same people studied over a period of time

Age at time of testing (y-axis: 10, 12, 14, 16, 18)

Year testing is conducted (x-axis: 0, 1998, 2000, 2002, 2004, 2006, 2008)

10 years old — 14 years old — 18 years old (longitudinal)

18 years old — 14 years old — 10 years old (cross-sectional)

---

research, go to http://link.brightcove.com/services/player/bcpid1460906593?bctid=22804415001. This longitudinal study can teach us many important lessons about resiliency, perseverance, self-esteem, and many other areas of interest. This opportunity to make generalizations based on research is precisely the goal toward which most scientific research aims.

Cross-Sectional Studies

Cross-sectional studies compare groups of individuals of various ages at the same time. For example, if you want to know how creative thinking changes or grows during adolescence, you could administer creativity tests to groups of 10-, 12-, 14-, 16-, and 18-year-olds and check on the differences of the average scores of the five groups. Gail Jaquish and Richard Ripple (1981) did this in a cross-sectional study of subjects ranging in age from 18 to 84! (They found that age differences accounted for little variance in creative thinking.)

As with each of the other research designs, challenges exist with this method. Although careful selection can minimize the effects of cultural change, it is possible that the differences you find may be due to differences in age cohort, rather than maturation. Age cohorts are groups of people born at about the same time. Each cohort has had different experiences throughout its history, and this fact can affect the results as well as the actual differences in age.

Sequential (Longitudinal/Cross-Sectional) Studies

A sequential study is a cross-sectional study done with the same groups of individuals, several times, over a period of time (such as administering creativity tests to the same five groups of youth, but at three different points in their lives). Therefore, the aforementioned problems may be allevi-

ated. Figure 1.4 shows an illustration of a sequential study. Although sequential studies are complicated and expensive, they may be the only type of study capable of answering important questions in the complex and fast-changing times in which we live.

Each data collection technique may be combined with each of the time-variable designs to create numerous variations that are appropriate for individual studies. Depending on the goals of research, different studies can be designed and later serve as models for future research. The level of control—the degree to which the investigator can control the relevant variables—and the level of inclusiveness—the degree to which all relevant information is included in data—are important considerations in research design and should inform your reading and application of knowledge.

UNDERSTANDING THE RESEARCH ARTICLE

As you continue your reading and work in lifespan development, you will undoubtedly review articles that shed light on the topic you're studying. Many of these articles present the results of an experiment that reflects the scientific method.

The typical research article contains four sections: the *Introduction,* the *Method* section, the *Results* section, and the *Discussion.* Let's take a look at each of these sections using a well-designed study, *The Effects of Early Education on Children's Competence in Elementary School,* published in *Evaluation Review* (Bronson, Pierson, & Tivnan, 1984).

cross-sectional studies
Studies that compare groups of individuals of various ages at the same time.

sequential (longitudinal/cross-sectional) studies
Cross-sectional studies done at several times with the same groups of individuals.

1. **The Introduction** The introduction states the purpose of the article (usually as an attempt to solve a problem) and predicts the outcome of the study (usually in the form of hypotheses). The introduction typically contains a review of the literature. In the introduction to the article by Bronson and associates, the researchers state that their intent is to determine the effects of an early education program on the performance of pupils in elementary school. They concisely review the pertinent research and suggest a means of evaluating competence.

2. **The Method section** The Method section informs the reader abut the subjects in the experiment (Who were they? How many? How were they chosen?), describes any tests that were used, and summarizes the steps taken to carry out the study. In this study, the subjects were 169 second-grade children who had been in an early education program and 169 other children who had not been in the early education program. A classroom observation tool was used to observe and record children's behaviors. The authors describe in considerable detail how they observed the pupils in this study.

3. **The Results section** In the Results section, the results are presented, together with the statistics that help us to summarize and interpret the data. Authors typically present their data in several clear tables and show differences between the two groups using appropriate statistics.

4. **Discussion** Finally, the authors of any research article will discuss the importance of what they found (or did not find) and relate their findings to theory and previous research. In the Bronson article, the authors report that the pupils who had experienced an early education program showed significantly greater competence in the second grade than those who had not been in an early education program. The authors conclude by noting the value of these programs in reducing classroom behavior problems and improving pupils' competence.

Research articles, while denser than most popular magazine articles, include much information that can be accessed in each of the specific sections. Note the important features of a research article and see how the results could help you better understand people's behavior at a particular age.

WHEN ARE RESEARCH REFERENCES TOO OLD?

For the rest of your life, you will be reading research—magazine or journal articles, chapters in books, newspaper reports, and so on. When should you decide that a reference is too old to be credible any longer? As

code of ethics A guiding set of principles for members of a particular group.

with so many aspects of social science, the answer is "it all depends." Guidelines exist, however, so let's try to understand them by looking at several sample references:

1. As many as one third of adolescents receive less than 70% of their minimum daily requirement for the most common minerals, such as calcium and iron (U.S. Department of Health, Education, and Welfare, 1996).

   Decision: Because eating habits of adolescents are likely to change with the times (depending, among other things, on the economic condition of the country), this statistic is unreliable, because more than ten years have passed since the data were collected.

2. Noise-induced hearing loss is recognized as the second most common cause of irreversible hearing loss in older persons (Surjan, Devald, & Palfalvin, 1973).

   Decision: Here is a study that is over 30 years old, but because there is no known reason to believe that aging factors have changed much over the years, if the study was well designed, we may still accept the results.

3. The major crisis in the first 1-1/2 years of human life is the establishment of basic trust (Erikson, 1963).

   Decision: This statement is not a research finding; rather, it represents Erikson's belief as reflected in his psychosocial theory of human development. It is therefore accurate because that is exactly what Erikson said.

ETHICS

Any research must abide by ethical standards to ensure the safety and integrity of all involved. Before researchers are supported in their work, for example, they must receive approval from the appropriate group that oversees scientific study at their institutions. Within the broader fields of science or psychology there are disciplines that focus on narrower areas within those fields, and many professions, organizations, and societies articulate a detailed **code of ethics** that guides the work of members of those groups. A code of ethics generally outlines guiding principles that address moral considerations and responsibilities, such as the ethics guidelines developed by the American Psychological Association (APA), which can be found at http://www.apa.org/ethics/code/index.aspx. Participants in any study must be informed of every aspect of their involvement, must be anonymous unless other terms of confidentiality are discussed, and must be debriefed once their role in the study has concluded.

CONCLUSIONS & SUMMARY

In this chapter, you've been urged to think about lifespan development as a rich, multilayered complex of interactions. The biopsychosocial model of development—the model that forms the structure of this book—was explained. This model can be used to help you grasp and retain the material and meaning of the chapters to come. Age groups that constitute the lifespan, and that are the focus of this book, were identified. As a result of reading about the strengths and weaknesses of different research methods, you should be more analytical and critical of the studies that are presented.

Lifespan study can aid us in adjusting to a society in which rapid change seems to be an inevitable process. By acquiring insights into your own development and recognizing the developmental characteristics of people of differing ages, you can hope to have more harmonious relationships with others.

How would you define and describe lifespan development?

- As psychologists defined childhood and agreed that development does not cease at adolescence but continues into adulthood and old age, lifespan psychology assumed an important place in developmental psychology.
- To understand development is to accept the positive and negative features of change.
- The timing of experiences, as well as the transitions during the lifespan, help us to gain insights into developmental processes.
- Development cannot be explained by age alone.

How have views of lifespan development changed over the years?

- Children today are seen as complex individuals who develop subject to the interaction of many external and internal factors.
- Conflicting interpretations of adolescence (storm, stress, or calm) continue to rage today.
- The adult years are no longer seen as a time devoid of change until decline sets in.

What are the different views of lifespan development?

- A biological interpretation of development emphasizes the powerful impact the genes have on development.
- The need for more sophisticated perspectives on development has highlighted the place of reciprocal interactions in development.

What role do biopsychosocial interactions play in lifespan development?

- Biopsychosocial interactions in human development refer to the interactions of biological, psychological, and social forces.
- Biopsychosocial interactions occur at multiple levels of the developing person, from the genetic to the environmental levels.
- Analyzing development from a biopsychosocial perspective helps to identify the complexities of human development.

What are the major issues in lifespan development?

- If it is to present a complete picture of development, any analysis of lifespan development must address key developmental issues, such as the importance of culture and development.
- Many psychologists believe that development occurs as a steady progression of small accomplishments (continuity); other psychologists believe that development occurs in spurts or stages (discontinuity).
- The controversies over stability versus change and nature versus nurture continue to stimulate debate among developmental psychologists.

What is the role of research in studying lifespan development?

- To explain the various ages and stages of development, we must use the best data available to enrich our insights and to provide a thoughtful perspective on the lifespan.
- Good data demand careful research methods; otherwise, we would be constantly suspicious of our conclusions.

- The most widely used research techniques include descriptive studies, manipulative experiments, and naturalistic experiments.
- Developmental psychologists also use four time-variable designs: one-time, one-group; longitudinal studies; cross-sectional studies; and sequential studies.

KEY TERMS

biopsychosocial interactions *5*

code of ethics *22*

continuity *16*

cross-sectional studies *21*

culture *13*

descriptive studies *17*

development *7*

discontinuity *16*

epigenetic view *13*

hypothesis *17*

lifespan development *5*

lifespan psychology *7*

longitudinal studies *19*

manipulative experiments *19*

naturalistic experiments *19*

one-time, one-group studies *19*

scientific method *17*

sequential (longitudinal/ cross-sectional) studies *21*

time-variable designs *19*

For REVIEW

1. Consider the biopsychosocial model presented in this chapter. How do you explain its potential value? Now think of an example in your own life, or in the life of someone you know, and describe how biological, psychological, and social factors interacted to produce a particular effect. Do you think the model helped you to explain that person's behavior?

2. Several issues were presented that thread their way through lifespan studies, such as culture and development and continuity versus discontinuity. Why do you think these are issues? Examine each one separately and defend your reasons for stating that each has strong developmental implications.

3. Throughout the chapter, the important role that the environment or context plays in development was stressed. What do you think of this emphasis? Think about your own life and the influences (both positive and negative) that those around you have had. Cite these personal experiences in your answer.

Chapter Review Test

Answers: 1a, 2a, 3c, 4d, 5c, 6b, 7a, 8a, 9a, 10d

1. Development is about
   a. change.
   b. age.
   c. gender.
   d. genes.

2. Development is
   a. a lifelong process.
   b. age focused.
   c. topically restricted.
   d. circular in nature.

3. Lifespan psychology assumes that development is
   a. unidimensional.
   b. chronologically explained.
   c. multidimensional.
   d. age limited.

4. Understanding childhood at any historical period depends on what _____ think of children.
   a. peers
   b. scientists
   c. siblings
   d. adults

5. A model that uses the interaction of biological, psychological, and social influences to explain development is the
   a. psychoanalytic.
   b. cognitive.
   c. biopsychosocial.
   d. behavioral.

6. One of the first outstanding theorists to recognize the importance of the early years was
   a. Skinner.
   b. Freud.
   c. Bandura.
   d. Hebb.

7. When we refer to the values, beliefs, and characteristics of a people, we are referring to
   a. culture.
   b. race.
   c. ethnicity.
   d. customs.

8. Adolescence begins in _____ and ends in _____ .
   a. biology, culture
   b. school, marriage
   c. structures, schema
   d. ego, superego

9. An example of a cross-sectional study is
   a. comparing individuals of various ages at the same time.
   b. continued observations of the same individuals.
   c. careful description by the researcher.
   d. one that requires no manipulation.

10. The typical research article contains four sections. Which item is not included in a research article?
   a. introduction
   b. method
   c. results
   d. author biography

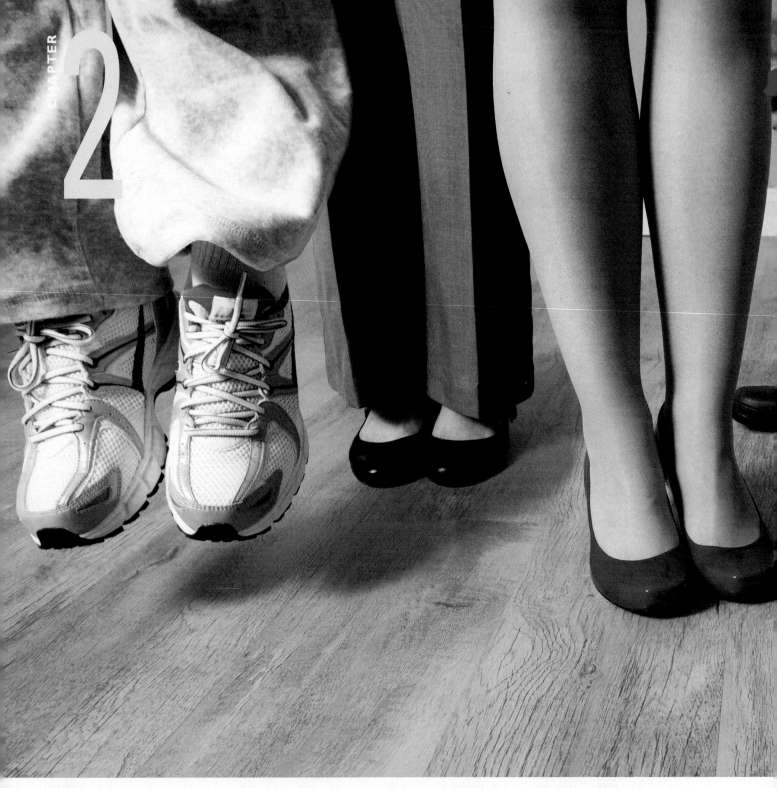

THEORIES OF
DEVELOPMENT:

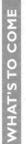

As You READ

After reading this chapter, you should be able to answer the following questions:

- How does psychoanalytic theory explain development across the lifespan?

- What is the relationship between psychosocial crises and lifespan development?

- How did Piaget explain cognitive development?

- What impact does culture have on lifespan development?

- What is the behavioral perspective on development?

- What is the status of current developmental theory?

INTERPRETING THE LIFESPAN

In this chapter, you'll read about several prominent developmental theories written by people who were curious about different aspects of lifespan development. As you will notice, the theories present one way of interpreting human development, and although no one theory is perfect, the driving force behind all the theories is their usefulness as invitations to consider lifespan development from different angles.

In a society that relies on scientific fact as truth that guides our behavior, what's the point of studying theories that suggest only "Maybe" and "Perhaps if . . ." are answers to the "Why?" of lifespan development? The answer is simple: Theories are essential for constructing meaning out of facts. They suggest explanations for phenomena. Good theories

- *help to organize a huge body of information.* Published studies on human development number in the tens of thousands, and the classic theories were written long before technological advances introduced websites, blogs, podcasts, and instant messaging as means of communicating and sharing ideas. The conclusions that research presents would be dizzying unless organized in some meaningful manner. A theory provides a way of examining facts and supplies "hooks" on which we can hang similar types of research findings. In this way, we build a lens through which to view development.

- *help to focus our search for new understandings.* Theories offer guideposts as we search for insights into the mysteries of human development.

- *help to explain how findings may be interpreted.* They offer a detailed guide that leads us to decide *which* facts are important and *what* conclusions we can draw.

- *help to identify major disagreements among scholars.* By highlighting these disagreements, theories offer testable ideas that can be confirmed or refuted by research.

When researchers are deciding what to study, they often begin with their emerging hypotheses and work toward formulating a theory. As we saw in Chapter 1, a hypothesis is a tentative explanation for a phenomenon that can be tested through research to see if indeed the explanation holds true in specific situations. For example, a researcher may notice that people in elevators tend to look up, down, or straight ahead rather than make eye contact with fellow riders. The researcher can test this hypothesis by riding in elevators and recording the behavior of fellow riders. The results of this investigation could lead to further assumptions about behavior that relate to social and/or psychological ideas. A researcher can develop a theory that people feel awkward about speaking in elevators because they do not wish to appear overly friendly and break social boundaries. **Theory,** then, refers to a belief or idea that develops based on information or evidence. A theory can inform research at the beginning of a study or take shape as the study unfolds. Theories allow people to make predictions about

theory A belief or idea that develops based on information or evidence; a proposed explanation for observed phenomena.

people's behavior. A person can predict that when she rides in an elevator, most often people will avoid eye contact. She can test the theory by smiling and blurting a hearty "Hi there!" every time someone gets on to see what, if anything, changes people's behavior. See what happens when you take your next ride in an elevator!

As you read the theories introduced in this chapter, you will notice the various approaches that theorists bring to their inquiry. Ultimately, the goal of any theory is to provide a framework for the study of human development that furthers scientific vision and leads to the application of that science for public policy and social programs, thereby contributing to the greater good of society.

A common criticism of theory is that it can feel removed from actual application of the ideas. This is referred to as the gap between theory and practice. It's therefore helpful to ground any discussion of theory in an actual example of the ideas in a real-life scenario. The following case study will serve as a launching pad for the use of theory as a way of examining lifespan development. After you have finished reading this chapter, we encourage you to reread and analyze the information in the following case study and interpret it according to a theory that strikes you as particularly interesting. You may believe that one theory explains one or more aspects of the situation well, while one of your classmates believes that a different theory is more applicable. Perhaps the answer lies in some unique combination of

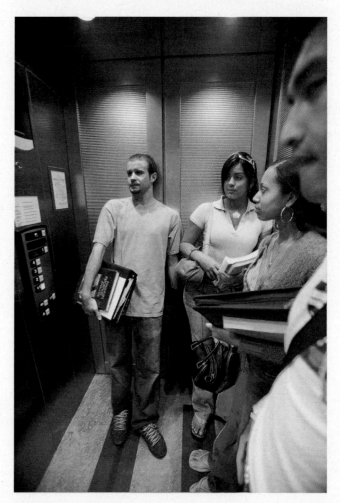

theories. There is no right or wrong answer; rather, as you and your classmates discuss various interpretations, you will gain a sense of how theory guides analysis of behavior.

Case Study: Amshula Khare

Amshula is 7 years old and the daughter of Indian immigrants. She attends the local public elementary school in her neighborhood and is finishing first grade. An only child, she often plays with her older cousins, and she's heard them speaking about tests that she'll have to take when she's in third and fourth grade. Her cousins use the word "fail" with dramatic and somber tones. Even though she enjoys school, the thought of failing the tests makes her very worried. She does not want to disappoint or embarrass her parents.

Amshula's parents do not speak English, and they work long hours at the family restaurant. Amshula goes to the restaurant after school and works on her homework in the kitchen. Because her help is needed at the restaurant, she does not have much time for playdates with peers or extracurricular activities.

At home, Amshula has begun to have stomachaches in the mornings before school. Her teacher, Mrs. Iskric, has noticed that Amshula often bites her nails and twirls her hair around her finger constantly. Amshula is a very serious student and tends to spend more time at desk work than center work with her peers. At recess, she can be found running around the blacktop, pausing to observe other children at play, or else she gathers rocks or sticks on the field by herself. Mrs. Iskric is concerned that Amshula is not forming close friendships and wonders whether Amshula is overly anxious.

Amshula's parents could not read the invitation to the school's open house, and even if they had read it, they would have had to miss it in order to work at the restaurant. Because they do not speak English, they are not familiar with the school's standard assessments and rely on their relatives for information about the typical progression through the school grades. Amshula's mother did attend the school's parent-teacher conference, but the school did not have a translator available, so she was unable to gain much information about Amshula's progress in school. Mr. and Mrs. Khare expect that Amshula will work in the family restaurant when she graduates from high school.

In this chapter, we explore the ideas of theorists who have guided thinking about lifespan development. A dis-

cussion of the present status of developmental theory and several issues related to the direction of developmental theory follows. Finally, you will learn how developmental systems theory and brain research reflect recent thinking regarding new directions in developmental analysis. As you read about these ideas, the overlap between biological, psychological, and social forces will become evident. Is it possible to separate one factor from the others as the most important contributor to lifespan development?

The **Freudian theory** *is one of the most important foundation stones for an edifice to be built by* future generations, *the dwelling of a freer and* **wiser humanity.**

THOMAS MANN (1939), GERMAN AUTHOR AND CRITIC

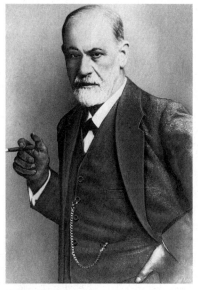

Sigmund Freud

Psychoanalytic Theories

Mention the word "psychoanalysis" to someone and the following images may spring to her mind: a couch, a therapist sitting in a chair holding pad and pen, the brain, and/or dreams. These images all relate to the ideas of one man who developed an approach to understanding human development that earned him the title "father of modern psychology." In more than 100 years of psychological research, no one has played a larger role than Sigmund Freud. Even his most severe critics admit that his theory on the development of personality is a milestone in the social sciences (Ferris, 1997). His ideas about the power of the unconscious, called **psychoanalytic theory**—the belief that we possess powerful ideas and impulses of which we're unaware but that exert a strong influence on our behavior—are a staple in any psychological discussion (Kahn, 2002). Freud's ideas no longer dominate developmental psychology as they did in the early part of the 20th century, due to interpretations

> **psychoanalytic theory**
> Freud's theory of the development of personality; emphasis on the role of the unconscious.

FIGURE 2.1

Freudian Stages of Development

1	2	3	4	5
The Oral Stage (0 to 1.5 years old)	**The Anal Stage** (1.5 to 3 years old)	**The Phallic Stage** (3 to 5 years old)	**The Latency Stage** (5 to 12 years old)	**The Genital Stage** (12 years old and older)
• The oral cavity (mouth, lips, tongue, gums) is the pleasure center. Its function is to obtain an appropriate amount of sucking, eating, and biting.	• The anus is the pleasure center. The function here is successful toilet training.	• The genitals are the pleasure centers in this stage and in the two remaining stages. The major function of this stage is the healthy development of sexual interest, which sometimes involves unconscious sexual desire for the parent of the opposite sex (called the *Oedipus complex* in males and the *Electra complex* in females).	• During this stage, sexual desire becomes dormant. Children tend to put energy into developing physical, intellectual, and social skills, such as sports and schoolwork.	• At this stage a surge of sexual hormones occurs in both genders, which brings about a recurrence of the phallic stage. People set about establishing relationships with others outside the immediate family.

by later theorists. However, his insistence on the early years as a vital period in human development remains a powerful concept when considering influences on human development (Crain, 2005).

FREUD'S THEORY

In Freud's view, development involves moving through five distinct stages, each one assigned to a specific age range and separate from the others: oral, anal, phallic, latency, and genital (see Figure 2.1). Each stage has a major function based on developmental wants or needs in that period of life and is linked to what Freud calls a pleasure center. The location of the pleasure center changes with development, and unless this pleasure center is satisfied (e.g., during breast-feeding or potty training), a person cannot resolve the inner conflicts relating to her wants or needs. Aspects of her personality remain at that stage (Freud's term *fixated*), and she is unable to become a fully mature person (Kahn, 2002). Conflicts arise in each stage, resulting in anxiety. Freud argued that the human personality uses **defense mechanisms** (psychological strategies to cope with anxiety or perceived threats) to deal with these crises.

Freud argued that at different stages of a person's development, personality is influenced by three distinct structures of the mind: the **id**, the **ego**, and the **superego**. They are fueled by the *libido*, Freud's term for psychic energy, which is similar to the physical energy that drives bodily functions. The characteristics of the three structures of the mind are as follows:

The id. This structure, the only one present at birth, contains

defense mechanisms Psychological strategies to cope with anxiety or perceived threats.

id Freud's structure of mind relating to our basic instincts; strives to secure pleasure.

ego Freud's notion of the central part of our personality; keeps id in check.

superego Freud's concept of our conscience; internal determinant of right and wrong.

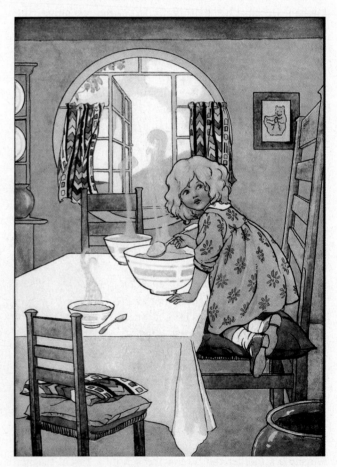

Several characters in beloved fairy tales exemplify the tension between Freud's mental forces as they encounter situations forcing them to decide between instant gratification and long-term gains.

all the basic instincts, such as the need for food, drink, comfort, and nurturance. The most primitive of the structures, it strives only to secure pleasure.

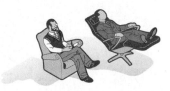

The superego. The superego is our conscience. Throughout infancy, we gain an increasingly clearer conception of what the world is like. Toward the end of the first year, we begin to internalize parental and societal standards of right and wrong, and we are expected to behave according to these values and beliefs.

The ego. The ego is the central part of our personality, the (usually) rational part that plans and keeps us in touch with reality, and keeps the id in check. Freud believed that the stronger the ego becomes, the more realistic and usually the more successful a person is likely to be (Lerner, 2002). The desires of the id and the demands of the superego are in constant battle, with the ego struggling to strike compromises between these two powerful forces.

Psychoanalytic theory has undergone many changes since Freud first proposed it, and as the significant role of culture in development has become increasingly apparent, social influences on development have assumed greater importance in psychoanalytic theory (Eagle, 2000; Westin, 2000). These social and cultural influences are precisely what propelled the theory of Erik Erikson, which will be presented in the next section. In spite of the diminished acceptance of Freud's ideas because of the heavy emphasis on sexual instincts, psychoanalytic theory has retained a solid core of support through the years. Recently, neuropsychologist Mark Solm (2004) argued strongly that although Freud's views (focusing on unconscious, invisible influences) took a backseat to brain research and the findings of neuroscientists in the 1980s (focusing on physical, visible biological phenomena), more current research has drawn renewed interest in the concepts of psychoanalysis.

For example, Eric Kandel, a 2000 Nobel Prize winner, called psychoanalysis the most coherent and intellectually satisfying view of the mind. With this statement, Kandel reflected the belief of several modern neuroscientists that some of Freud's conclusions enforce the research results of current experiments. Cognitive neuroscientists, for example, identify different memory systems as *explicit* or

Career Apps

As a teacher, how might you use fairy tales to help children grapple with their own personal fears or concerns?

implicit, which complements Freud's notion of *conscious* and *unconscious* memory.

As you can imagine, these ideas have not gone unchallenged. J. Allan Hobson, a professor of psychiatry at Harvard Medical School, argued just as forcefully that scientific investigations of Freud's concepts reveal errors in major parts of his theory. For example, most neuroscientists agree that the ego–id struggle does *not* control brain chemistry. To illustrate the wide gulf separating believers from nonbelievers, Hobson (2004) states that psychoanalytic

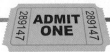

FEATURED MEDIA

Psychoanalysis on the Screen

Spellbound (1945) – What twists and surprises emerge as an amnesia patient, accused of murder, attempts to regain his memory with the help of psychoanalysis? Can the woman who loves him protect his identity?

High Anxiety (1977) – What lengths would the administrator of a psychiatric hospital go to in order to solve a murder mystery? Can he conquer his personal anxieties stemming from childhood that have begun to interfere with his life?

Grosse Pointe Blank (1997) – You're a professional hit man, plagued by old, unresolved problems, returning home for your 10-year high school reunion. How do you face the love of your life and that thing called growing up?

In Treatment (2008) – This television series explores what happens when a psychotherapist's personal psychological crises run parallel to, and sometimes intersect with, those of his clients.

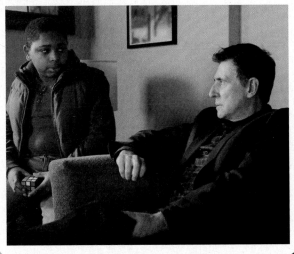

theory is indeed comprehensive, but if it is terribly off the mark, then its comprehensiveness is hardly of any value. Perhaps the "truth" or validity of Freud's theory is less important than its impact on an evolving appreciation of biopsychosocial influences. Threads of Freud's theory are tightly woven into the work of other prominent theorists, such as Erikson.

ERIKSON'S PSYCHOSOCIAL THEORY

Influenced by Freud, but searching for a different perspective, Erik Erikson developed a **psychosocial theory** of development that emphasizes the impact of social experiences on stages of human development. His seminal work, *Childhood and Society* (1963), is a perceptive and at times poetic description of human life.

Erikson's view of human development flowed from his extensive study of people living in an impressive variety of cultures: Germans, East Indians, the Sioux of South Dakota, the Yuroks of California, and wealthy adolescents in the northeastern United States (Erikson, 1959, 1968). His ideas also stem from intensive studies of historical figures such as Martin Luther (Erikson, 1958) and Mahatma Gandhi (Erikson, 1969). Erikson's theory continues to attract considerable attention and thus remains a vital interpretation of human development.

According to Erikson, human life progresses through a series of eight stages (see Table 2.1). Each of these stages is marked by a **life crisis** that must be resolved so that the individual can move on. Erikson used the term *crisis* to signify a time of both increased vulnerability and heightened potential.

Let's look at each stage more closely.

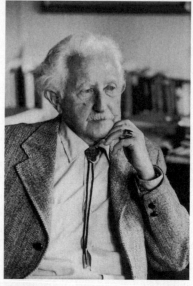

Erik Erikson

1. *Basic trust versus mistrust* (birth to 2 years old). In the first stage, infants develop a sense of basic trust. For Erikson, trust has an unusually broad meaning. To the trusting infant, it is not just that the world is a safe and happy place but that it is an orderly, predictable place. Infants learn about causes and effects. Trust flourishes with warmth, care, and discipline.

2. *Autonomy versus shame and doubt* (2 to 3 years old). When children are about 2 years old, they move into the second stage, characterized by the crisis of autonomy versus shame and doubt. Children begin to feed and dress themselves, and toilet training usually begins during these years. Toilet training is not the only accomplishment of the period; children of this age usually start acquiring self-control.

TABLE 2.1

Erikson's Psychosocial Theory of Development

Age	Stage	Psychosocial Crisis	Psychosocial Strength	Environmental Influence
Birth to 2 years	Infancy	Basic trust vs. mistrust	Hope	Maternal
2–3 years	Early childhood	Autonomy vs. shame and doubt	Willpower	Both parents or adult substitutes
3–5 years	Preschool, nursery school	Initiative vs. guilt	Purpose	Parents, family, friends
5–12 years	Middle childhood	Industry vs. inferiority	Competence	School
12–18 years	Adolescence	Identity vs. identity confusion	Fidelity	Peers
18–25 years	Young adulthood	Intimacy vs. isolation	Love	Partners, spouse/lover, friends
25–65 years	Middle age	Generativity vs. stagnation	Care	Family, society
65 years and older	Old age	Integrity vs. despair	Wisdom	All humans

3. *Initiative versus guilt* (3 to 5 years old). The third crisis, initiative versus guilt, begins when children are about 4 years old. Building on their ability to control themselves, children acquire some influence over others in the family and begin to successfully manipulate their surroundings. They don't merely react, they also initiate. Erikson believed that play is particularly important during these years, to support a child's identity and as a safe way to reduce tension by dealing with problems in a symbolic way (Csikszentmihalyi & Rathunde, 1998).

4. *Industry versus inferiority* (5 to 12 years old). The fourth stage corresponds closely to the child's elementary school years. The crisis extends beyond imitating ideal models to acquiring necessary information and skills of the culture. Children expand their horizons beyond the family and begin to explore the neighborhood. Children should experience a sense of accomplishment in creating and building; otherwise, they may develop a lasting sense of inferiority.

5. *Identity versus identity confusion* (12 to 18 years old). The main task of the adolescent is to achieve a state of identity. Erikson, who originated the term **identity crisis,** used the word in a specific way. In addition to thinking of identity as the general picture one has of oneself, Erikson referred to it as a state toward which one strives. In a state of identity, the various aspects of self-image would be aligned.

6. *Intimacy versus isolation* (18 to 25 years old). In the sixth stage, intimacy with others should develop. By intimacy, Erikson means the essential ability to relate one's deepest hopes and fears to another person and to accept in turn another person's need for intimacy.

7. *Generativity versus stagnation* (25 to 65 years old). Generativity means the ability to be useful to self and to society, thus leading to a sense of personal fulfillment. In this stage, individuals strive to make the world a better place for posterity in general and for one's own children in particular. Many people become mentors to younger individuals, sharing their knowledge and philosophy of life. When people fail in generativity, they begin to stagnate, to become bored and self-indulgent, unable to contribute to society.

8. *Integrity versus despair* (65 years old and older). To the extent that individuals have been successful in resolving the first seven crises, they achieve a sense of personal integrity. Adults with a sense of integrity accept their lives as having been well spent. They feel a kinship with people of other cultures and of previous and future generations. They have a sense of having helped to create a more dignified life for others. If, however, people look back over their lives and feel they have made the wrong decisions, they see life as lacking integration. Despair is the result of the negative resolution of this crisis. Individuals often hide their

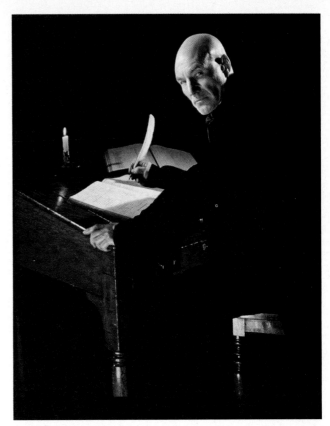

Patrick Stewart in Scrooge.

terror of death by appearing contemptuous of humanity in general and of those of their own religion or race in particular. The character Ebenezer Scrooge in Charles Dickens's classic novel *A Christmas Carol* is a perfect example of a person experiencing despair, someone who—before forced to examine his life—cares nothing for those around him.

> **identity crisis** Erikson's term for those situations, usually in adolescence, that cause us to make major decisions about our identity.

Erikson's eight stages cover age periods that extend beyond the age-related stages Freud proposed, and many people find Erikson's theory intuitively makes a lot of sense.

CONTRIBUTIONS AND CRITICISM OF PSYCHOANALYTIC THEORIES

Over the years, psychoanalytic theory has contributed much to the study of lifespan development and generated much debate. Some noteworthy contributions include

- an emphasis on the early years of life as critical to human development,

- the influence of the unconscious aspects of the mind on behavior,

- that personal fears may be confronted in symbolic terms (e.g., fairy tales), and

- that changes occur throughout the entire lifespan.

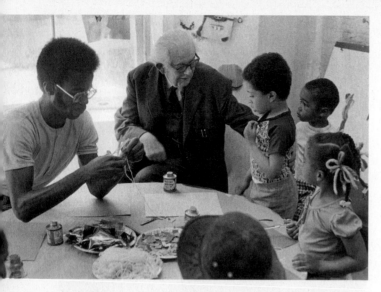

Much of Piaget's work developed based on his systematic observations.

Criticism includes the following:

- Unconscious thoughts or reconstructed memories may not be reliable sources of influence on development.

- Negative aspects of human development are overemphasized, particularly sexual desires.

- Although the roles of family and culture are deemed highly influential, there is a bias toward Western culture as the norm against which all other cultures are evaluated.

Cognitive Theories

Unlike psychoanalytic theories, which stress the unconscious or invisible workings of the mind, cognitive theorists such as Jean Piaget and Lev Vygotsky chose to focus on people's conscious thought processes. Other theorists agree with information-processing theory, which considers actions from a more mechanical standpoint.

PIAGET'S COGNITIVE DEVELOPMENTAL THEORY

The Swiss psychologist Jean Piaget's (1896–1980) training as a biologist had a major impact on his thinking about cognitive development. While working in Paris, field-testing questions for a standardized intelligence test, Piaget became fascinated with the thought processes that led children to make incorrect answers in reasoning tests. This caused him to turn his attention to the analysis of children's developing intelligence. Rather than focusing on test scores, Piaget focused on the process by which children actively construct meaning in their environments. Piaget was the first psychologist to systematically study cognitive development and to argue that thought processes influence human behavior in distinctly different ways throughout the lifespan.

object permanence
The realization that objects continue to exist even when they cannot be seen, heard, or touched.

cognitive structures
Piaget's term to describe the basic tools of cognitive development.

Have you ever been in a restaurant and wondered why a very young infant who accidentally knocks a toy off her highchair tray makes no attempt to find it, whereas a slightly older infant will try to find the toy or even purposefully drop a toy repeatedly and expect someone to pick it up? This apparently simple behavior, and many other behaviors like it, fascinated Piaget, who developed his theory of development based on systematic, close observations of his own children. In the example above, the older infant is exhibiting an understanding of **object permanence,** the realization that objects continue to exist even when they cannot be seen, heard, or touched. In Piaget's theory, object permanence is an important developmental accomplishment of an infant's first 2 years of life. Piaget viewed development as consisting of four distinct, increasingly sophisticated stages of mental representation that individuals pass through on their way to adulthood.

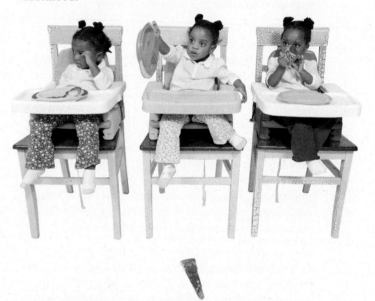

Piaget's Stages

Piaget believed that development occurs as we develop increasingly effective **cognitive structures,** mental representations that enable us to organize and adapt to our world. He also believed that individuals form more sophisticated cognitive structures as they pass through four stages: the *sensorimotor stage* (birth to 2 years old); the *preoperational stage* (2 to 7 years old); the *concrete operational stage* (7 to 11 years old); and the *formal operational stage* (11 years old and older). (See Table 2.2.) Piaget believed that cognitive structures begin as responses to concrete phenomena—babies know only what they can touch, taste, or see. Our ability to use symbols and to think abstractly increases with each stage until we are able to manipulate abstract concepts and consider complex hypothetical alternatives.

Piaget stated that we are able to form cognitive structures because we have inherited a method of intellectual functioning that permits us to respond to our environ-

TABLE 2.2
Piaget's Stages of Cognitive Development

Stage	Age	Major Feature
Sensorimotor	Birth to 2 years	Infants' sensory experiences with the environment form patterns that lead to cognitive structures; object permanence develops.
Preoperational	2 to 7 years	Use of symbols; rapid language growth.
Concrete operational	7 to 11 years	Can reason about physical objects.
Formal operational	11+ years	Abstract thinking leads to reasoning with more complex symbols.

ment. At the heart of this method is the mechanism of **adaptation.**

Piaget believed that adaptation consists of **assimilation** and **accommodation.** When we assimilate something, we incorporate it; we take it in. Think of eating; we take food into the structure of our mouths and change it to fit the shape of our mouths, throats, and digestive tracts. We take objects, concepts, and events into our minds similarly, incorporating this new information to fit our existing mental structures. For example, you are now studying Piaget's views on cognitive development. These ideas are unique and will require effort to understand them. You may attempt to comprehend them by fitting them to the cognitive structures you now possess.

Humans also change as a result of accommodation, that is, the adaptation of existing ways of understanding to new information. Just as the food we eat produces biochemical changes, the stimuli we incorporate into our minds produce mental changes. While we change what we take in, we are also changed by it.

adaptation One of the two functional invariants in Piaget's theory.

assimilation Piaget's term to describe the manner in which we incorporate data into our cognitive structures.

accommodation Piaget's term to describe the manner by which cognitive structures change.

perspectives on Diversity

Angels All Around Us

The idea of angels—beings that protect us, guide us, or provide for us—has been accepted across cultures for thousands upon thousands of years. Whether the term is most often used to describe earthly creatures or heavenly messengers, there is universal appreciation of (if not blatant belief in) angels among different nationalities, cultures, and ethnicities. It is striking that the concept of angels seems to defy rational thinking. For example, some young children may believe that the tooth fairy turns teeth into treasure in the form of coins or cash. Some young children may believe that Santa Claus delivers gifts to their homes once a year. Children's thought processes develop to a point where they eventually realize that these "angels" are not real. Yet some adults believe in religious angels who, for example, acted as messengers relating to specific biblical events, record our present-day good or bad actions, or are responsible for earthly elements of wind, fire, and water.

As you read the two examples that follow, think about how the concept of angels incorporates aspects of assimilation and/or accommodation, and how we actively construct meaning in order to make sense of new ideas or experiences.

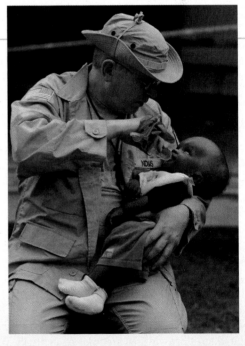

1. A woman's car won't start and she is parked in a New York underground parking garage, where she can't pick up a cell phone signal to call for assistance. A parking attendant brings over a portable battery charger and brings her battery to life.
2. An earthquake in Haiti devastates the homes and lives of hundreds of thousands of people. Learning of the event and the tragic aftermath through Twitter feeds and Facebook or blog posts, millions of people around the world donate resources to the relief effort.

Thus, the adaptive process is the heart of Piaget's explanation of learning. As we encounter new information, we try to strike a balance between assimilation and accommodation, a process that is called **equilibration.** By continued interaction with the environment, we correct these mistakes and change our cognitive structures (we have accommodated) into organized patterns of thought and action, which Piaget referred to as **schemes.**

Try thinking of Piaget's theory in the following way: Stimuli come from the environment and are filtered through the activities of adaptation and assimilation. For example, you may have had your own idea of what intelligence is, but now you change your structures relating to intelligence because of your new knowledge about Piaget. Your content or behavior changes because of the changes in your cognitive structures. The following summarizes Piaget's cognitive process:

Environment
(filtered through)
↓

Assimilation and Accommodation
(produce)
↓

Cognitive Structures
(which combine with behavior to form)
↓

Schemes
(organized patterns of thought and action)

VYGOTSKY'S SOCIOCULTURAL THEORY

The work of the Russian psychologist Lev Vygotsky (1896–1934) has attracted considerable attention because of his emphasis on social processes. Born in Russia in 1896, the same year as Piaget, Vygotsky was educated at Moscow University and quickly turned his attention to educational psychology, developmental psychology, and psychopathology. For Vygotsky, the clues to understanding mental development lie in children's social processes. He proposed that development depends on children's interactions with the adults around them.

Tragically, tuberculosis ended Vygotsky's life in 1934. His work today, because of its cultural emphasis, is more popular than it was in his lifetime. In contrast to Piaget, who believed that children function as "little scientists" investigating their own hypotheses as they make sense of the world, Vygotsky turned to social interactions to explain children's cognitive development.

Vygotsky identified dual paths of cognitive development—*elementary processes,* which are basically biological, and *psychological processes,* which are essentially sociocultural (Vygotsky, 1978). Children's behaviors emerge from the intertwining of these two paths. For example, brain develop-

equilibration Piaget's term to describe the balance between assimilation and accommodation.

schemes Piaget's term for organized patterns of thought and action.

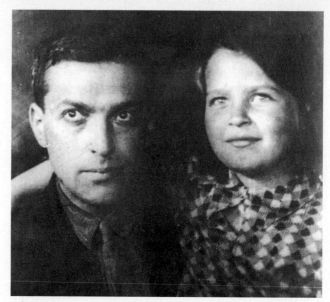

Lev Vygotsky

Through others, *we become* ourselves.

LEV VYGOTSKY

ment provides the mechanism for the appearance of external or visible speech (evidence of a child's thinking), which gradually becomes the internal speech children use to guide their behavior.

Three fundamental themes run through Vygotsky's work: the unique manner in which he identified and used the concept of development; the social origin of mind; and the role of speech in cognitive development.

1. At the heart of Vygotsky's theory is his belief that elementary biological processes are qualitatively transformed into higher psychological functioning by developmental processes. In other words, such behaviors as speech, thought, and learning are biological at the core, yet are manifest in the context of psychological functions.

2. To understand cognitive development, Vygotsky believed we must examine the social and cultural processes shaping children. Vygotsky argued that any function in a child's cultural development appears twice, on two planes: first, in an interpsychological category (social exchanges with others), and, second, within the child as an intrapsychological category (using inner speech to guide behavior).

What happens to transform an external activity to an internal activity? For Vygotsky, the answer lies in the phenomenon of internalization—when we observe something (behaviors, customs, rules) and then make it part of our own repertoire over time.

Respect for Culture

A telling example of culture's importance occurred when several American psychologists went to Rwanda to help with the massive psychological problems caused by the savagery and violence the people had experienced (Seppa, 1996). They found that traditional Western therapeutic methods, such as individualized therapy, were useless and that successful efforts in Africa helped restore social supports and relationships. They also discovered that urging patients to "talk it out" simply did not work. Using song, dance, and storytelling, which their patients found natural and comforting, proved to be more successful.

Can you think of other examples (from history, current life, or TV/film) where people worked successfully with and within a culture rather than imposing a foreign culture?

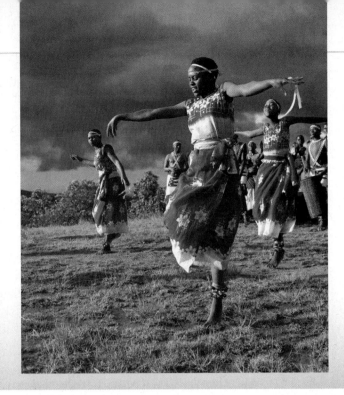

3. Although Vygotsky lacked hard data to explain it, he believed that speech is one of the most powerful tools humans use to progress developmentally. He wrote, "The most significant moment in the course of intellectual development . . . occurs when speech and practical activity, two previously completely independent lines of development, converge" (Vygotsky, 1978, p. 24). Speech allows us to ask questions, explain our thoughts, feelings, and actions, and connect with other members of family and society.

Vygotsky's concept of the **zone of proximal development (ZPD)** exemplifies the influence of social interaction and connections with others on cognitive development. Vygotsky described a range of ability for a given task, where the bottom of the range represents the actual ability a child might have on a given day, and the top of the range represents the level of ability a child might reach after working with a teacher, mentor, or peer. The social interaction will result in benefits that the child would not have experienced if he or she had worked alone. The ZPD is not limited to children. At any age we may learn a new skill and greatly benefit from support or guidance from a more experienced person.

Contemporary researcher Barbara Rogoff has investigated the role of culture in learning, specifically cultural variation in learning processes such as observation. Rogoff's work complements that of Vygotsky, and she shares Vygosky's interest in topics such as collaboration, social interaction, and the influence of mentoring on learning. Her book *Apprenticeship in Thinking* (1991) examines cognitive development in a sociocultural context and is noteworthy because it draws from a variety of her strengths as a contemporary female researcher. Rogoff's work is distinctive for drawing from a variety of disci-

plines, including anthropology, cultural psychology, and research on communication, and contributes to a body of knowledge and solid data about the influence of social and cultural forces.

Table 2.3 summarizes the key differences between Piaget's and Vygotsky's theories.

> **zone of proximal development** Vygotsky's term for a range of ability in a given task, where the higher limit is achieved through interaction with others.
>
> **information-processing theory** Cognitive theory that uses a computer metaphor to understand how the human mind processes information.

INFORMATION-PROCESSING THEORY

Distinct from the theories of Piaget and Vygotsky for several reasons, **information-processing theory** contributes another lens through which to consider human thinking. This theory is not attributed to one individual but, rather, is a broader way of examining cognitive development using the computer as a metaphor. Neither Piaget nor Vygotsky could have imagined computers as we know them today, let alone the important influence that computers would

Career Apps

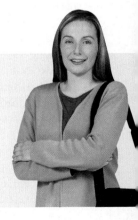

As an Early Head Start home visitor*, how might you demonstrate respect for children's and families' cultures in terms of language and literacy, religious practices, decisions about medical treatment, and family dynamics?

*Early Head Start is a federally funded community-based program for low-income families with infants and toddlers.

TABLE 2.3

Key Differences Between Theories: Piaget and Vygotsky

	Piaget	Vygotsky
Perspective	Individual child constructs view of world by forming cognitive structures—"the little scientist."	Child's cognitive development progresses by social interactions with others—"social origins of mind."
Basic Psychological Mechanism	Equilibration—child acts to regain equilibrium between external stimuli and the current level of cognitive structures.	Social interaction encourages development through the guidance of skillful adults.
Language	Emerges as cognitive structures develop.	Begins as preintellectual speech and develops into sophisticated form of inner speech; one of the main forces of cognitive development.
Learning	Assimilation and accommodation lead to equilibrium.	Results from the interaction of biological elementary processes and sociocultural interactions.
Problem Solving	Child independently searches for data needed to change cognitive structures, enabling child to reach solution.	Two aspects of problem solving—key role of speech to guide "planful" behavior and joint efforts with others.

have on psychologists' understandings of cognition. Just as computers perform operations based on their hardware and software, the human brain performs operations based on cognitive structures and thought processes (Bjorkland, 2005).

Information-processing theory is not a stage theory but, rather, a processing capacity. Throughout our lifespan, we develop an increasing capacity for processing information. We are therefore able to perform more complicated tasks as we acquire the knowledge and skills needed to do so. For example, a young child may need to pay careful attention as she learns to tie her shoes. With practice and repetition, the child will soon need to pay less attention to the task and is later able to tie her shoes with minimal effort. The same may be said for a teenager learning to drive a car—at first the teen must pay close attention to every hand and foot movement as she coordinates the car's equipment. With practice and experience, the teen will be able to drive with minimal effort, perhaps singing along to favorite tunes on the radio. As you can see, the age of an individual does not matter as much as the specific task. An adult can be an expert or a novice at a task in the same way a child is an expert or novice.

Experts on the subject of information-processing theory, such as D. E. Broadbent (1954) and Robert Siegler (1996, 2006), have evolved specific positions on the theory. While Broadbent's work emphasizes the role of selective attention, Siegler's work focuses on the increasing variety of mental processes that we have to draw upon as we age. Consistent with a computer model, information-processing theorists agree that humans perceive, encode, represent, store, and retrieve information. The process repeats itself from situation to situation, and the more strategies we have at our disposal, the quicker and more successfully we are able to think.

CONTRIBUTIONS AND CRITICISM OF COGNITIVE THEORIES

Cognitive theories have contributed to a greater understanding of human development. Some key contributions include:

- a view of people as active participants in constructing knowledge and meaning,

- conscious efforts to understand the world lead to advances in development, and

- viewing biological structures as influenced by social forces, which, in turn, influence our biology.

Some criticisms of cognitive theories include:

- an underestimation (on Piaget's part) of the cognitive skills of infants and young children, and

- lack of attention to individual variation in cognitive development, especially based on cultural and family background.

The Behavioral Approach

A strictly behavioral explanation of human development argues that only what can be observed and measured may be scientifically studied. This approach takes us into the world of learning and learning theory. Some of its best-known proponents are Ivan Pavlov (1849–1936) and John Watson (1878–1958) for their work with classical conditioning, B. F. Skinner (1904–1990) for his insights into the role of reinforcement, and Albert Bandura (b. 1925), who called our attention to the power of modeling in development.

PAVLOV'S AND WATSON'S CLASSICAL CONDITIONING

Behavioral theorists argue that development is observable behavior that can be learned over time. Pavlov had observed that dogs would salivate when they ate food. He also noticed that they would begin to salivate when they heard certain sounds (such as a food cupboard door opening or closing) or saw certain things (such as a person retrieving a food dish) associated with eating. He designed a famous experiment in which the ringing of a bell was paired with food being presented to dogs. Over time, the dogs learned to salivate merely at the ringing of the bell. Pavlov's experiment is noteworthy because he showed that an involuntary response (salivating) could be elicited through a specific learning process. Pavlov called this learning **classical conditioning.**

John Watson shared an interest in classical conditioning but focused on human beings rather than animals. Watson conducted a famous experiment in which he conditioned an infant ("Little Albert") to fear a white rat. Every time Albert played with the rat, a loud noise was made behind him, startling him and causing him to cry. Over time, as play with the rat was paired with the loud noise, Albert began to cry at the mere sight of the rat. Unfortunately, ethical codes of conduct of the sort that exist today were not considered at the time of this experiment. Albert would not have been subjected to repeated upset in a modern version of this study; yet the significance of Watson's work must be acknowledged for the attention it brought to human behavior and the ways in which we are conditioned in our everyday lives.

SKINNER'S OPERANT CONDITIONING

Convinced of the importance of reinforcement, Skinner developed an explanation of learning that stressed the consequences of behavior—the effects of actions are all-important. **Reinforcement,** defined as anything that makes a response more likely to happen in the future, has proven to be a powerful tool in the developing, shaping, and control of behavior in numerous contexts. Prominent in American psychology for over 60 years, B. F. Skinner inspired and stimulated research and theory.

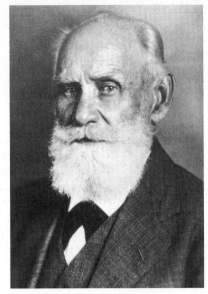
Ivan Pavlov

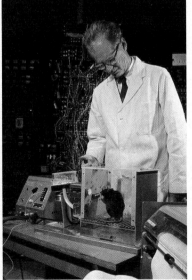
B. F. Skinner

Skinner preferred the term *reinforcement* to *reward* and identified two kinds of reinforcement. **Positive reinforcement** refers to any event that, when it occurs after a response, makes that response more likely to happen in the future. **Negative reinforcement** is any event that, when it ceases to occur after a response, makes that response more likely to happen in the future. Note that both types of reinforcement make a response more likely to happen. Giving a child candy for doing the right thing is positive reinforcement. Ceasing to twist your brother's arm when he gives you back your pen is negative reinforcement. The presence or absence of the stimulus causes increase or decrease in behavior. Thus human development is the result of the continuous flow of learning that comes about from the operant conditioning we receive from the environment every day.

In Skinner's theory, the concept of **operant conditioning** has a large influence on learning. Operant conditioning refers to our behavior or actions that we do voluntarily, and how the use of consequences can modify or shape such behavior. A simple example from everyday life is the notion of a "customer reward program." Many stores, restaurants, and credit cards offer customers points that they can use on future visits or to acquire other items. The more you shop at that store, the more points you acquire. You are rewarded for your purchases, and the likelihood that you will repeat your shopping behavior is greater with this incentive. Skinner argued that the environment (parents, teachers, peers) reacts to our behavior and either reinforces or eliminates that behavior. Consequently, the environment holds the key to understanding behavior.

Skinner argued that if the environment reinforces a certain behavior, it's more likely to result the next time that stimulus occurs. His famous "Skinner box" became renowned for making visible the power of reinforcement on lab rats' behaviors. Skinner devised a box in which rats would receive food pellets when they pushed a certain lever (see

classical conditioning The learning process in which a neutral stimulus produces an involuntary response that is usually elicited by another stimulus.

reinforcement Anything that increases the likelihood a response will occur in the future.

positive reinforcement An event that increases the likelihood of a desired response in the future.

negative reinforcement An event that, when it ceases to occur, makes that response more likely to happen in the future.

operant conditioning The use of consequences (reinforcement, punishment) to modify or shape voluntary behavior or actions.

FIGURE 2.2

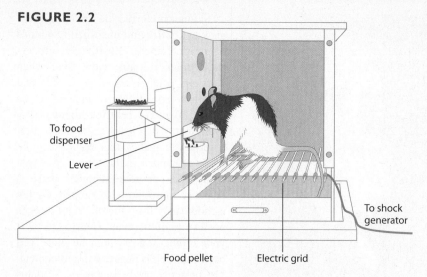

To food dispenser

Lever

To shock generator

Food pellet   Electric grid

Figure 2.2). The rats' behavior indicated that they learned to push the lever in order to acquire more food.

Skinner also used the terms *punishment* and *extinction* in his discussion of operant conditioning. **Punishment** refers to a decrease in behaviors when an unpleasant response follows the behavior. **Extinction** is the systematic way in which behaviors are conditioned out of a person's behavior. In a human scenario, if a teacher repeats a particular question, a student is more likely to give the right answer, because that response was reinforced (the student feels happy and proud). If the response is punished, the response is less likely in the future (the student feels sad and humiliated). If the response is simply ignored, it also becomes less likely in the future (the student learns that her effort is not recognized).

Skinner's ideas about change in human behavior have been enhanced by the work of Albert Bandura, who expanded the behaviorist view to cover social behavior.

Social learning theory has particular relevance for development. As Bandura noted, children do not always do what adults tell them to do but rather what they see adults do. If Bandura's assumptions are correct, adults can be a potent force in shaping the behavior of children because of what they do.

The importance of models is seen in Bandura's interpretation of what happens as a result of observing others:

Children may acquire new responses, including socially appropriate behaviors.

Observation of models may strengthen or weaken existing responses.

Observation of a model may cause the reappearance of responses that were seemingly forgotten.

If children witness undesirable behavior that is either rewarded or goes unpunished, undesirable behavior may result. The reverse is also true.

Bandura, Ross, and Ross (1963) studied the relative effects of live models, filmed human aggression, and filmed cartoon aggression on preschool children's aggressive behavior in the classic Bobo doll experiment. The filmed human adult models displayed aggression toward an inflated doll; in the filmed cartoon aggression, a cartoon character displayed the same aggression. Later, all the children who observed the aggression were more aggressive than children in the control group. This experiment has serious implications for how modeling can be a powerful force in development. Children are influenced by live models, as well as by behaviors they observe in the media.

punishment Process by which an unpleasant response is paired with an undesired behavior to decrease the likelihood of that behavior occurring in the future.

extinction The systematic process in which behaviors are de-conditioned or eliminated.

modeling Bandura's term for observational learning.

observational learning Bandura's term to explain the information we obtain from observing other people, things, and events.

social (cognitive) learning Bandura's theory that refers to the process whereby the information we glean from observing others influences our behavior.

BANDURA'S SOCIAL COGNITIVE LEARNING

Albert Bandura, one of the chief architects of social learning theory, has stressed the potent influence of **modeling** on personality development (Bandura, 1997). He called this **observational learning.** In a famous statement on **social (cognitive) learning theory,** Bandura and Walters (1963) cited evidence to show that learning occurs through observing others, even when the observers do not imitate the model's responses at that time and get no reinforcement. For Bandura, observational learning means that the information we get from observing other people, things, and events influences the way we act (Bjorklund, 2005).

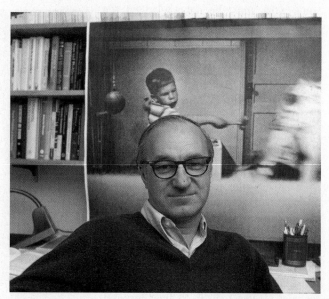

Albert Bandura

Does Spanking Lead to Violence?

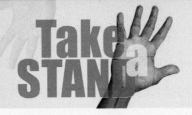

The debate over spanking (a.k.a., corporal punishment) has led to arguments linking spanking to more or less violence when children grow into adulthood. Each of these arguments relates to aspects of behavioral theory in terms of reinforcement and modeling.

Argument A: If spanking *is NOT* used as a method of discipline, children will grow into more violent adults and more criminal behavior will result from a lack of control.

Argument B: If spanking *IS* used as a method of discipline, children will grow into more violent adults because they have learned that violence is an appropriate way to express feelings.

Argument C: *NOT* spanking children will lead to a decrease in violent and criminal acts, in addition to a reduction in cases of depression, anxiety, and substance abuse, because children will learn other ways of negotiating and resolving conflicts.

Do you think spanking is a useful form of punishment for children? If so, what are the appropriate boundaries for spanking behavior? Who should determine whether or not spanking is acceptable—families, doctors, or human service agencies?

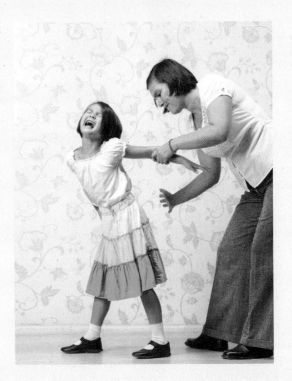

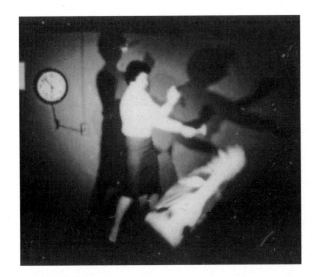

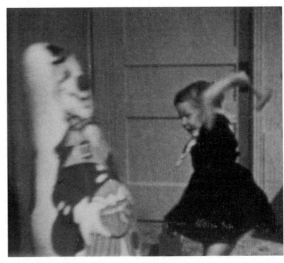

Another example of the power of Bandura's ideas is seen in the concept of **self-efficacy**—a person's belief that she can behave in a certain way to achieve a desired goal. Bandura and colleagues (2001) believe that a child's sense of self-efficacy helps him to produce desired outcomes that might otherwise elude him. Unless children—and adults—believe that their actions will attain desired goals, they have little incentive to act and certainly will not persist in the face of difficulty. Bjorklund (2005) believes that Bandura's ideas testify to the significance of the interaction between a child's cognitive and social worlds.

Because the important role of biology in human development was dismissed, operant conditioning eventually lost its appeal to developmental biologists (Cairns & Cairns, 2006). The idea of a bioecological model of human development became more widely accepted in the mainstream of modern science.

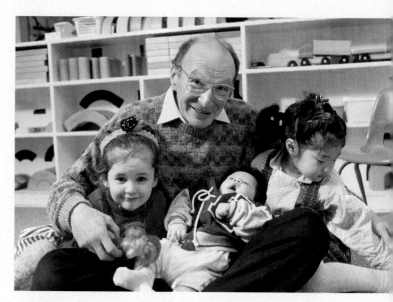

Uri Bronfenbrenner

A Bioecological Model

Physical, cognitive, and social factors interact in ways that we are only beginning to comprehend. For example, psychologists recognize the importance of **reciprocal interactions** in development. Reciprocal interactions are people's responses to those around them that cause them to change; their responses to us then change, which in turn produces new changes in us. These don't rely exclusively on either heredity or environment. Rather, the interactions between the two help describe and explain developmental changes that occur from birth, if not sooner.

Thanks to the systems analysis of Uri Bronfenbrenner (1917–2005), we now realize that there are many environments (also called systems) acting on us. Bronfenbrenner's perspective is called the **bioecological model,** defined as the continuity and change in the biopsychosocial characteristics of human beings, both as individuals and as groups. The bioecological model contains four major components. The first component, *proximal processes,* refers to the reciprocal interactions between a person and the environment (often called the *context* of development). Feeding and playing with a child, peer play, and school learning with teachers are all examples of proximal processes. Bronfenbrenner and Morris (1998, 2006) refer to proximal processes as the primary engines of development.

The second component is the *person* involved, especially an individual's temperament or disposition that activates the proximal processes. Third is the person's *context,* those environmental features that either foster or interfere with development. Finally, developmental changes occur over *time,* the fourth component of the bioecological model. Bronfenbrenner realized that most theories represent development in snapshots of developmental periods, so to speak. He recognized that the passing of time greatly influences people throughout their lives as they interact with their surroundings.

Bronfenbrenner visualized the environment as a set of nested systems, each inside the next, as shown in Figure 2.3.

self-efficacy A person's belief that she can behave in a certain way to achieve a desired goal.

reciprocal interactions People's responses to those around them that cause them to change; their responses then change, which in turn produces new changes.

bioecological model The continuity and change in the biopsychosocial characteristics of human beings, both as individuals and as groups.

microsystem The home or school.

mesosystem The relationship among microsystems.

He identified the innermost environmental system as the **microsystem** (for example, the home or school). Next is the **mesosystem,** which refers to the relationship among microsystems. A good example is seen in a child's school achievement. Those children who are fortunate enough to be in a family that maintains positive relationships with the school tend to do well in their classwork.

The **exosystem,** Bronfenbrenner's next level, is an environment in which the developing person is not actually present but that nevertheless affects development. For example, a teenager has a friend whose parents, unlike her own parents, are relaxed about curfews, don't pressure their daughter to complete assignments, and so on. These different parenting practices may eventually cause conflict between the teen and her parents. The **macrosystem,** Bronfenbrenner's final level, is the blueprint of any society, a kind of master plan for human development within that society. Think for a moment about the different experiences that people in the mainland Chinese society have encountered when compared to the experiences of American citizens.

These systems do not remain isolated from one another but interact over time (sometimes called the *chronosystem*). An example is a child whose father has just lost his job (changes in the exosystem), which then causes the family to move to another location with different friends and schools for the child (changes in the micro- and mesosystems). These examples illustrate how a bioecological anal-

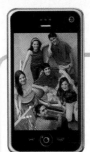

TECH TRENDS

Theory Clips

The popularity of sites such as YouTube (www.youtube.com) and TeacherTube (*www.teachertube.com*) has prompted the use of video as a tool to gain insights into theorists and their ideas. The following examples are but a few that are available for viewing:

Erikson – mnemonic device for remembering the eight stages of Erikson's theory:

http://www.thepsychfiles.com/200808/episode_67-mnemonic-device-for-eriksons-eight-stages-of-development/

Piaget and conservation tasks:

http://teachertube.com/viewVideo.php?video_id=55837&title=Piaget_Conservation_Tasks

Bandura and the Bobo doll experiment:

http://www.youtube.com/watch?v=vdh7Mngntnl

Overview of Bronfenbrenner's theory:

http://www.youtube.com/watch?v=me7l03olE-g

FIGURE 2.3

Bronfenbrenner's Ecological Theory

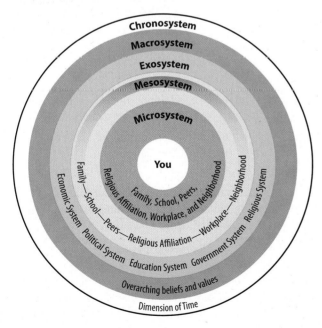

ysis emphasizes the role of context in development.

Supporting the importance of acknowledging complex interactions between systems, Rutter (2002b) has presented a threefold argument stressing that, although genes are at the heart of all psychological traits, it is the interaction of biological, psychological, and social influences that explains behavior.

exosystem Environment in which the developing person is not present but that nevertheless affects development.

macrosystem The blueprint of any society.

1. Given today's remarkable scientific advances, there is little disagreement about the influence of genes. But even from a biological perspective, the real challenge is to discover how genetic influences and brain functions, for example, are altered by experience.

2. Emerging genetic evidence clearly illustrates the significance of *nongenetic* influences. As Rutter notes, even with those traits that are most powerfully influenced by genetic forces, environmental effects are far from trivial.

3. Finally, the same genetic factors may be involved in different types of childhood psychopathology, for example, anxiety and depression.

Developmental Theory: Current Status and Future Directions

A persistent criticism of traditional theorists such as Piaget and Freud is that they were simply too one-dimensional to explain the complexity of development. That is, they focused on only one aspect of development. For example, Piaget focused solely on cognitive development, and Freud spent his lifetime delving into the role of the unconscious in development. But as Lerner (1988) noted, in current developmental theories, the person is not simply "biologized, psychologized, or sociologized." Such focused viewpoints, however much they help clarify the processes involved in development, present an inadequate portrayal of the richness and vigor of the human lifespan. The nuances of human development cannot be captured by theories limited to one facet of development: motor, cognitive, or language. To address this situation, psychologists have proposed a developmental systems theory, one that encompasses previously hard-won knowledge and searches for explanations in the relationships among the multiple levels that contribute to development (Lewis, 2000). According to this view, to describe and understand the changes that take place over the lifespan, we must pay attention to all the levels at which change can occur and focus on the interactions among these changes.

INTERACTIONS AMONG LEVELS OF DEVELOPMENT

Developmental psychologists currently analyze activity at four levels: genetic, neural, behavioral, and environmental (Gottlieb, 1997; Gottlieb, Wahlsten, & Lickliter, 2006). With close attention paid to the interactions among these levels, the biopsychosocial nature of development is illustrated as new understandings (and new questions) continue to emerge.

Genes produce a particular physical makeup that contributes to a person's behavior, helping that individual to select a particular environment (peers, activities, and such). But the environment also acts to influence behavior, physical status, and even genetic activity. In other words, each level interacts with all other levels.

DEVELOPMENTAL SYSTEMS THEORY

It's clear that heredity and environment produce results in a complex, interactive manner that supports the idea of reciprocal interactions. It appears that there are no simple cause-and-effect explanations of development. All humans—children, adolescents, and adults—experience a constant state of reorganization as they move through the life cycle (Lerner, Fisher, & Weinberg, 2000).

developmental systems theory Set of beliefs leading to the conclusion that we construct our own views of the world.

life course theory Theory referring to a sequence of socially defined, age-graded events and roles that individuals enact over time.

Developmental systems theory was popularized by Richard Lerner (1991, 1998, 2002, 2006) and Gilbert Gottlieb (1997). The current version attributed to Gottlieb, Douglas Wahlsten, and Robert Lickliter (2006) argues that all of our characteristics (biological, psychological, and social) function by reciprocal interactions with the environment (a.k.a., context). In this way, developmental systems theory leads to the belief that we *construct* our view of the surrounding world.

Lerner (2002) emphasized that developmental systems theory requires three levels of analysis:

1. Knowledge of the characteristics of those being studied

2. Understanding of a person's context and a justification for why this portion of the context is significant for analysis

3. Conceptualization of the relationship between individual characteristics and the portion of the context

Exchanges between individuals and the multiple levels of their complex contexts propel development (Horowitz, 2000; Lerner & Ashman, 2006). (See Figure 2.4.) The crucial aspect of development is therefore the changing relationship between our own complexity and a multilayered context. No single level of organization is seen as the primary or the ultimate causal influence on behavior and development (Dixon & Lerner, 1999). Although developmental systems theory exemplifies current changes in the search for developmental explanations, other ideas continue to emerge.

UNIQUE THEORIES OF DEVELOPMENT

While all of the theories discussed so far have a distinct approach to understanding human development, the following theories do not fall into one of the broader theoretical categories but, rather, stand alone as influential in the field. **Life course theory,** proposed by Glen Elder, refers to a sequence of socially defined, age-graded events and roles that individuals enact over time. Life course researchers must

• change from studying children alone to a strategy that focuses on aging over the entire life course;

• rethink how human lives are organized and evolve over time, while searching for patterns of constancy and change;

• relate individuals' life course to an ever-changing society, stressing the developmental changes brought about by this interaction (Elder & Shanahan, 2006).

Evolutionary developmental psychology is an explanation of development that assumes our physiological and psychological systems resulted from evolution by selection. In 1859, Charles Darwin published *On the Origin of Species,* in which he concluded that natural selection is the basic principle of change. Evolutionary theory suggests

FIGURE 2.4
Developmental Contextual Model

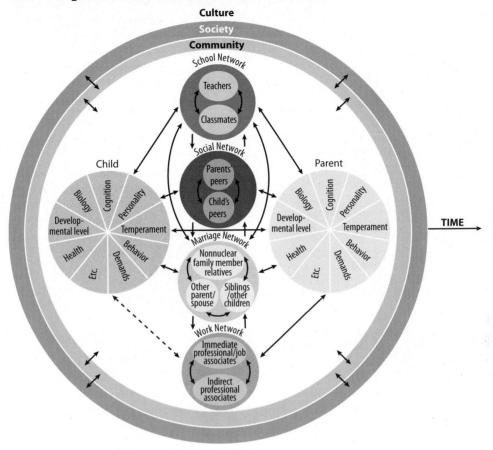

that psychological mechanisms evolved to bring about specific adaptive functions. It's the study of how our genes are expressed during development and how the context of development influences the expression of genetic action. **Evolutionary developmental psychology** can be defined as the use of principles of Darwinian evolution, particularly natural selection, to explain human development. It involves the physiological and psychological mechanisms that underlie universal development.

Evolutionary developmental psychology has also received support from what has been called the cognitive revolution. Widely and wildly popular with psychologists, studies of cognition provided respectability to explanations of behavior that were not immediately visible (Geary & Bjorklund, 2000). Evolutionary psychology brings together revolutionary ideas in science—the cognitive revolution that began in the 1950s and 1960s, which helped us to understand why we have the kind of mind we do, and the change in evolutionary biology that explained the ability of living things to adapt by selection. Thus the physiological and psychological mechanisms needed for healthy development are those that survive the process of natural selection. Biology is not our destiny, and environmental input does impact development.

Humanistic psychologist Abraham Maslow's hierarchy of needs (1987), while not a distinctly developmental theory, emphasizes the importance of growing and developing as a person to achieve one's potential. According to Maslow, there are five types of needs: physiological (hunger and sleep), safety (security, protection, stability, and freedom from fear and anxiety), love and belonging (need for family and friends), esteem (positive opinion of self and also by others), and self-actualization (doing all that we think we are capable of doing). (See Figure 2.5.) In Maslow's estimation, only approximately 2% of the world population will ever reach this highest level of needs being met and utilized.

What does Maslow's theory look like in everyday life? Examples of Maslow's theory in action are as follows:

Physiological needs. A child comes to school without eating breakfast in the morning and must summon the energy and focus to accomplish the same tasks as his peers. (How can the child generate the energy and focus required to succeed in the classroom?)

Safety needs. A single parent gets laid off from work and is forced to choose between paying for the

> **evolutionary developmental psychology** Explanation of development that rests on the assumption that our physiological and psychological systems resulted from evolution by selection.

FIGURE 2.5

Maslow's Hierarchy of Needs

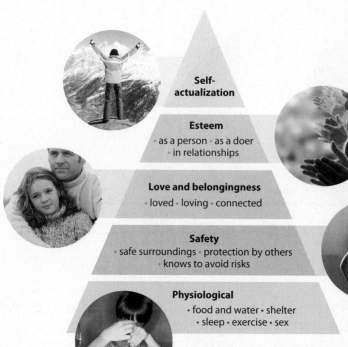

Self-actualization

Esteem
· as a person · as a doer
· in relationships

Love and belongingness
· loved · loving · connected

Safety
· safe surroundings · protection by others
· knows to avoid risks

Physiological
· food and water · shelter
· sleep · exercise · sex

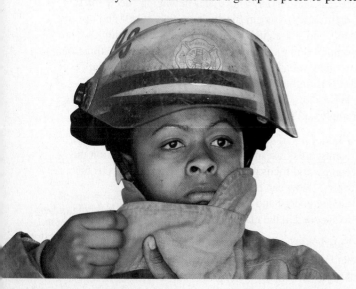

support and stimulation as she transitions into her new community?)

Self-esteem needs. A grandfather invites his family on a group vacation to celebrate his 40th wedding anniversary, affording him the chance to function as the patriarch of the group. (How does one express pride and authority among a group of people who have grown over time and have developed different expectations for his role as father and grandfather?)

Self-actualization. A Hollywood celebrity decides to leave his mansion in the Hollywood hills and dedicate two years of his life to working with African children who have lost parents to AIDS. (How might he reconcile the creative energy required for his work as an actor and high-profile personality with the realistic demands on his energy, time, and persona in this specific context?)

In an effort to be all we can be, we must consider the needs that must be met on different levels in order for anyone to achieve the ultimate source of satisfaction and generativity. Table 2.4 summarizes the theories of development we have discussed in this chapter.

heating bill and buying groceries for his family, knowing that whichever choice he makes will lead to severe problems for his loved ones. (How can this dad feel like he's contributing to society and a source of pride to his children?)

Love and belonging needs. A mother moves to a new city and, even though she works part-time and has a loving spouse, feels lonely as she cares for her toddler each day. (How can she find a group of peers to provide

FROM NEURONS TO NEIGHBORHOODS

The study done in 2000 by the National Research Council Institute of Medicine and published in the book *From Neurons to Neighborhoods: The Science of Early Childhood Development,* edited by Jack Shonkoff and Deborah Phillips, has been highly regarded as an attempt to synthesize nearly 50 years of early childhood development with the goal of improving policies aimed at raising and educating young children. The following 10 statements, taken from the study, synthesize extensive research and investigation, resulting in powerful arguments for the role and responsibility of science and effectively bringing theory into practice.

1. Human development is shaped by a dynamic and continuous interaction between biology and experience.

2. Culture influences every aspect of human development and is reflected in childrearing beliefs and practices designed to promote healthy adaptation.

3. The growth of self-regulation is a cornerstone of early childhood development that cuts across all domains of behavior.

4. Children are active participants in their own development, reflecting the intrinsic human drive to explore and master one's environment.

5. Human relationships, and the effects of relationships on other relationships, are the building blocks of healthy development.

TABLE 2.4

Comparing Theories of Development

Pscyhoanalytic	Psychosocial	Cognitive	Cultural	Behavioral	Contextual
Major Figures					
Freud	Erikson	Piaget	Vygotsky	Skinner, Bandura	Lerner
Major Ideas					
Passage through the psychosexual stages	Passage through the psychosocial stages	Development of cognitive structures through stages of cognitive development	Social processes embedded within a culture influence development	Power of operant conditioning; role of modeling in development	Development occurs as an individual's characteristics interact with that person's context
Essential Features					
Id, ego, superego; psychosexual stages	Psychosocial crises; psychosocial stages	Formation of cognitive structures; stages of cognitive development	Social processes	Reinforcement of responses; observational learning modeling	Interaction among multiple levels of development
Source of Developmental Problems					
Conflict during development leads to fixation, regression, and personality problems	Inadequate resolution of psychosocial crises	Weak formation of cognitive structures	Environmental support lacking or insufficient	Lack of reinforcement, incorrect pairing of stimuli and responses	Faulty exchanges between the individual and the multiple levels of the context
Goal					
Sexually mature individual	A sense of personal integrity	Satisfactory formation and use of cognitive structures	Recognition and use of social processes to guide development	Acquisition of conditioned acts to fulfill needs	Satisfactory relationships between the individual and a multilayered context

6. The broad range of individual differences among young children often makes it difficult to distinguish normal variations and maturational delays from transient disorders and persistent impairments.

7. The development of children unfolds along individual pathways whose trajectories are characterized by continuities and discontinuities, as well as by a series of significant transitions.

8. Human development is shaped by the ongoing interplay among sources of vulnerability and sources of resilience.

9. The timing of early experiences can matter, but, more often that not, the developing child remains vulnerable to risks and open to protective influences throughout the early years of life and into adulthood.

10. The course of development can be altered in early childhood by effective interventions that change the balance between risk and protection, thereby shifting the odds in favor of adaptive outcomes.

One of the most important outcomes of this extensive work is that the researchers who conducted the study brought critical issues in human development to light and identified immediate policy efforts that would address critical needs for children. Because young children are often undervalued or ignored in the policy arena, *From Neurons to Neighborhoods* is evidence that society's investment in children will have long-term benefits for all citizens.

Any interpretation of human development is subject to scrutiny and must be considered in the context of history. As you consider the stages of lifespan development in the chapters that follow, the theoretical foundation laid in this chapter will guide you as you pursue your own inquiry and emerging hypotheses. The interactions between biology, psychology, and social forces will continue to emerge as the primary source of development over time.

CONCLUSIONS & SUMMARY

In this chapter, several interpretations of development were introduced to help you understand and integrate developmental data. The theories presented here have played or are playing major roles in our understanding of human development, and additional theories will be presented throughout the text. Now that you have become familiar with the major theories in human development, consider the case study of Amshula Khare presented at the beginning of the chapter. What strikes you about Amshula's story, and what connections to theory do you make at this time?

How does psychoanalytic theory explain development across the lifespan?

- Freud considered the unconscious mind to be the key to understanding human beings.
- Important information in the unconscious mind is kept hidden through an array of defense mechanisms.
- The mind is divided into three constructs—the id, the ego, and the superego—each of which appears at different stages of a child's development.
- Personality development is divided into five instinctive stages of life—oral, anal, phallic, latency, and genital—each stage serving a major function.
- Failure to pass through a stage of development results in fixation, which halts a person from becoming fully mature.

What is the relationship between psychosocial crises and lifespan development?

- Erikson believed that human life progresses through eight "psychosocial" stages, each one marked by a crisis and its resolution.
- Although the ages at which one goes through each stage vary, the sequence of stages is fixed. Stages may overlap, however.
- A human being must experience each crisis before proceeding to the next stage. Inadequate resolution of the crisis at any stage hinders development.

How did Piaget explain cognitive development?

- Piaget focused on the development of the cognitive structures of the intellect during childhood and adolescence.
- Organization and adaptation play key roles in the formation of structures.
- Piaget believed that cognitive growth occurred in four discrete stages: sensorimotor, preoperational, concrete operational, and formal operational.

What impact does culture have on lifespan development?

- Lev Vygotsky, a leading commentator on the role of culture in development, emphasized the significance of social processes to bring about satisfactory growth.
- Vygotsky believed that the capacity to learn depends on abilities of the child's teachers as well as on the child's abilities.
- The difference between the child's ability to learn independently and to learn with help is called the zone of proximal development.

What is the behavioral perspective on development?

- Pavlov, Watson, and Skinner believed that the consequences of behavior are critical.
- Skinner's paradigm involves three steps: a stimulus occurs in the environment; a response is made in the presence of that stimulus; and the response is reinforced, punished, or extinguished.
- Bandura has extended Skinner's work to the area of social learning, which he calls observational learning.

What is the current status of developmental theory?

- Interactions among the various levels of development are the focus of current developmental research.
- Lerner's developmental contextualism concentrates on the exchanges between an individual's levels of developmental and the context to explain developmental processes.

KEY TERMS

accommodation 35

adaptation 35

assimilation 35

bioecological model 42

classical conditioning 39

cognitive structures 34

defense mechanisms 30

developmental systems
theory 44

ego 30

equilibration 36

evolutionary developmental
psychology 45

exosystem 43

extinction 40

identity crisis 33

id 30

information-processing
theory 37

life course theory 44

life crisis 32

macrosystem 43

mesosystem 42

microsystem 42

modeling 40

negative reinforcement 39

object permanence 34

observational learning 40

operant conditioning 39

positive reinforcement 39

psychoanalytic theory 29

psychosocial theory 32

punishment 40

reciprocal interactions 42

reinforcement 39

schemes 36

self-efficacy 42

social (cognitive) learning 40

superego 30

theory 28

zone of proximal
development 37

For REVIEW

1. What is your reaction to the statement "The perceived truth of a theory depends on its perceived benefit to society"?

2. Skinner criticized the other theorists discussed in this chapter for believing they can describe what goes on in the human mind. After all, he said, no one has ever looked inside one. What's your position?

3. If, as Erikson argued, identity is a state toward which we strive, how do heredity and the environment work (independently or together) to influence our sense of identity?

Chapter Review Test

1. Freud believed that development entails moving through psychosexual stages. Difficulty at any stage can cause a person to become
   a. fixated.
   b. operational.
   c. negatively reinforced.
   d. displaced.

2. Bronfenbrenner's theory of development is called the
   a. environmental search model.
   b. generic trace model.
   c. bioecological model.
   d. reinforcement model.

3. The psychosocial crisis of industry versus inferiority must be resolved during
   a. the school years.
   b. early childhood.
   c. adolescence.
   d. adulthood.

4. Piaget's theory of cognitive development focused on the formation and development of
   a. zones of proximal development.
   b. reinforcement schedules.
   c. cognitive structures.
   d. modeling strategies.

5. Although both Piaget and Vygotsky devoted their lives to studying cognitive development, Vygotsky placed greater emphasis on
   a. cognitive structures.
   b. social interactions.
   c. sensitive periods.
   d. observational learning.

6. Skinner carefully analyzed the role of reinforcement in development and distinguished it from
   a. cognitive structures.
   b. reward.
   c. operations.
   d. needs.

7. The great value of observational learning is that a person need not overtly react to learn
   a. mental operations.
   b. new responses.
   c. ego identity.
   d. schedule of reinforcements.

8. Lerner's analysis of development depends on analyzing
   a. multiple levels of development.
   b. schedules of reinforcement.

   c. identity stages.
   d. cognitive stages.

9. The resurgence of interest in biological explanations of development is due to
   a. government subsidies.
   b. the influence of learning theorists.
   c. recent genetic research.
   d. studies of prenatal development.

10. More complex explanations of development depend on the idea of
    a. genes.
    b. reciprocal interactions.
    c. naturalistic research.
    d. stimulus–response experiments.

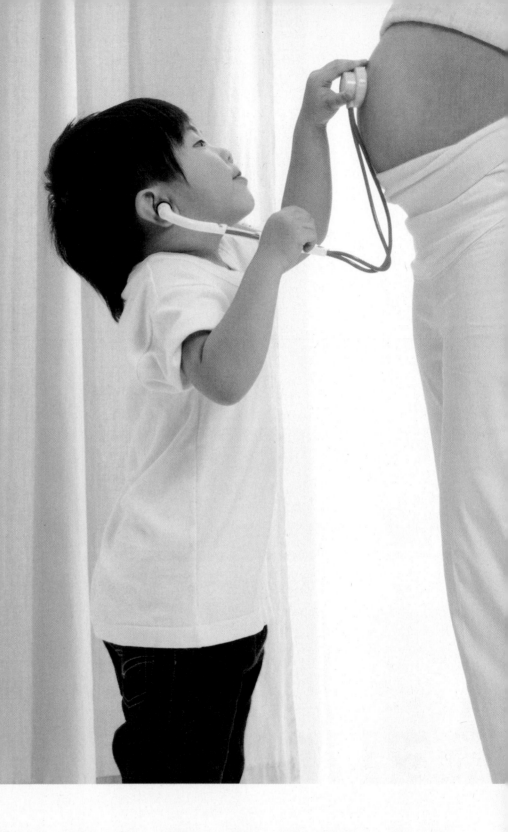

PREGNANCY

As You READ

After reading this chapter, you should be able to answer the following questions:

- How does heredity work, and why doesn't it work well all the time?
- How does fertilization, both natural and assisted, occur?
- What are the stages of the prenatal period?
- What are the major types of prenatal tests?
- What influences prenatal development, and what precautions can be taken?

AND PRENATAL DEVELOPMENT

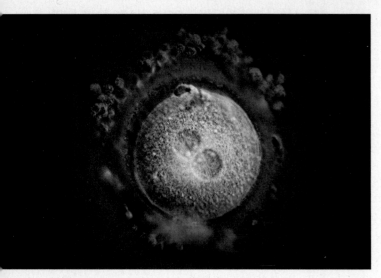

Close-up look at a zygote.

The Biological Basis of Development

I t's hard to imagine, but at conception you were but a fertilized egg, or **zygote**—not much bigger than the period at the end of this sentence. From our microscopic beginnings we travel along a developmental path—one that is rooted in biology, but affected by psychological and social forces. In this chapter you will learn about our genetic makeup and how heredity and the environment work together (and sometimes at odds) to influence pregnancy and the prenatal environment.

Chromosomes, DNA, and Genes

After the sperm and egg unite, the entire genetic code required to grow into a person made of trillions of cells is activated. Three structures work closely together to coordinate our biological makeup—chromosomes, DNA, and genes. Each of these plays a critical role in the development of a human being. At the center of each cell in the human body is a nucleus that contains chromosomes. **Chromosomes** are structures in the cell nucleus that are composed of DNA and proteins. They are often described as "threadlike" or "rodlike," or as a clever 7-year-old noted, "tiny versions of *The Very Hungry Caterpillar*"!

Every human cell (excluding egg or sperm cells) has 22 matching chromosome pairs, plus a 23rd pair of sex chromosomes that determine whether a person is male or female. When scientists study chromosomes,

zygote The cell that results when an egg is fertilized by a sperm.

chromosomes Threadlike structures in the cell that come in 23 pairs (46 total) and contain the genetic material DNA. Each parent contributes half of each chromosome pair.

DNA (deoxyribonucleic acid) A molecule with the shape of a double helix that contains genetic information.

gene A segment of DNA that is a unit of hereditary information.

they number the pairs from longest to shortest (1 to 22) plus the last pair of sex chromosomes, for a total of 23 pairs, or 46 total chromosomes. The 23rd pair is made up of two X chromosomes if the person is female (XX), and one X and one Y chromosome if the person is male (XY). Each parent contributes half of each chromosome pair, so an individual's total biological heritage comes from the combination of two parents' chromosomes. Keep in mind that it is the male's X- or Y-carrying sperm that determines the sex of the future zygote—since the female's egg contains only X chromosomes.

The significance of the chromosomes lies in the material they contain. Chromosomes are composed of **DNA (deoxyribonucleic acid),** which contains critical genetic information. **Genes** are specific segments of DNA that direct cells to reproduce and combine to build proteins. DNA resembles a long and winding ladder—called a *double helix*—and the rungs of the DNA ladder consist of pairs of genes. Each chromosome contains thousands of genes, yet at the most basic level, genes consist of only four building blocks,

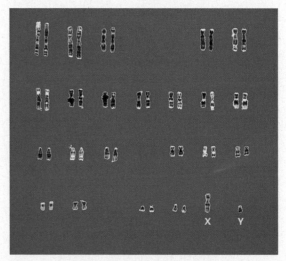

(a)

Chromosome structure of males.

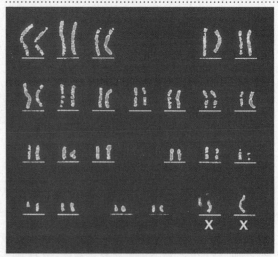

(b)

Chromosome structure of females.

FIGURE 3.1

Structure of a Cell

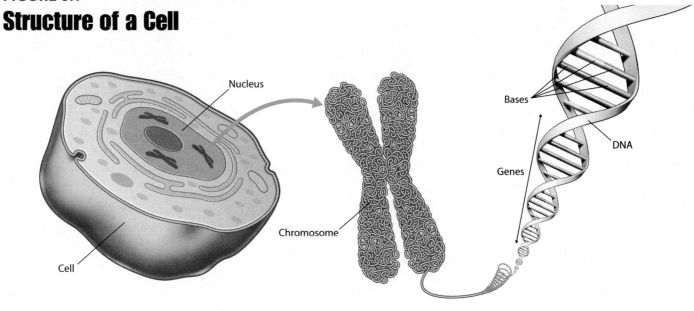

the chemical bases adenine (A), guanine (G), cytosine (C), and thymine (T). To determine the specific function of any gene, researchers first identify the exact order of the four chemical bases—A G C T—of the gene. (See Figure 3.1.) Estimates are that the entire human **genome** contains about 3 billion letters and is often referred to as the text of a book. Reading this book at the rate of one letter every second, you would spend 11 years finishing it (Shreeve, 2005).

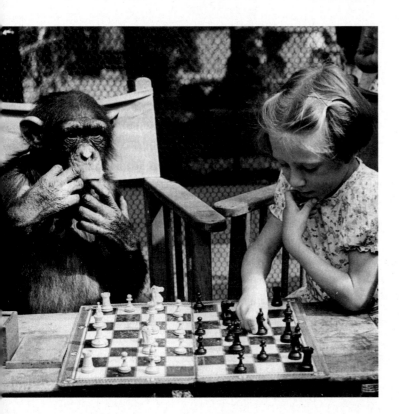

Every pair of genes ultimately determines the specific traits we inherit, from hair and eye color to skin shade, the tendency toward baldness, blood type, and so on. Although a single pair of genes determines some traits, other traits require a combination of several pairs of genes in a specific sequence. Our **genotype** (the genetic makeup of an individual that is invisible to the naked eye) is expressed as a **phenotype** (an individual's observable characteristics or traits, such as eye color and height).

When you look around a room full of people, it may appear that everyone is vastly different from each other, but the amount of genetic material shared between human beings is astounding—approximately 99.1% (Gibbons et al., 2004)! Therefore, it is only a relatively miniscule amount of genetic material that determines the unique traits that set one person apart from another. Even more surprising are research findings that have determined approximately 98–99% of human DNA to be identical to that of chimpanzees!

The differences between humans, chimpanzees and other mammals, molds, and bacteria are more than biological. Environmental circumstances affect the way that the genes function and express themselves. For example, some hormones act as a trigger to activate a gene. If hormones are impacted by a person's nutrition or use of medication, this could affect a gene's function. Genes have been shown to affect behavior in ways that range from food preferences to fussiness. Ultimately, it is the collaboration between multiple factors that results in a person being who they are.

genome All of the hereditary information needed to maintain a living organism.

genotype A person's genetic makeup that is invisible to the naked eye.

phenotype A person's observable characteristics or traits.

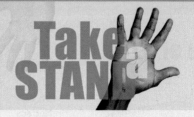
As critical as genes are to life itself, who owns them? There's a gene in your body that is crucial for early spinal cord development—and it belongs to Harvard University! Incyte Corporation of Delaware has the patent for a gene of a receptor for histamine, a substance that is released during an allergic reaction. Nearly half the genes involved in cancer are patented. The owners of patents then charge royalties to researchers who want to study the gene. The United States Supreme Court has held that living things are patentable as long as they incorporate human intervention—therefore, as long as they are made by humans (Stix, 2006). As of today, universities, corporations, government agencies, and nonprofit organizations have patents for about 20% of the human genome.

Is it right for genes to be owned? Who should decide who owns biological material that is shared by all? What are some of the implications of gene ownership?

MITOSIS AND MEIOSIS

In terms of collaboration, two processes occur that ensure genes get passed along from one generation to the next—mitosis and meiosis. These processes are two specific kinds of cell division that occur during the human journey from one cell to trillions of cells. Before mitosis and meiosis occur, two important cells—egg and sperm—combine to form the zygote that will ultimately become the new human being. **Mitosis** is the process in which the zygote's nucleus, including the chromosomes, duplicates itself and divides (see Figure 3.2). Much like a zipper unzipping, the strands of DNA split apart lengthwise. Each chromosome half combines with the bases (A, G, C, T) needed to form a new and complete copy of DNA. The two copies of DNA move to opposite sides of the cell, and the cell divides. Two cells are formed, each containing the same DNA as the original cell, with 23 pairs of chromosomes. This process continues as more and more cells are created. It is during this process that a **mutation** can occur, either through accident or because of environmental influences, such as radiation. A mutation refers to some change in DNA that impacts the arrangement of the genes. For example, when the chemical bases A, G, C, and T are pairing up, a mutation can occur that adds an extra base, deletes a base, or exchanges one base for another. As you can imagine, a tiny blip in the DNA sequence can have a ripple effect as strands of DNA duplicate and form new pairs of the DNA zipper. A change in DNA can impact changes in every aspect of a person's life, such as appearance, behavior, and internal functions.

Meiosis is a different kind of cell division, whereby only the sex cells (sperm cells for men, egg cells for women) duplicate, splitting into cells with 23 chromosomes, rather than 46 (see Figure 3.3). During meiosis, the 46 chromosomes line up in the sex cell nucleus, and then the DNA strands unzip in the same manner as during mitosis. The difference is that, whereas in mitosis the strands of the

FIGURE 3.2
Mitosis

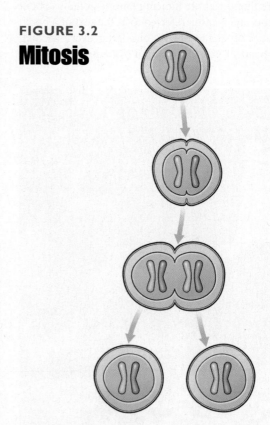

A mitotic division is a cell division in which each new cell receives the same number of chromosomes as a parent cell—46.

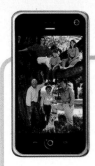
FIGURE 3.3
Meiosis

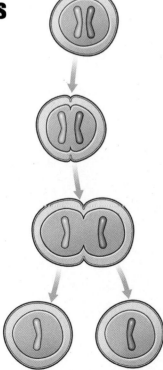

A meiotic division is a cell division in which each new cell receives half of the chromosomes as a parent cell—23.

ladder duplicate and reunite to form new ladderlike DNA structures, in meiosis the strands of the DNA ladders remain halved. As the cell divides, one member of each pair of chromosomes goes into the new cell. As members of each pair of chromosomes are separated, it is pure chance which chromosome in the pair goes into which new cell. This is a critical part of human variation that helps with the survival of our species, because new combinations of genes are created by the exchange of chromosomes during cell division. The division that reduces the number of chromosomes ensures that male and female sex cells can combine in fertilization to result in the necessary number of chromosomes.

Hereditary Disorders

As mentioned above, mutations sometimes occur. Such hereditary abnormalities occur at the level of the chromosomes or the genes. Either source of the abnormality affects the entire genetic process.

CHROMOSOMAL DISORDERS

Several human disorders are due to alterations in chromosome number. The cause of chromosomal disorders is often attributed to chance (given that so many cell divisions occur) or by damage to the DNA. Older eggs and sperm have a greater likelihood of containing damaged DNA, which often contributes to disorders such as Down syndrome.

Down syndrome is caused by the presence of an extra copy of chromosome 21, resulting in 47 chromosomes rather than 46. In a large majority of cases, the syndrome results from a failure of the 21st pair of chromosomes to separate during meiosis, so that an individual receives three of these chromosomes instead of two. An individual with Down syndrome has distinctive facial features, small hands, a large tongue, and possible functional difficulties such as cognitive deficits, heart defects, and an increased risk of leukemia. The incidence of Down syndrome is closely related to the mother's age, as the graph in Figure 3.4 shows. Under age 30, the ratio is only 1 in 1,700 births; once a woman reaches the age of 45, the incidence increases to 1 in 30 (Watson, 2003).

Research during the past 40 years has led to improvements in life expectancy, overall health, and quality of life for people with Down syndrome. Innovative educational programs, early intervention techniques, and specific therapies have promoted higher-quality functioning and socialization and have helped to reduce stereotypes about the condition.

Other disorders are linked to an abnormal number of the sex chromosomes—the 23rd pair of

mitosis Cell division in which the number of chromosomes remains the same (46).

mutation A change in DNA, affecting the genes, that occurs during mitosis by accident or because of environmental factors.

meiosis Cell division in which the number of chromosomes is halved to 23.

Down syndrome Chromosomal disorder caused by an extra copy of chromosome 21.

FIGURE 3.4

Age-Related Prevalence of Down Syndrome

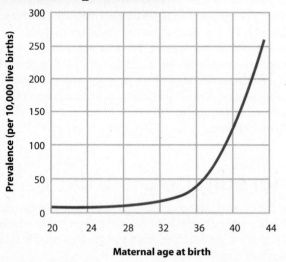

Source: Morris, J., Mutton, D., & Alberman, E. (2005). Corrections to maternal age-specific live birth prevalence of Down syndrome. Journal of Medical Screening, 12(4), 202.

Klinefelter syndrome Chromosomal disorder in males caused by an XXY chromosomal pattern.

XYY syndrome Chromosomal disorder in males caused by an extra Y chromosome.

fragile X syndrome Chromosomal disorder caused by an impaired X chromosome.

Turner syndrome Chromosomal disorder in females caused by an XO chromosomal pattern.

chromosomes (XX for females, XY for males). In **Klinefelter syndrome,** a male possesses an XXY pattern rather than the normal XY. Those affected typically have small testes, reduced body hair, possible infertility, and language impairment. Klinefelter occurs in about 1 in 600 male births and its effects may be lessened by injections of testosterone (Handelsman & Liu, 2006). In **XYY syndrome,** affected males have an extra Y chromosome, which may cause above-average height and possibly increased aggression (Briken et al., 2006).

In 1970 a condition called **fragile X syndrome** was identified. In this disorder, the end of the X chromosome looks ready to break off. Fragile X syndrome appears in about 1 in 2,500 male births and about 1 in 5,000 female births. It affects males more severely than females and characteristically leads to learning disabilities and developmental delays in speech and communication skills (Hartl & Jones, 2005).

Females occasionally lack an X chromosome and possess what is called an XO pattern rather than XX. This condition, called **Turner syndrome,** occurs in about 1 in 2,500 female births and is characterized by short stature, infertility, and webbed neck (Carel, 2005).

GENETIC DISORDERS

Some abnormalities are the result of harmful or malfunctioning genes. However, some genetic disorders may go unnoticed in a person's life because other genes compensate for the problem (Hartl & Jones, 2005). The presence and functioning of every gene found in the human body has been the subject of much research, speculation, and debate (see Figure 3.5). No one fully understands all of the mysteries that lie in human genes, and why certain combinations result in disorders while other combinations result in healthy functioning, but we're getting closer to gaining a more complete understanding. Even as this is being written, new genetic discoveries are being announced daily, due in large part to the Human Genome Project.

Tay-Sachs disease, which is caused by a recessive gene, affects Jews of Eastern European origin. Those with Tay-Sachs disease lack an enzyme that breaks down harmful fatty material in the central nervous system (CNS). At birth, the children appear normal, but mental and motor deterioration begins by the age of 6 months, and death usually occurs by the age of 4 or 5. About 1 in 30 Jews of Eastern European origin carries the defective gene. Today there are reliable genetics tests that identify carriers and assess the genetic status of a fetus (Curtis & Barnes, 1998).

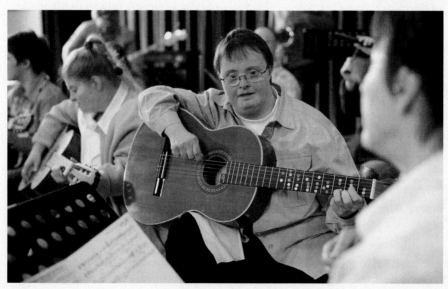

perspectives on Diversity

The Human Genome Project

It is obvious that human beings are different in many ways: height, weight, eye color, skin color, hair texture, and so on. What is less obvious is how very similar we are.

The goal of the Human Genome Project has been to determine the sequence of the 3 billion bases that make up human DNA and maps the genes of the human genome. On June 26, 2000, Dr. Francis Collins, director of the National Genome Research Institute, and Dr. J. Craig Venter, president of Celera Genomics, jointly announced that they had completed a "rough draft" of the genes of the human genome. Three years later, the finished version appeared—a developmental blueprint for the genetic makeup of the human species.

As a result of this impressive work, scientists found that humans have approximately 25,000 genes—many fewer than the estimated 100,000 genes scientists believed necessary to carry out all the activity humans require. Because the genes are the result of combinations of approximately 3 billion units of DNA, genes do not program proteins in a one-to-one correspondence, making human genes quite flexible and complex. In fact, we have many more proteins than genes, which supports the notion that genes collaborate with other structures to create proteins.

The implications of the Human Genome Project range from the altruistic to the unethical. In the most ideal sense, the results of this work could mean improved quality of life for humankind and new career opportunities as knowledge grows. Some of the major areas of ethical concern are

- Who will have access to personal genetic information?
- How will genetic information be used?
- Who oversees the genetic information (ownership and control)?
- Will genetic testing be able to predict human behavior or potential?
- What are the implications for diversity (physical, cultural, social)?

We know that genes and heredity are only one piece of the human development puzzle. Biopsychosocial interactions result in the life experience of each individual, so learning about human genes can only take us so far in understanding human life.

FIGURE 3.5

Number of Genes—Comparing Several Species

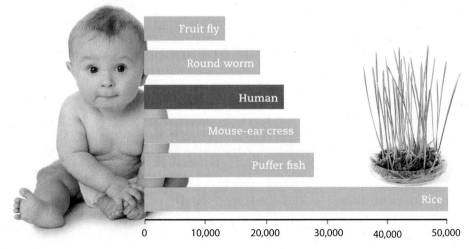

Fruit fly
Round worm
Human
Mouse-ear cress
Puffer fish
Rice

0   10,000   20,000   30,000   40,000   50,000

Approximate number of genes in select organisms

Source: Adapted from Pennisi, E. (2005). Why do humans have so few genes? Science, 309, 80. http://www.sciencemag.org/cgi/reprint/309/5731/80.

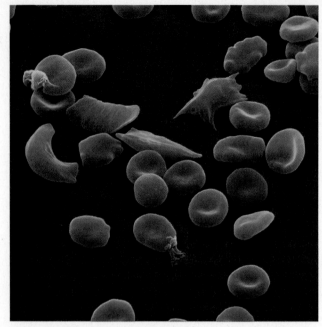
Sickle cells among normal, red blood cells.

Sickle-cell disease, which mainly afflicts people of African descent, is a blood disorder in which red blood cells take on a distorted, sickle shape. Because of this shape, the cells have trouble passing through blood vessels. Cells tend to clump, producing oxygen starvation and severe pain. In the most common form of the disease, the body reacts to eliminate these abnormal cells, causing anemia. Approximately 10% of the U.S. African-American population carries the defective gene, and sickle-cell anemia affects approximately 1 in every 5,000 people.

In the United States, **cystic fibrosis (CF)** is an inherited disease in which the lungs, intestines, and pancreas become clogged with thick mucus, causing breathing and digestive problems. It is caused by a mutation in a single gene. CF is the most severe genetic disease, affecting about 1 in 2,000 children. About 1 in 30 individuals is a carrier, or has the gene but shows no symptoms of the disease. About 30,000 children and adults have CF in the United States, and it kills more children than any other genetic disease (Ball & Bindler, 2006). The CF gene has been identified, however, and has made possible the detection of carriers.

Phenylketonuria (PKU), an inherited disease, is also caused by a mutation in a single gene. In phenylketonuria, the enzyme needed to break down the amino acid phenylalanine is lacking. Phenylalanine accumulates and eventually affects the nervous system, causing mental retardation and brain damage. Most states now require infants to be tested at birth. If PKU is present,

Tay-Sachs disease
Genetic disorder caused by the lack of an enzyme that breaks down fatty material in the CNS.

sickle-cell disease Blood disorder resulting in abnormal hemoglobin.

cystic fibrosis (CF) Chromosomal disorder producing a malfunction of the exocrine glands.

phenylketonuria (PKU) Inherited disease caused by a gene mutation.

spina bifida Genetic disorder resulting in the failure of the spinal column to close completely.

infants are placed on a diet low in phenylalanine and must remain on the diet for the rest of their lives. This disorder provides an example of the biopsychosocial influence on development. Biology (genes) dictates whether someone is a carrier, but the diet determines whether or not the disorder develops (social).

Another example that shows a biopsychosocial influence is **spina bifida,** failure of the spinal column to close completely. This genetic defect is caused by the interaction of several genes with possible environmental factors. During the formation of the nervous system, if the developing neural tube does not close, spina bifida results (biology). Studies have shown that if women take extra folic acid when they are pregnant, the number of cases of spina bifida decreases (Blackman, 1997).

Many other diseases also have, or are suspected of having, a strong genetic origin, including diabetes, epilepsy, heart disorders, cancer, arthritis, and some mental illnesses. Some couples wish to learn more about their genetic heritage and the likelihood that their offspring may be at risk for genetic abnormalities. Genetic counselors gather information from couples using medical tests (such as blood tests) and interviews about family histories and current lifestyle practices to create a profile for couples. If the outlook is not favorable, some couples prefer to adopt children rather than have biological children who could be at risk for health problems. It is believed that in many cases, genetic, environmental, medical, and lifestyle factors interact to produce problems for children and families.

The Fertilization Process

Although advances in technology continue to develop, the nuts and bolts of making babies haven't changed. What have changed are the opportunities for planning and intervention, which have increased dramatically. Terms like *assisted reproductive technology* and *in vitro fertilization* have become part of the vernacular. In the end, however, it all begins with a sperm and an egg.

MENSTRUAL CYCLE

Beginning at puberty and typically continuing throughout the reproductive years, females experience monthly sexual cycles, involving activity of the brain's hypothalamus, the pituitary gland, ovaries,

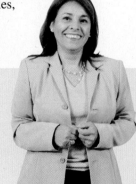

Career Apps

As a genetic counselor, what questions might arise for you as you advise a couple who wish to have children but have a family history of Tay-Sachs disease and one partner has recently been laid off from her job?

uterus, vagina, and mammary glands (Moore & Persaud, 2003). The process of **ovulation** triggers a chemical reaction that inhibits the ripening of further eggs. It also prepares the uterine lining for a potential fertilized ovum.

If fertilization does not occur, the prepared uterine lining is shed in menstruation, and the entire process begins again. The monthly cycle during which the egg is released is known as the menstrual cycle. As a woman approaches the end of her reproductive years, these last ova have been present for at least 40 years. This may explain why the children of older women are more susceptible to genetic abnormalities. The eggs have been exposed to environmental hazards (such as radiation) too long to escape damage (Muller et al., 2000).

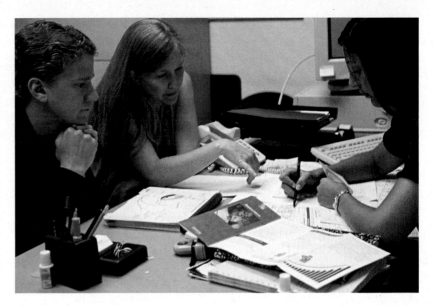

EGG

Egg cells are produced in a woman's ovaries (see Figure 3.6). Estimates are that about 2 million eggs will be available during a woman's reproductive years, and of these only about 400 will be released (Leifer, 2003). Because only one mature egg is required each month for about 35 years, the number far exceeds the need.

Once the egg is released from the ovary, it passes into one of two **fallopian tubes,** which conduct the egg from the ovary to the uterus. Fertilization occurs in the first part of the fallopian tube. After the union of sperm and egg takes place, it's only a matter of hours (about 24–30), before the single cell begins to divide rapidly. The fertilized egg must now pass through the remainder of the fallopian tube to reach the uterus, a journey of about 3 to 4 days to travel 5 or 6 inches. The fertilized egg attaches itself to the uterine wall during **implantation.**

SPERM

The sole objective of sperm cells is the delivery of DNA to the egg. Sperm are produced in a man's testes and contain half the number of chromosomes (23) found in body cells (46). Sperm remain capable of fertilizing an egg for about 24 to 48 hours after ejaculation (Moore & Persaud, 2003). A normal male ejaculation typically results in anywhere from 100 to 650 million sperm (Campbell & Reece, 2005). Of the more than 200 million sperm that enter the vagina, only about 200 survive the journey to the woman's fallopian tubes, where fertilization occurs.

ovulation The process in which the egg bursts from the surface of the ovary.

fallopian tube Either of a pair of tubes that join the ovary to the uterus.

implantation Attachment of the fertilized egg to the uterine wall.

fraternal twins Twins who develop from two eggs fertilized by separate sperm; individuals do not share identical genetic makeup.

Multiples

Occasionally, often for reasons unknown, multiple babies are born. The most common type of multiples occurs when a woman's ovaries release two eggs (rather than one) and both are fertilized by separate sperm. These twins are called **fraternal,** or dizygotic, and their genes are no more

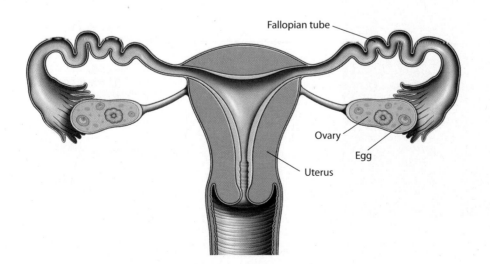

Fallopian tube

Ovary

Egg

Uterus

FIGURE 3.6

From Ovulation to Implantation

The relationship of ovary, egg, fallopian tube, and uterus

Source: From Travers, J. F. (1982). The growing child. *Glenview, IL: Scott Foresman and Co.*

alike than those of siblings born of the same parents but at different times. About two thirds of all twins are fraternal. The increase in number of twins born in recent decades has been influenced by many factors, such as fertility medications and assistive fertility technologies (Russell et al., 2003). In the United States, twins occur in about 1 in 85 pregnancies. Recent figures show that 137,085 twins were born in 2006. The rate of fraternal twin births, however, varies considerably from country to country. For example, the rate of fraternal twins is 1 in 500 in Asia, but 1 in 20 in certain African countries (Moore & Persaud, 2003).

Less frequently, multiples develop from a single fertilized egg that divides after conception. Two embryos, each in its own amniotic sac, develop within one chorionic sac (fluid-filled sac containing the embryo). This process leads to **identical,** or monozygotic, twins whose genes are identical; that is, they share the same genotype.

Researchers often use twins as a comparison group to explore the influence of genetics on development. Because identical twins share the same genetic material, it is assumed that the environment accounts for any differences between them. In a study that includes both identical twins and other siblings, for example, a researcher can estimate the relative influence of genes and environments on behavioral differences among people. Researchers can focus on topics such as personality, anxiety, or other behaviors to gain insights into the role of genetics on development. The assumption is that if identical twins behave similarly and nonidentical siblings behave differently, chances are biology has a major influence on that

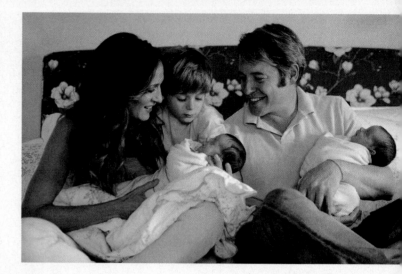

phenomenon. However, because the environment itself may be influenced by the fact that some children are identical twins (many families emphasize the "sameness" of twins through clothing, furniture, and other household items), it is not accurate to believe that genetics alone account for all research findings.

Fertility: Challenges and Opportunities

Although the typical fertilization process is the normal process for most women, there are exceptions. **Infertility** is defined as the inability to conceive a child after 1 year of unprotected sexual intercourse. Many people, attempting to overcome this problem, turn to medical and/or adoption procedures.

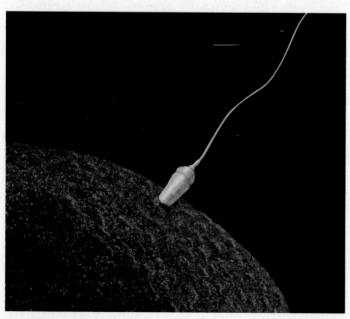

The moment of fertilization
Sperm = 5 microns, ovum = 397 microns, 1 inch = 25,400 microns.

FIGURE 3.7
Fertility Rates

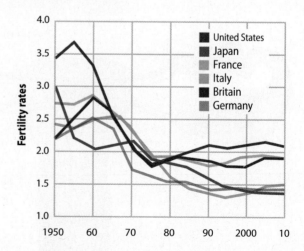

Source: World Population Prospects, United Nations, 2009.

CAUSES OF INFERTILITY

The American Society for Reproductive Medicine estimates that infertility affects about 6.1 million people in the United States, about 10% of the reproductive population. Low sperm count and inactive sperm are the most common problems for men, and irregular (or lack of) ovulation is cited as problematic for women. Males must deposit a sufficient number of normal sperm near a woman's cervix that can survive the acidic vaginal environment and swim toward the egg (Leifer, 2003). Females must regularly produce normal eggs and possess a uterine environment that will sustain a pregnancy.

Sexually transmitted diseases (STDs) may cause infertility or lead to conditions that can result in infertility. Also, a growing number of women are delaying childbearing. Older women are more likely to become infertile if they have had abdominal surgery or have experienced endometriosis, the growth of endometrial tissue outside the uterus.

If a couple or an individual finds that they are indeed infertile, their hopes of parenthood may still become a reality, since many assisted reproductive techniques are now available.

ASSISTED REPRODUCTION TECHNOLOGIES

Many forms of **assisted reproduction technologies (ART)** are now available (Gardner et al., 2004; Leifer, 2003; Marrs, Bloch, & Silverman, 1997).

- **In vitro fertilization (IVF).** The most familiar term for fertility treatment, fertilization occurs in a petri dish. A woman's eggs are surgically extracted and placed in a solution containing blood serum and nutrients. Treated sperm are added to the solution, where fertilization occurs. The fertilized egg is transferred to a fresh solution, where it remains for 5 to 7 days. The best embryos (typically one or two) are selected for transfer into the woman's uterus, where implantation may occur.

- **Intrauterine insemination (IUI).** Although in vitro fertilization is probably the best-known ART procedure, IUI is by far the most widely used one, often because of favorable health insurance policies. Potential users of IUI, whereby sperm is injected into a woman's uterus, have the option of using sperm from the prospective father or donor sperm, depending on the situation.

- **Gamete intrafallopian transfer (GIFT).** Sperm and egg are surgically placed in a fallopian tube with the intent of achieving fertilization in a more natural environment.

- Sperm and egg donation. Males and females sometimes donate or sell their sperm and eggs. Today hundreds of sperm banks operate in the United States, storing and/or selling sperm, which are frozen in liquid nitrogen at −190 °C and remain potent for years. Women who will donate or sell their eggs are in great demand.

- **Surrogate mother.** A surrogate mother is a woman who becomes pregnant (usually by IUI or IVF) for the purpose of carrying the fetus to term for another woman.

assisted reproduction technologies External fertilization procedures; fertilization occurs with help outside the woman's body

in vitro fertilization (IVF) An ART technique in which fertilization occurs in a petri dish and the resulting embryos are transferred to the woman's uterus.

intrauterine insemination (IUI) An ART technique in which sperm are injected directly into the uterus as part of the fertilization procedure.

gamete intrafallopian transfer (GIFT) An ART technique in which sperm and egg are surgically placed in a fallopian tube with the intent of achieving fertilization.

surrogate mother A woman who carries another woman's fetus.

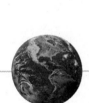 *perspectives on* **Diversity**

Worldwide Birth Dearth

A special report in *The Economist* in 2009 reported that in Germany about 25% of women in their 40s have remained childless. The concern, shared by other developed countries around the world, is that as the population ages, it is necessary to have a younger generation to balance the aging population and achieve population stability. In more than 70 countries, fertility is currently below replacement level, which is 2.1. The graph in Figure 3.7 shows the fertility rates of the United States and five other countries.

Efforts are being made in various countries to entice women to have children, such as offering child-care assistance and financial supports. The reality of raising children today, even from a purely economical standpoint, makes the decision complex. Children can be viewed as a liability rather than an asset, especially when parents are faced with the costs of child care and education, not to mention food, diapers, and clothing.

Consider what incentives might work across geographic locations to increase the number of women who would want to have babies. Similarly, what ideas might citizens in different countries have about what makes them more or less likely to have children?

adoption The process of voluntarily taking a child of other parents as one's own.

closed adoption Adoption procedures in which the biological parents know nothing about the adopting parents.

open adoption Adoption procedure in which biological parents have considerable input into the adoption process.

germinal period First two weeks following fertilization.

blastocyst The fertilized egg when it reaches the uterus (about 7 days after conception).

placenta Supplies the embryo with all its needs, carries off all its wastes, and protects it from harm.

umbilical cord Contains blood vessels that go to and from the mother through the arteries and veins supplying the placenta.

amniotic sac Fluid-filled uterine sac that surrounds the embryo/fetus.

More than 3 million babies have been born using IVF and other assisted reproductive technologies since the world's first IVF baby was born in 1978.

ADOPTION

Many people remain childless in spite of several attempts at natural or assisted fertilization, resulting in the pursuit of other channels to welcome a baby into their home. **Adoption,** the process of voluntarily taking a child of other parents as one's own, offers a viable option. The poem "Motherbridge of Love" celebrates the bond between a mother and child and offers the perspective of both the adoptive mother and biological mother:

Regardless of race, ethnicity, socioeconomic or marital status, sexual orientation, or religion, people who decide to adopt face stiff competition from other adults. Single parenthood is widely accepted today, and more single women are able to support their children. The increasing use of contraception and the legality of abortion have impacted the number of available children in the United States, leading to heightened interest in children from other nations. Although more children are available for adoption than often thought, the waiting period for healthy infants may run into years.

In the United States, more people who wish to become parents are turning to international adoption and adopting children whose race or abilities differ from their own. Census figures indicate that about 25,000 children were obtained through international adoption in 2009. The majority of these children come from China (about 7,500) and Russia (about 6,000).

Adoption procedures were formerly closed (**closed adoption**), and biological parents were completely removed from the life of their child once the child was officially adopted. The bonds between birth parent(s) and child were legally severed. Although closed adoption was designed with good intentions, it robs the child of a personal history and can increase emotional upset.

Today, however, when a pregnant woman approaches an adoption agency, she has options. She can insist that her child be raised by a specific kind of couple and can ask to see her child several times a year after the adoption. This process is

Once there were two women who never knew each other. One you do not know. The other you call Mother.

"MOTHERBRIDGE OF LOVE" (2007)

called **open adoption.** Open adoption may help a child to overcome the sense of loss that can accompany adoption (Leon, 2002), but it can also complicate the realities of raising the child. Adoptive parents must accept the idea that their children will want to know more about their biological parents (Brodzinsky & Pinderhughes, 2002).

Prenatal Development

The prenatal period can be divided into three fairly distinct stages of development: germinal, embryonic, and fetal. Table 3.1 summarizes the milestones of development in these stages.

GERMINAL PERIOD

The **germinal period** extends through the first 2 weeks. The zygote takes the form of a fluid-filled ball of cells called a **blastocyst.** During the second week, the blastocyst becomes firmly implanted in the wall of the uterus. The inner cell layer develops into the embryo itself, and the **placenta,** the **umbilical cord,** and the **amniotic sac** develop from the blastocyst's outer layer of cells. The placenta supplies the embryo with all its needs, carries off all its wastes, and protects it from harm. The placenta has two

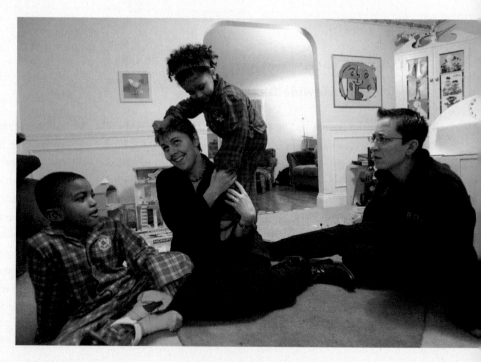

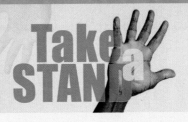

A New Ice Age

On Mother's Day 2001, a woman's eggs were extracted as part of her routine IVF process. A total of 61 eggs were retrieved, fertilized with her husband's sperm, and frozen in lots of five for future use. When the time arrived to transfer the embryos, an embryologist selected one lot of five frozen embryos, which were thawed, and the three most robust embryos were chosen and transferred into her uterus. A healthy baby boy was born 9 months later!

About a year after the birth of their son, the couple decided to try a second round of IVF in hopes of a second child. An embryologist selected another lot of five frozen embryos. Of these five, two were selected for transfer, because of their robustness and because the woman had success the first time. The woman gave birth to a healthy baby girl 9 months later.

The siblings, born over 2 years apart, were conceived on the same day in 2001, along with many other potential siblings. It was sheer chance that those two lots of five were selected by the two embryologists and that one was chosen first and one second.

Research indicates that children born from frozen embryos are as healthy as babies born naturally (European Society for Human Reproduction and Embryology, 2009). Who has the most influence over births that result from assisted technology—the parents or the medical professionals? How much control is desirable in orchestrating the births of children?

---

separate sets of blood vessels, one going to and from the baby through the umbilical cord, the other going to and from the mother through the arteries and veins supplying the placenta.

EMBRYONIC PERIOD

Perhaps the most remarkable change in the **embryonic period** (weeks 3–8) is cellular differentiation. Three distinct layers form in the embryo: the ectoderm, which will give rise to skin, hair, nails, teeth, and the nervous system; the mesoderm, which will give rise to muscles, skeleton, and the circulatory and excretory systems; and the endoderm, which will give rise to lungs, liver, and pancreas.

Around the 3rd week, the first signs of the nervous system appear. The mesoderm sends a chemical signal to the ectoderm, and a process called *neural induction* leads to the formation of the neural plate and the rest of the nervous system. A groove forms in the neural plate and begins to fold in on itself, leading to the creation of the neural tube. The top of the tube expands into the brain, and the rest will become the spinal cord. The nerve cells at this stage are called *neurons,* and they begin to leave the neural tube and travel to their destination in the developing brain. This process of cell migration typically starts during the 7th prenatal week. The neurons now begin forming 1,000 trillion connections in a child's brain, and a pruning process sets in, which is nature's way of ensuring survival of the fittest neurons. From these beginnings, a familiar image of the

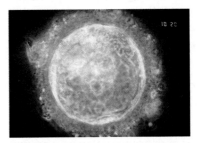

The blastocyst as seen in an ultrasound.

embryonic period 3rd through the 8th week following fertilization.

organogenesis Process by which organs are formed; occurs around 6 to 7 weeks of pregnancy.

brain appears. The top of the neural tube leads to the formation of the two cerebral hemispheres and the four lobes of the cerebral cortex.

The heart begins to beat around week 4—the embryo's first detectable movement. During the 5th week, eyes and ears begin to emerge; body buds give clear evidence of becoming arms and legs; and the head area is the largest part of the rapidly growing embryo.

During the 6th and 7th weeks, fingers begin to appear on the hands, the outline of toes is seen, and the beginnings of the spinal cord are visible. In this period the organs are formed—a process called **organogenesis.** After 8 weeks, 95% of the body parts are formed and general body movements are detected.

It's stunning to realize how quickly development occurs. The neuroscientist Marian Diamond (1999) summarizes the rapid growth this way: If fertilization occurred on Monday, by Thursday the embryo would consist of 30 cells clustered

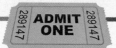
FEATURED MEDIA

Films About Pregnancy

Baby Mama (2008) – What lengths will a successful single businesswoman go to so that she can have the baby she longs for? What are the boundaries between a surrogate mother and the future parent?

Juno (2007) – What does a 16-year-old high school junior do when she finds out she's pregnant after having sex with her best friend?

Knocked Up (2007) – Can a one-night stand turn into a sincere and fulfilling lifelong family commitment?

Then She Found Me (2007) – How does a teacher come to terms with her own adoptive mother and biological mother as she strives to conceive a child of her own and sustain a romantic relationship?

placenta. The placenta itself never actually joins with the uterus but, instead, exchanges nourishment and waste products through the walls of the blood vessels (Moore & Persaud, 2003). The mother-to-be begins to experience some of the noticeable effects of pregnancy: the need to urinate more frequently, morning sickness, and increasing fullness of breasts.

FETAL PERIOD

The **fetal period** extends from the beginning of the 3rd month to birth. During this time, the fetus grows rapidly in both height and weight. The sex organs appear, and it is possible to determine the baby's sex. Visible sexual differentiation begins, and the nervous system continues to increase in size and complexity.

By the 4th month, the fetus is about 8 to 10 inches in length and weighs about 6 to 8 ounces. The 4th to the 5th month is usually the peak growth period. During this time, the mother begins to feel movement. The fetus now swallows, digests, and discharges urine. Growth is rapid during the 4th month to accommodate an increasing oxygen demand. The fetus produces specialized cells: red blood cells to transport oxygen and white blood cells to combat disease. The fetus is now active—sucking, turning its head, and pushing with hands and feet—and the mother is acutely aware of the life within her.

By the end of the 5th month, the fetus is 10 to 12 inches long, weighs about a pound, and sleeps and wakes, even choosing a favorite sleep position. Rapid growth continues in the 6th month, with the fetus gaining another few inches and a pound, but growth typically slows during the 7th month. Viability, the ability to survive if born, is attained.

During fetal testing, the fetal heart rate changes and movement increases, suggesting that the fetus has sensed tactile stimulation. Muscular development of the eyes

together. By Saturday, this cluster of cells (the blastocyst) would have started nestling into the woman's uterine wall. By Tuesday of the following week, the endoderm, mesoderm, and ectoderm would be emerging. Again, remember that all this happens before the woman misses her first period.

At the end of the embryonic period, a discernible human being with arms, legs, a beating heart, and a nervous system exists. It receives nourishment and discharges waste through the umbilical cord, which leads to the

fetal period Period that extends from beginning of the 3rd month to birth.

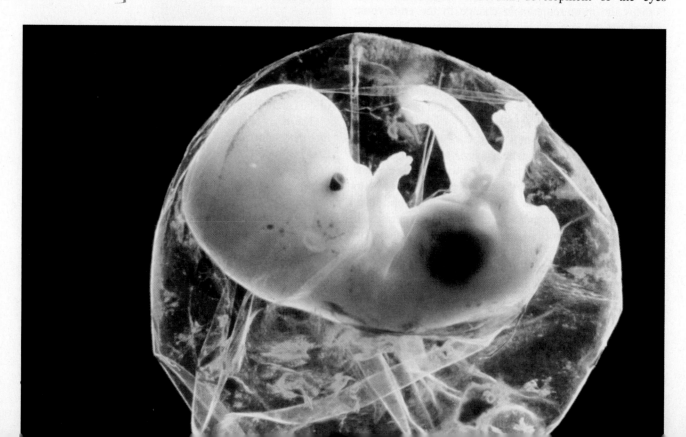

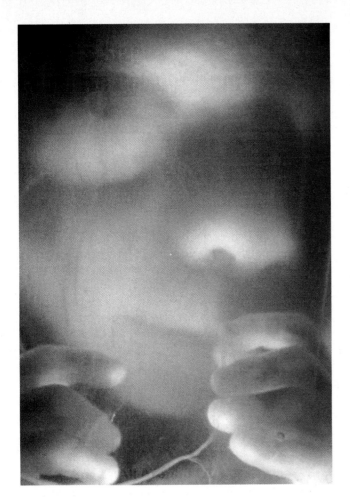

TABLE 3.1

Milestones in Prenatal Development

Age	Accomplishment
3 weeks	Nervous system begins to form
4 weeks	Heart begins to beat
5 weeks	Head continues rapid growth
8 weeks	Almost all body parts are differentiated
12 weeks	Possible to visually determine baby's sex
	Growth of head slows
	Formation of red blood cells by liver slows
14 weeks	Begins to coordinate limb movements
	Slow eye movements occur
16 weeks	Ultrasound shows clearly defined bone structure
20 weeks	Possible to hear heartbeat with stethoscope
	Baby covered by fine downy hair called lanugo
	Fetal movements called quickening are felt by mother
21 weeks	Rapid eye movements commence
	Substantial weight gain
24 weeks	Fingernails can be seen
28 weeks	Eyes open and close
	Lungs capable of breathing
32 weeks	Skin pink and smooth
	Chubby appearance
38 weeks	Nervous system can carry out some integrative functions
	Reacts to light
	Usually assumes upside-down position as birth approaches

Source: Leifer, 2003; Moore & Persaud, 2003; Olds, London, & Ladewig, 1996.

enables the fetus to move its eyes during sleep. From about the 16th week, the fetus is sensitive to any light that penetrates the uterine wall and the amniotic fluid. Toward the end of pregnancy, a bright light pointed at the mother's abdomen causes the fetus to move. The fetus begins to swallow amniotic fluid early in the pregnancy, and researchers have attempted to demonstrate that fetuses can taste and exhibit other sensory functions.

This description of fetal life leads to an inevitable conclusion: Given adequate conditions, the fetus at birth is equipped to deal effectively with the transition from its sheltered environment to the world outside the uterus.

Prenatal Testing

Some women have a greater chance of developing difficulties during pregnancy or delivering a child with problems. Similar to genetic counseling, the rapidly expanding field of fetal diagnosis not only identifies problems but also offers means of treatment.

ULTRASOUND

Ultrasound is a noninvasive procedure that uses sound waves to produce an image that enables a physician to detect structural abnormalities, to guide other procedures, to confirm fetal viability, and to determine the amount of amniotic fluid (Leifer, 2003). Useful pictures can be obtained as early as 7 weeks.

AMNIOCENTESIS

Amniocentesis involves inserting a needle through the woman's abdomen, piercing the amniotic sac, and withdrawing a sample of the amniotic fluid. The fluid sample provides information about the child's sex and almost 70 chromosomal abnormalities (Moore & Persaud, 2003). If required, amniocentesis is done after the 15th week of pregnancy.

ALPHA-FETOPROTEIN (AFP) TEST

In fetuses with neural tube problems, AFP (a protein produced by a baby's

ultrasound Use of sound waves and special equipment to produce an image that enables a physician to detect internal structural abnormalities.

amniocentesis Fetal testing procedure that involves inserting a needle through the woman's abdomen, piercing the amniotic sac, and withdrawing a sample of amniotic fluid.

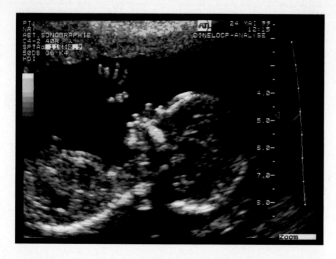

liver) escapes from the spinal fluid (Jasper, 2000), and then passes into the mother's bloodstream. Babies with spina bifida show a raised level of AFP, which may be detected in the mother's blood. A low level of AFP can indicate Down syndrome. The blood test (done when the mother is 15–17 weeks pregnant) does produce false positives, however, which raises the issue of further testing. Pairing the results of the AFP with an ultrasound provides more accurate information.

CHORIONIC VILLI SAMPLING (CVS)

The outer layer of the embryo is almost completely covered with chorionic villi, fingerlike projections that reach into the uterine lining. A catheter is inserted through the vagina to the villi, and a small section is suctioned into the tube. **Chorionic villi sampling (CVS)** is an excellent test to determine the fetus's genetic structure and may be done as early as 9 to 10 weeks. Results are available in 3 hours to 7 days, as compared with 2 to 4 weeks for amniocentesis.

Critical Interactions: Biology and the Environment

At birth an infant has already had 9 months of prenatal living, with all the benefits and harm that can result from biological and environmental influences. The embryonic period can be hazardous for the newly formed organism. During these weeks, embryonic tissue is particularly sensitive to any foreign agents, especially beginning at the 3rd or 4th week of the pregnancy. Estimates are that about 30% of all embryos are aborted at this time without the mother's knowledge and that about 90% of all embryos with chromosomal abnormalities are spontaneously aborted.

Many women currently experience the benefits of the most up-to-date and superior prenatal care. Diet, exercise,

and rest can be designed to meet the needs of each individual. When women, especially pregnant teenagers, do not receive prenatal care the rates of prenatal loss, stillbirths, and newborn mortality substantially increase. Organizations such as Children's Defense Fund (http://www.childrensdefensefund.org) and Early Head Start (http://www.ehsnrc.org) provide resources for and media attention to prenatal development that not only benefit pregnant mothers directly, but also have a powerful impact on and implications for prenatal development.

NUTRITION AND EXERCISE

Because a fetus depends on its mother for nourishment, most women today are keenly aware of the need to have a proper diet that will help them give birth to a healthy baby. Good nutrition helps women sustain healthy pregnancies. Healthy habits throughout pregnancy not only attend to maternal and fetal needs, but also carry over after the baby is born. Doctors usually recommend dietary supplements, such as additional protein, iron, calcium, sodium, fiber, folic acid, and vitamins. According to the 2005 Dietary Guidelines for Americans, a healthy diet emphasizes fruits, vegetables, whole grains, and low-fat or fat-free milk. It also includes lean meats, poultry, fish, beans, eggs, and nuts, as well as foods low in saturated fats, sodium, and cholesterol.

Women need to evaluate their weight and nutritional habits well before becoming pregnant. In a typical pregnancy, a woman will gain 25 to 35 pounds, while the newborn baby usually weighs only 7 to 8 pounds. Additional weight is distributed among the uterus (2.5 lbs), the breasts (1.5–3 lbs), the placenta (1–1.5 lbs), and other areas. Women who are overweight or underweight before pregnancy may need to follow different nutritional guidelines, depending on health, nutritional status, and other factors (Balcazar & Mattson, 2000; Grodner, Long, & DeYoung, 2004).

As long as the woman is physically able, moderate exercise during the prenatal period contributes to mental health and general fitness. The American College of Obstetricians and Gynecologists suggests that pregnant women do not engage in intense exercise and avoid exercise that could affect balance.

EMOTIONS AND SENSE OF SELF

The primary focus for pregnant women involves their new role as a mother, including developing maternal identity and competency. The classic work of Ruth Rubin (1984) attempts to explain the stressful emotional road many pregnant women travel. Rubin believed that women must master four tasks in the transition to motherhood. They must (1) transition from a focus on themselves to a focus on the unborn child, (2) ensure the acceptance of the child by significant persons in the family, (3) establish a bond with the unborn child that grows into a relationship during the milestones of pregnancy, and (4) commit to the realities of "giving of themselves"—the strenuous physical toll preg-

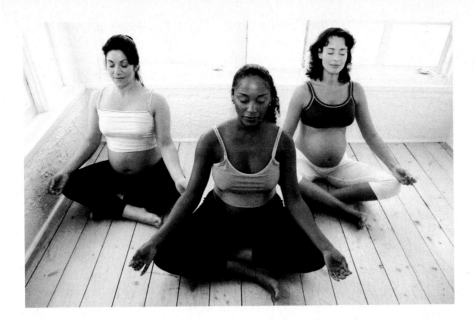

Current advances in technology can provide an endless stream of information to families of all constellations, but they also contribute to anxiety when new parents are presented with "expert" opinions. Often, cultural traditions (what to eat, how to ward off bad luck) contribute more substantially to a positive experience with pregnancy and birth.

CULTURE

The United States is a culturally diverse nation that claims to encourage newcomers to share our way of life, yet even under the best of conditions, the path for many can be difficult. Even within specific racial or ethnic groups, tremendous cultural variation appears. Cross-cultural data indicate dramatically different variations among different cultures in the experience of pregnancy. Being sensitive to cultural differences is important and beneficial to health-care providers in their treatment of a woman and her family (Greenfield, Suzuki, & Rothstein-Fisch, 2006).

To ensure that a woman's journey through the prenatal months is as safe and satisfying as possible, some basic ideas must be recognized. For example, communication assumes paramount importance—not only language but also such behaviors as body language and tone of voice. How does the woman's family, as members of a particular culture, view the pregnancy? Is it seen as a natural, expected occurrence that doesn't require constant medical care? Does the woman's status change as a result of the pregnancy? Are there cultural dietary considerations that should be addressed? Are there spiritual beliefs that health-care providers should be aware of?

nancy takes on their bodies and the emotional roller coaster of excitement and anxiety.

Rubin believed that mastering these tasks prepares a woman for the subsequent demands of motherhood. We could also ask, How do women *and* men negotiate the change in roles that is about to occur? How will they balance work and parenting, share domestic responsibilities, and come to terms with the profound changes in their lives? Traditional roles of one partner taking care of domestic responsibilities and the other taking care of work outside the home don't sit well with many contemporary couples. Recognizing the importance of family responsibilities, more flexible work policies, and access to high-quality, affordable child care would help reduce the tension couples experience.

Juno: Most Fruitful Yuki?
What is . . . Oh my god, she's
a pregnant superhero!

—FROM *JUNO*, WRITTEN BY DIABLO CODY

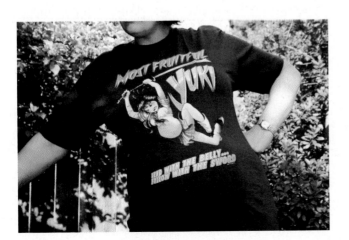

TERATOGENS

In spite of good intentions, all pregnancies expose mother and child to various health risks. **Developmental risk** is a term used to identify children whose well-being is in jeopardy. Such risks involve a range of biopsychosocial conditions. It is clear that the earlier the damage (a toxic drug or maternal infection) occurs in a child's life, the greater the chance of negative long-term effects.

A major concern relating to developmental risk involves substances that greatly influence the prenatal environment. **Teratogens** are any environmental agents that cause harm to the embryo or fetus. They fall into two classes: infectious diseases and different types of chemical substances (see Table 3.2). Most of these are avoidable risks. For example, about

developmental risk Risk to children's well-being involving a range of damaging biopsychosocial conditions.

teratogens Any environmental agents that harm the embryo or fetus.

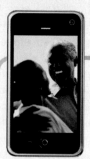
effects can take a toll on a child's behavior and psychological well-being. This can impact parent–child relationships, as well as teacher–pupil and peer relationships, for example. There is great potential for biopsychosocial consequences of teratogens that cannot be discounted or taken lightly.

Infectious Diseases

Some diseases that are potentially harmful to the developing fetus and acquired either before or during birth are grouped together as the **STORCH** diseases (Blackman, 1997): **s**yphilis, **t**oxoplasmosis, **o**ther infections, **r**ubella, **c**ytomegalovirus, and **h**erpes. HIV/AIDS is a disease that can be passed from mother to baby during pregnancy, labor, and delivery. The potential risk of the disease lies in the timing of infection. Estimates are that about 15% of all women experience some type of infectious disease during pregnancy (Arenson & Drake, 2007).

SYPHILIS

Syphilis is a sexually transmitted infection that, if untreated, may affect the fetus. It makes no difference whether the mother contracted the disease during pregnancy or many years before. About 25% of infected fetuses die during or after the second trimester, and another 25% die soon after birth. Those who survive may be affected by serious problems such as blindness, mental retardation, and deafness. Because of advances in antibiotic treatments, the incidence of syphilis has steadily decreased, although there has been a recent upsurge due to an increase in numbers of cases among adolescents (Leifer, 2003).

TOXOPLASMOSIS

Toxoplasmosis is caused by a parasite that is transmitted to humans by many animals, especially cats, or occasionally from raw meat. In fact, pregnant cat owners should avoid contact with kitty litter to avoid contracting toxoplasmosis. Usually harmless in adults, the infection can cause serious problems for the fetus, including spontaneous abortion, premature delivery, and neurological problems such as mental retardation, blindness, and cerebral palsy. Low birth weight, an enlarged liver and spleen, and anemia also characterize the disease. The incidence of toxoplasmosis is about 1 per 1,000 live births (Moran, 2000).

20% of pregnant women continue to smoke cigarettes; more than 13% of pregnant women report drinking alcohol; and about 5.5% of pregnant women admit to using illicit drugs (Arenson & Drake, 2007).

Depending on the age of exposure to particular teratogens, the effects are more or less serious. Medical research has identified specific periods when an embryo's or fetus's critical organs are developing and is therefore susceptible to harm that ranges from minor defects to major abnormalities (see Figure 3.8). For example, teratogens can damage the embryo's heart during the first few weeks of development, but the ears are not at such serious risk of damage until several weeks later. Generally speaking, the embryo is at greater risk than the fetus because the groundwork for virtually all body parts is established during the embryonic period.

Some effects of teratogens are not visible to the naked eye, however, and manifest themselves in other ways that may be delayed for months or even years. Some harmful health

STORCH diseases syphilis, **t**oxoplasmosis, **o**ther infections, **r**ubella, **c**ytomegalovirus, **h**erpes.

syphilis Sexually transmitted disease that, if untreated, may adversely affect the fetus.

toxoplasmosis Infection caused by a parasite; may cause damage to a fetus.

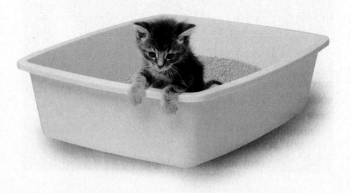

TABLE 3.2

Teratogens: Their Effects, and Time of Risk

Agent	Possible Effects	Time of Risk During Pregnancy
Infectious Diseases		
HIV/AIDS	Growth failure, low birth weight, developmental delay, death from infection	Before conception, throughout pregnancy, during delivery, during breast-feeding
Rubella	Mental retardation, physical problems, possible death	First 3 months, may have effects during later months
Syphilis	Fetal death, congenital syphilis, prematurity	From 5 months on
CMV	Retardation, deafness, blindness	Uncertain, perhaps 4 to 24 weeks
Herpes simplex	CNS damage, prematurity	Potential risk throughout pregnancy and at birth
Chemical Substances		
Alcohol	Fetal alcohol syndrome (FAS), growth retardation, cognitive deficits	Throughout pregnancy
Aspirin	Bleeding problems	Last month, at birth
Cigarettes	Prematurity, lung problems	After 20 weeks
DES	Cancer of female reproductive system	From 3 to 20 weeks
LSD	Isolated abnormalities	Before conception
Lead	Death, anemia, mental retardation	Throughout pregnancy
Marijuana	Unknown long-term effects, early neurological problems	Throughout pregnancy
Thalidomide	Fetal death, physical and mental abnormalities	The first month
Cocaine	Spontaneous abortion, neurological problems	Throughout pregnancy

OTHER INFECTIONS

Other infectious diseases include influenza, chicken pox, and several rare viruses. Recent concern about swine flu (H1N1) has brought attention to the increased risk of severe illness and death that pregnant women face. Pregnant women are four times more likely to be hospitalized and have an unusually high death rate associated with the illness. Of the 266 U.S. swine flu deaths that the CDC had detailed, as of July 2009, 15 of them were among pregnant women (approximately 6%). For this reason, immunizations for both H1N1 and seasonal flu are recommended for pregnant women.

RUBELLA (GERMAN MEASLES)

Rubella (also known as German measles) is an infectious disease generally characterized by a rash, fever, and swollen lymph nodes. The disease, however, is extremely dangerous to a fetus during the first trimester and can result in serious defects including congenital heart disorder, cataracts, deafness, and/ or mental retardation. In 2006, only 11 new cases of rubella were reported (CDC, 2008). Any woman who had German measles as a child cannot assume that she is immune, so a woman who wishes to become pregnant should take a blood test. If immunity is not found, the woman can receive a vaccination before she becomes pregnant that will protect her and the fetus.

CYTOMEGALOVIRUS (CMV)

Cytomegalovirus (CMV) is a widespread infection that is often unrecognized in pregnant women because the symptoms are mild. It can cause damage to the fetus, ranging from mental retardation to blindness, deafness, and even death. Most babies are not affected by the virus, and 90% of those who are infected show no symptoms at birth. However, approximately 8,000 children each year develop lasting disabilities caused by CMV, such as hearing or vision loss and learning disabilities.

GENITAL HERPES

Genital herpes is a virus that is passed on to the fetus during delivery through the birth canal. The infant develops symptoms during the first week following birth. The eyes and the nervous system are most susceptible to this disease. About one third of infected babies die, and of those who survive, one fourth suffer some form of brain damage. If genital herpes is detected, the baby can be delivered by cesarean section (through an incision in the mother's

rubella (also known as German measles) An infectious disease that can cause serious birth defects. If a woman contracts the disease during pregnancy, extremely dangerous to a fetus during the first trimester.

cytomegalovirus (CMV) A widespread infection, often unrecognized in pregnant women, that can cause severe fetal damage.

genital herpes Infection that can be contracted by a fetus during delivery; the infant can develop symptoms during the first week following the birth.

Career Apps

As a professional translator, what challenges might you face with increasing use of visual technology, such as computers and the Internet, particularly in light of the cost of such tools for populations who might not have the means to use them?

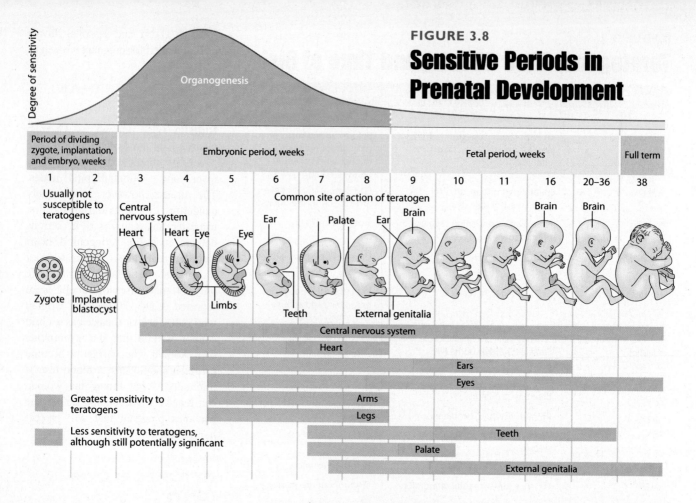

FIGURE 3.8
Sensitive Periods in Prenatal Development

abdomen) to prevent exposure to the infection.

HIV/AIDS

AIDS (acquired immune deficiency syndrome) is caused by the **human immunodeficiency virus (HIV)**. The human body, once infected with HIV, experiences a reduction in cells that are vital to our immune system and begins producing antibodies to battle the HIV. HIV, which is present in the bloodstream and genital secretions, can be transmitted when blood or secretions come into contact with mucous membranes (in various parts of the human body) or breaks in the skin (such as cuts or needle punctures).

An infected mother can pass the HIV virus to the fetus during pregnancy, during labor and delivery, and after birth, occasionally through breast milk. Statistics show that only one in four babies born to mothers infected with HIV develops AIDS. These figures are directly related to the amount of the virus the mother is carrying; that is, the more extensive the infection in the mother, the greater the chance the baby will be born with the virus. Consequently, treatment with zidovudine ZDV (formerly called azidothy-

midine [AZT]) or other drugs early in the pregnancy may help to prevent the transmission of the virus.

Estimates are that an infected mother transmits HIV from 30% to 50% of the time. Thus, 50–70% of fetuses remain unaffected. When the virus is transmitted, a condition called *AIDS embryopathy* may develop, which causes growth retardation, small head size (microcephaly), flat nose, and widespread, upward-slanted eyes, among other characteristics. AIDS is also associated with higher rates of preterm disease, low birth weight, and miscarriage. Because AIDS has a shorter incubation period in fetuses than in adults, symptoms may appear as early as 6 months after birth and include weight loss, fever, diarrhea, and chronic infections. Once symptoms appear, babies rarely survive more than 5 to 8 months.

TABLE 3.3
Some HIV/AIDS Statistics

- *People diagnosed with AIDS in U.S. in 2007:* 1,018,428 (9,209 children)
- *People living with HIV/AIDS in U.S.:* 454,747 (889 children under age 13)
- *AIDS deaths in U.S. 2007:* 14,110
- *Total number of AIDS deaths in U.S.:* 583,298 (4,891 children under age 13)

Prescription and Nonprescription Drugs

Drugs that are prescribed during pregnancy can have serious effects on the fetus. For example, the acne drug isotretinoin (Accutane) and the psoriasis drug acitretin (Soriatane) are known to cause birth defects, including heart defects, facial deformities such as cleft lip and missing ears, and mental retardation. The drug **thalidomide,** originally prescribed as a sleeping pill and an antinausea medication for pregnant women, produced tragic consequences. In the 1960s, physicians noticed a major increase in children born with either partial or no limbs. In some cases, feet and hands were directly attached to the body. Other outcomes were deafness, blindness, and cognitive deficits. In tracing the cause of the outbreak, investigators discovered that the mothers of these children had taken thalidomide early in their pregnancies. As little as a single dose of thalidomide early on in pregnancy was capable of damaging the fetus. The current use of the drug to treat multiple myeloma, AIDS, and tuberculosis remains controversial.

DES (diethylstilbestrol), a synthetic hormone, is another example of a teratogenic drug. In the late 1940s and 1950s, DES was given to pregnant women to prevent miscarriage. Researchers later found that the daughters of the women who had received this treatment were more susceptible to vaginal and cervical cancer. These daughters also experienced more miscarriages when pregnant than would be expected. Recent suspicions have arisen about the sons of DES women, who seem to have more disorders of their reproductive systems.

People are quick to recognize street drugs or prescription drugs as potentially harmful, but they don't always consider over-the-counter drugs, dietary supplements, or herbal remedies as dangerous. Many women use a prescription drug during the first weeks of pregnancy because they don't know they're pregnant. For example, in 2007 more than 120 women became pregnant while taking Accutane, commonly prescribed for acne. Some form of screening for prescription and illegal drug use is often done at the first prenatal visit.

We know that prescription and nonprescription drugs pass through the placenta and affect the growing embryo and fetus, and that certain prenatal periods are more susceptible to damage than others, such as the embryonic period. To keep pregnancy as safe as possible, a woman should begin by avoiding any drugs known to cause damage to a fetus and checking with her physician before taking over-the-counter medications. Substances that are not prescribed, such as illegal drugs, also have serious effects on the fetus.

ILLEGAL DRUGS

Cocaine, methamphetamine, marijuana, and heroin are well-known illegal drugs that act on the nervous system. People typically use them to alter moods, perceptions, and

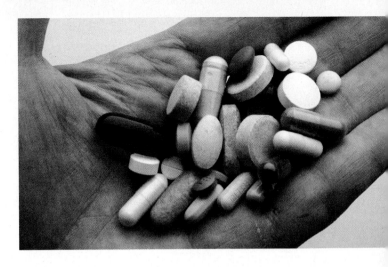

states of consciousness. Cocaine and methamphetamine are stimulants, which means that they speed up a person's nervous system. Babies born to mothers who used these stimulants during pregnancy may have low birth weight, behavioral problems, and impaired motor development. Marijuana use, which typically causes relaxation and heightened senses in adults, has been less documented in term of the prenatal effects on newborns. Some research shows that children whose mothers used marijuana during pregnancy experience problems with memory and depression. Heroin, a highly addictive drug made from morphine (a natural substance extracted from poppy plants), causes many behavioral problems in infants born to mothers who used the drug during pregnancy. These babies experience the same withdrawal symptoms as adults—tremors, sleep difficulty, impaired motor control. Most pregnant women who use illegal drugs do not consider the enormous risk they pose to their unborn child.

SMOKING

Smoking is probably the most common environmental threat to pregnancy. Tobacco use negatively affects everything about the reproduction process: fertility, conception, pregnancy, fetal development, labor, and delivery. Babies of mothers who smoke may have breathing difficulties and low resistance to infection, and they can suffer long-lasting health effects after birth, such as asthma.

Maternal smoking produces a condition called intrauterine growth retardation (IUGR). The birth weight of neonates whose mothers smoked during pregnancy is about 7 ounces less than that of babies whose mothers did not smoke. If mothers stop smoking before the 16th week of pregnancy, their babies show a great improvement in their birth weights.

> **thalidomide** Popular drug prescribed during the early 1960s that was later found to cause a variety of birth defects when taken by women early in their pregnancies.
>
> **DES (diethylstilbestrol)** A synthetic hormone that was administered to pregnant women in the late 1940s and 1950s supposedly to prevent miscarriage. It was later found that the daughters of the women who had received this treatment were more susceptible to vaginal and cervical cancer.

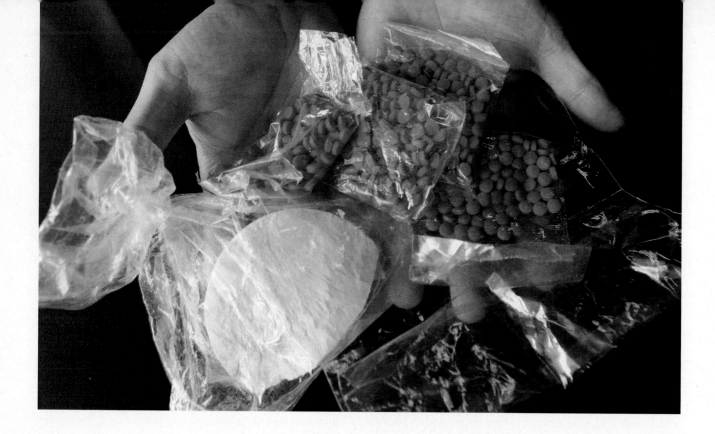

ALCOHOL

When a pregnant woman consumes alcohol, it crosses the placenta to the fetus. Because of this, drinking alcohol can harm the baby's development. Prenatal exposure to alcohol has been linked to so many problems that even moderate drinking is discouraged for pregnant women. Different levels of alcohol affect people differently, so it is hard to come up with safe drinking standards. To date, no safe amount of alcohol consumption during pregnancy has yet been established (Arenson & Drake, 2007).

fetal alcohol syndrome (FAS) The condition of babies whose mothers drank alcohol during pregnancy that is characterized by growth deficiencies, physical abnormalities, and CNS dysfunction.

One of the most severe effects of drinking during pregnancy is **fetal alcohol syndrome (FAS),** a condition characterized by growth deficiencies, physical abnormalities, and central nervous system dysfunction. FAS is one of the most common known causes of mental retardation and is the only cause that is entirely preventable. In the United States, the FAS prevalence rate is estimated to be between 0.2 and 2.0 cases per 1,000 live births.

CONCLUSIONS & SUMMARY

In this chapter, you have seen how a human being begins a journey through the lifespan. Nature's detailed choreography of prenatal development provides a remarkably complex yet elegant means of ensuring the survival of generations. Once conception occurs, uniting the genetic contribution of mother and father, the developmental process is under way, sheltering the fetus for the first 9 months in the protective cocoon of the womb.

What kinds of development occur during the prenatal period?

- The germinal period is the time when the fertilized egg passes through the fallopian tube.
- The embryonic period is a time of rapid development and great sensitivity.
- The fetal period is a time of preparation for life outside the womb.
- The senses develop during the prenatal months and are ready to function at birth.

What influences prenatal development and what precautions should be taken?

- Developmental risk is a term that applies to those children whose welfare is in jeopardy.
- Teratogens are those agents that cause abnormalities.
- Infectious diseases and chemical agents are the two basic classes of teratogens.
- Today AIDS is recognized as a potential danger for newborns.
- Maternal nutrition and emotions are important influences during pregnancy.
- Advancing technology has provided diagnostic tools for the detection of many fetal problems.

KEY TERMS

1. The various assisted reproductive technologies (ART) give people chances to have children that didn't exist years ago. How are opportunities afforded by ART examples of biopsychosocial interactions? Explain which plays a bigger role in fertility—nature or nurture.

2. Why is the discovery of DNA so important in our lives? Can you think of anything you have read or seen in the media that derives from this discovery?

3. What are some ethical considerations regarding frozen embryos? Should frozen embryos be available for adoption? If so, what policies would help regulate the adoption process?

Chapter Review Test

1. In vitro fertilization takes place
   a. in the fallopian tube.
   b. in the uterus.
   c. outside the woman's body.
   d. in the ovary.

2. Each sex cell carries a total of __ chromosomes.
   a. 23
   b. 24
   c. 47
   d. 46

3. Which of the following populations is more likely than the others to be afflicted with sickle-cell anemia?
   a. European Americans
   b. African Americans
   c. Asian Americans
   d. Hispanic Americans

4. Down syndrome is caused by
   a. the body's failure to break down amino acids.
   b. the fragile X syndrome.
   c. a deviation on the 21st pair of chromosomes.
   d. an XO pattern.

5. The Human Genome Project is an endeavor to identify and map
   a. certain substances within cells.
   b. all human genes.
   c. cell divisions.
   d. teratogens.

6. The first 2 weeks following fertilization are called the ___ period.
   a. embryonic
   b. fetal
   c. germinal
   d. pregnancy

7. Which of the following statements is true?
   a. The earlier the damage, the greater the chance of negative long-term effects.
   b. The fetus is safe from all harm while in the womb.
   c. Babies are usually born on the day predicted.
   d. A fetus hears no sound until birth.

8. In a typical pregnancy, a woman will gain about ____ pounds.
   a. 25 to 30
   b. 30 to 35
   c. 35 to 40
   d. 40 to 45

9. _____ is a technique in which a needle is inserted through a pregnant woman's abdomen and into the amniotic sac in order to obtain a fluid sample.
   a. Ultrasound
   b. Chorionic villi sampling
   c. Amniocentesis
   d. Nonstress test

10. Mental retardation, central nervous system dysfunction, and growth deficiencies can be symptoms of
    a. fetal alcohol syndrome (FAS).
    b. Rh factor.
    c. prematurity.
    d. anoxia.

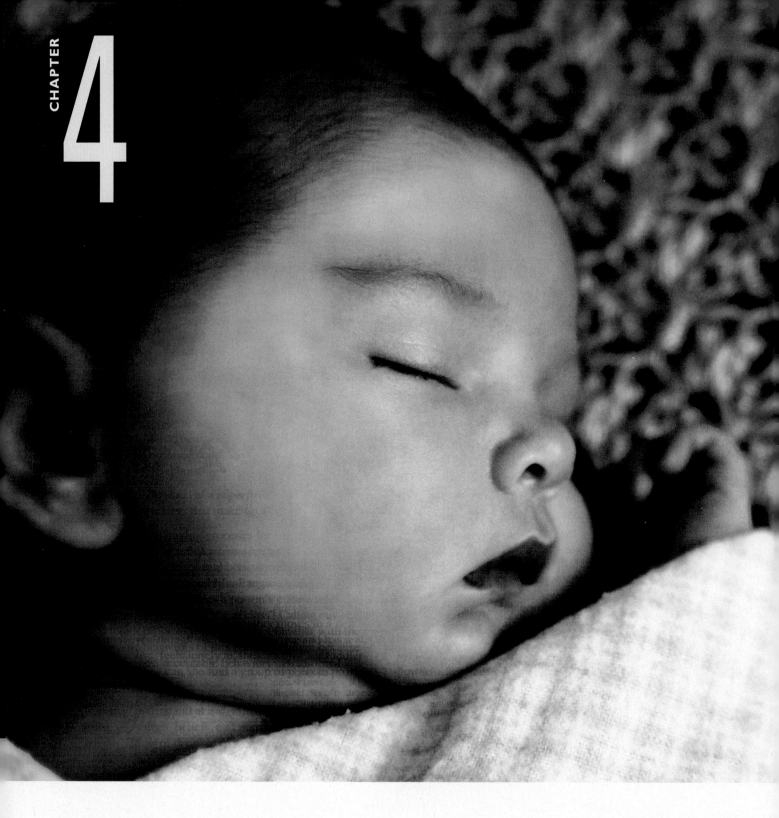

BIRTH AND THE

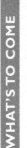
As You READ

After reading this chapter, you should be able to answer the following questions:

- What is the typical flow of the birth process, and what are some possible difficulties?

- What are some of the methods of childbirth?

- What are some challenges that can arise during childbirth, and what are some medical interventions?

- What are the characteristics of newborns?

- How do individuals and families adjust after the birth of a child?

NEWBORN CHILD

The 9-month experience of approximately 4 million American women each year typically culminates at birth (Guyer et al., 1999). No one knows exactly what causes labor to begin or why it begins about 280 days after the first day of the last menstrual period. What we do know is that birth practices over the years have changed remarkably and vary by culture.

Before the 20th century, few babies were born in hospitals. Most women gave birth at home, and medical intervention was not the primary force in childbirth. As concern about safety and sanitation grew, the number of babies born in hospitals increased rapidly, until the middle of the 20th century, when almost 80% were hospital births. Medical advances also meant that women received increasingly heavy medication for pain relief until the realization that the effects of drugs can be dangerous for the developing fetus. In the 1960s, an expanding use of childbirth techniques known as natural childbirth helped to minimize reliance on medication. Changes continue to this day, with more women seeking to employ more natural means of treatment and support during all stages of pregnancy and birth.

When a person is born, one of the greatest biopsychosocial shifts occurs (Cole, 1999). From the wet, warm prenatal environment, the newborn enters a drier, colder world. The newborn must breathe and eat on its own. For the first time, the newborn encounters other human beings. Parents can suddenly see and touch their child, and the interactions that foster a particular parent–child relationship begin.

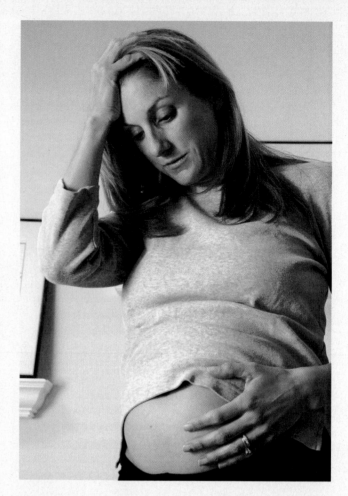

The Birth Process

As women enter the last weeks of pregnancy, wheels are set in motion according to what nature dictates. For example, in most cases the baby will position itself in a head-down position, where the head is resting comfortably in the mother's pelvic region. Mothers-to-be may hear their doctor describe this situation as the dropping or lightening of the baby. Women tend to feel less pressure on their chest and diaphragm, which is a welcome sensation after several weeks of expanding girth.

Many women experience false labor pains as pregnancy progresses, and these pains sometimes occur as early as the second trimester. Experts explain such pains, called **Braxton-Hicks contractions,** as relatively mild and a sort of training for the muscles and mind before real contractions begin. Real labor pains are more intense and more painful than Braxton-Hicks contractions. It's not uncommon for couples to rush to the hospital, anticipating the birth of their child, only to learn that the delivery will likely not occur for several weeks.

Once the birth process truly begins, marked by distinctive signals and events, biopsychosocial factors interact and set the stage for multifaceted lifetime development. For example, the baby may secrete hormones that, in turn, cause the mother's body to secrete hormones that initiate uterine contractions. During labor, the woman's pituitary gland secretes **oxytocin,** a hormone that has been linked to caregiving behaviors and bonding (Febo, Numan, & Ferris, 2005). Interestingly, fathers' hormone levels have been shown to change in various ways relating to different aspects of fatherhood and caregiving, so the biopsychosocial effects of birth are not limited to mothers before, during, and after the big event (Berg & Wynne-Edwards, 2001; Storey et al., 2000).

Stages in Labor and Delivery

A woman usually becomes aware of the beginning of labor by one or more of these signs:

- *Blood and/or mucus from the vagina.* As the cervix softens before labor, the mucous plug that had sealed the uterus and prevented infection is sometimes expelled with a small amount of blood. This usually means labor will begin within 24 to 48 hours (Arenson & Drake, 2007).

- *Amniotic fluid passing from the ruptured amniotic sac through the vagina.* Commonly known as "water breaking," this occurs before labor much less often than when labor is well under way.

Braxton-Hicks contractions Relatively mild muscle contractions that occur before real contractions begin.

oxytocin Hormone secreted by the pituitary gland that stimulates uterine contractions; has been linked to bonding between caregivers and infants.

- *Uterine contractions accompanied by significant discomfort.* Although every woman's tolerance of pain varies, there is a marked difference between mild contractions that last about 10 seconds and the stronger, regularly spaced contractions that last longer, occur every few minutes, and thus signal the onset of childbirth.

While the actual amount of time before a baby's arrival is not clear or consistent among women, three clear and distinct stages of labor are certain.

The first stage is called the **dilation** stage. The opening of the mother's cervix must increase in diameter in order for the baby to pass through and enter the world. Dilation is what causes most of the pain associated with labor. In the first stage (the longest of the three stages), the opening of the cervix dilates to about 10 centimeters (4 inches) in diameter. The dilation process and accompanying labor pains may last for several hours, and if the birth is a woman's first, the duration is longer than it will be with subsequent deliveries. When labor begins, the duration of each contraction increases to about 60 seconds as labor continues, and the baby's head starts to move into the birth canal (opening of the vagina).

The second stage is the **expulsion** stage. Once the cervix is fully dilated, the baby no longer meets resistance, and the contractions push it along the birth canal. The expulsion phase generally lasts an average of 1½ hours for first births and about half that time for women who have previously given birth. Most partners, if present, describe the appearance of the head of the baby (called crowning) as an amazing experience. Once crowning has occurred, the baby typically emerges in a matter of minutes. If this second stage of labor is prolonged—with no evidence of a prob-

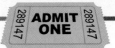

FEATURED MEDIA

Films About the Birth Process

The Business of Being Born (2008) – Should births be viewed as a natural process or treated as a medical situation? Surprising facts regarding historical and current practices of the child birth industry are interwoven with actual birth stories.

Junior (1994) – What would happen if men could conceive and deliver babies? What comic pitfalls and realizations could influence the process?

Star Trek (2009) – How does the moment of one baby's birth influence the rest of his life and the lives of infinite beings throughout the galaxy?

lem—surgical intervention typically remains unnecessary. Occasionally, women spend 5 or 6 hours (or more) in this stage in a normal first birth.

Many doctors will typically use massage and lubrication in an attempt to widen the vaginal opening, but if the birth canal is still hindering the baby's safe passage, a procedure known as an **episiotomy** may be used to facilitate the birth process. This refers to a surgical cut in the vaginal opening that allows for the baby to pass through the birth canal. Because most episiotomies are easily stitched and quick to heal, they are thought to be a helpful procedure that reduces vaginal tearing and other complications related to a baby's shoulder width or declining heart rate. However, having an episiotomy may cause pain and infection after delivery, and the American College of Obstetricians and Gynecologists supports the position of restricted, not routine, use of episiotomy. The number of episiotomies performed has dropped in the past few decades (Goldberg et al., 2002), as the use of massage and other techniques has increased women's preference for more-natural strategies to widen the vaginal opening.

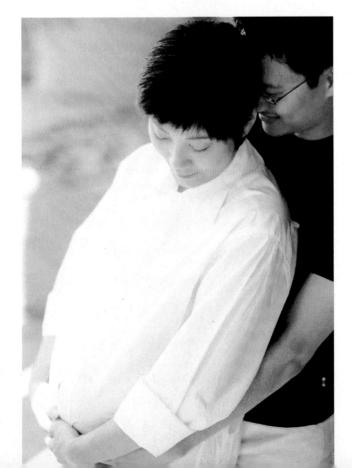

As the baby's head emerges from the mother's body, different procedures are used to prepare the baby for entry into a dramatically different environment. For example, warm blankets are at the ready to nestle the baby and lessen the shock of transition from the warm uterus to the different temperature and sounds of the birth environment. Parents' preference for method of delivery

dilation The first stage of the birth process, during which the opening of the cervix dilates to about 4 inches in diameter.

expulsion Stage 2 of the birth process; the baby passes through the birth canal.

episiotomy A surgical cut made to widen the vaginal opening.

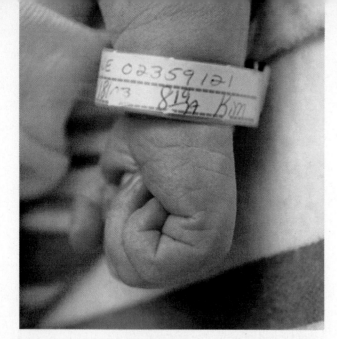

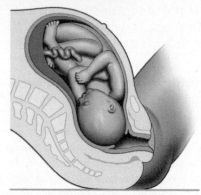

FIGURE 4.1

The Stages of Birth

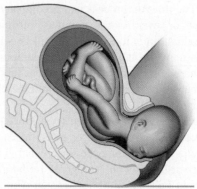

Stage one: Baby positions itself

Stage two: Baby begins to emerge

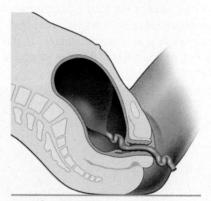

Stage three: Placenta is expelled

influences the type of procedures used, and precautions are taken to ensure that the baby's breathing is promoted and risk of infection is limited. By the time the baby has been weighed and measured, has had footprints taken, and has been given an ID bracelet to match the mother's, the mother has moved into the third and final stage of birth.

Called the **afterbirth** stage, this final stage is marked by the delivery of the placenta, the remaining umbilical cord, and other membranes. This stage may last only a few minutes or more than an hour. If the spontaneous delivery of the placenta is delayed, a doctor may remove it. The woman's body now acts to terminate any excessive bleeding. Figure 4.1 illustrates the stages of the birth process.

Methods of Childbirth

A woman's choices for childbirth practices will vary depending on her culture, the society of which she is a part, and her individual temperament. Whereas childbirth was once limited to the home and was a relatively family-centered experience, over the course of many decades delivery has moved to hospitals and other birth facilities for reasons related to hygiene and technology. For example, in the 1960s and 1970s, women whose mothers were sedated during childbirth in the 1930s and 1940s began to choose alternative methods of delivery. Instead of accepting heavy drugs that could potentially harm the baby and dull the mother's sensations during labor, mothers began to seek birth centers and techniques that focused on natural methods.

NATURAL CHILDBIRTH

Many mothers wish to create the most natural, peaceful environment possible during delivery. Methods to reduce mothers' pain and anxiety about delivery have increased in recent years, and many people argue that special tools and medications are not

afterbirth Stage 3 of the birth process in which the placenta and other membranes are discharged.

Childbirth *is more admirable than conquest,* more **amazing** *than self-defense, and as* courageous *as either one.*

GLORIA STEINEM, MS. MAGAZINE (1981)

perspectives on Diversity

Cultural Variations of the Birth Process

Although the biological processes involved in labor and birth are similar everywhere, the experience of giving birth varies from culture to culture. Values and expectations determine procedures and identify behaviors, emotions, and reactions to be expected. For example, the Hmong women of Laos may attempt to avoid any internal examination during labor and prefer to give birth in a squatting position; some Native American women remain upright, and Pueblo women may kneel, during the birth process. Vietnamese women attempt to maintain self-control and even keep smiling during labor, while the Ibo of Nigeria consider childbirth as an illness. Japanese women usually will not ask for pain relief. Arabic women are extremely concerned with modesty and try to keep their bodies covered as much as possible. Knowing these cultural variations and preferences leads to more considerate treatment by those supporting the woman during childbirth.

As Rogoff (2003) noted, birth involves cultural practices surrounding labor and delivery (e.g., medications for the mother, different birthing positions, and degree and kind of support). Rogoff explained how a cultural innova-

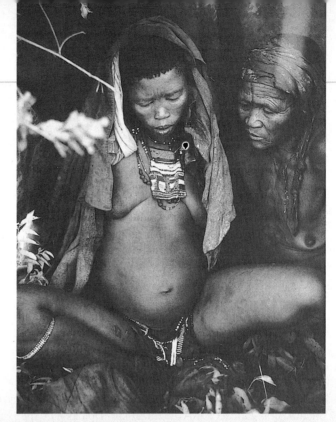

tion (cesarean section) saves a child whose head may be too large for the mother's birth canal. Thus, the genes for large heads are preserved and passed on from generation to generation. It's clear that cultural technologies can contribute to nature and that resulting biological changes, in turn, can produce cultural adaptations.

---

needed for women to experience a successful birth experience. Breathing and relaxation techniques are a big part of the process of **natural childbirth,** sometimes called **prepared childbirth.** Massage, hypnosis, and acupuncture are other options that women explore before and during delivery. The idea is that such techniques will reduce or eliminate the need for pain medication and give the woman more control over and awareness of her body. Other techniques, such as water births (delivering the baby in a tub of warm water), have become more popular as women strive to re-create the environment that the baby has been living in for the past 9 months.

One of the best-known natural childbirth methods is the **Lamaze method.** This method requires that the mother work with a partner before and during the delivery process to learn the techniques they will use during delivery. The partner coaches the mother by timing contractions and providing emotional and physical support. The use of specific breathing and relaxation exercises is intended to increase a woman's feelings of control during delivery and reduce anxiety and pain.

natural childbirth (or **prepared childbirth**) Term to describe techniques women use prior to and during the birth process to create the most natural experience possible during delivery

Lamaze method Natural childbirth method that stresses breathing and relaxation with the support of a partner.

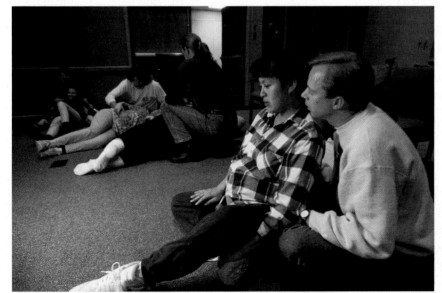

MIDWIVES AND DOULAS

Support during labor and delivery can take many forms. Women have relied on midwives and doulas during the birth process for thousands of years, and many women feel more confident with women trained in these areas than they do with licensed medical doctors. In the United States, a **midwife** is a woman who has been specially trained in delivering babies and spends time with pregnant women before and during delivery. Midwives who have trained as nurses in addition to midwifery are called nurse-midwives, and those who train without nursing training are called direct entry midwives. A midwife who has met specific requirements for midwife certification is able to call herself a certified professional midwife (CPM). Individuals who are interested in using a midwife should investigate potential midwives to ensure that a particular midwife meets all of the future parents' needs and expectations.

A **doula** is a woman who provides physical and emotional support for mothers before, during, and after delivery, which includes providing information as needed to help mothers make educated decisions. *Doula* stems from a Greek word meaning "woman who serves." In order to work as professional doulas, women must be certified by an organization called DONA International. Doulas can specialize in birth practices or postpartum period (the period from delivery to approximately 6 weeks after a woman delivers her baby) practices. Most often, midwives and doulas work together with medical professionals to ensure the safety of the birth while giving the mother as much possible control over her delivery.

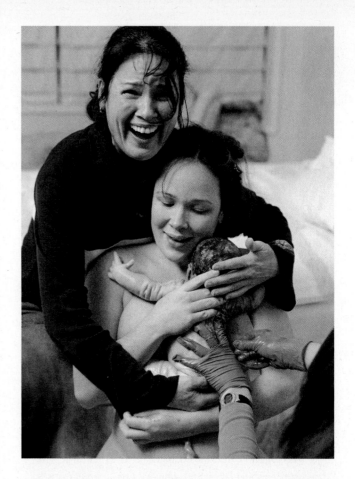

midwife A woman trained in delivering babies; typically a nurse.

doula A woman trained as a caregiver to provide ongoing support to pregnant women before, during, and after delivery.

analgesics Mild medications used to alleviate pain; may be used before and during labor.

anesthetics Stronger medications used during labor to control pain; can numb mother to pain in the various stages of labor.

HOME DELIVERY

Many women who seek the assistance of midwives and doulas often express interest in delivering their babies in the comfort and familiar surroundings of their own home. Interest in home deliveries has risen in the past 30 years, although research indicates that home deliveries carry greater risks for both baby and mother (Pang et al., 2002). Only a very small number of deliveries, approximately 1% of births in the United States, occur at home (Studelska, 2006). Medical doctors facilitate some home births, but most home births are not attended by physicians. If the mother is in good health and the likelihood of complications is low, home deliveries are generally safe for both mother and baby. However, if there is any doubt as to the well-being of mother or baby, the most appropriate place for delivery to occur is a hospital.

USE OF MEDICATION

Hospitals provide a safe setting for the use of medication, and doctors and nurses help inform decisions that mothers make about which medication is best for them at specific points in the birth process. **Analgesics** are drugs used to alleviate pain and can be administered in small doses to help the mother relax during labor. Analgesics range from over-the-counter brands of acetaminophen, such as Tylenol, to tranquilizers and narcotics, such as Demerol. **Anesthetics** are stronger forms of medication and can be used to control pain in the various stages of labor. For example, a mother may be given local anesthetics to numb specific areas of the body, such as an epidural block that numbs the body from the waist down. Gen-

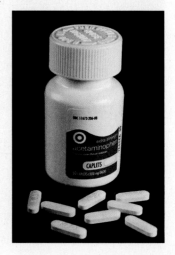

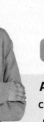

Career Apps

As a nurse-midwife, what strategies could you use to encourage family participation during labor and delivery?

eral anesthetics are not often used today, although women received them for years in the early 20th century. General anesthetics put mothers to sleep so that they experience little to none of the actual delivery, and the use of these anesthetics requires longer recovery time.

CESAREAN SECTION

One situation that requires the use of anesthetics, local and rarely general, is a procedure called a **cesarean section.** If the baby cannot come through the birth canal successfully, surgery is performed to deliver the baby through the mother's abdomen. An incision is made in the mother's abdomen and the baby is delivered directly from the uterus. (The term *cesarean* derived from the historical figure Julius Caesar, who is believed to have been delivered in the same manner.) Conditions suggesting a cesarean (also called a C-section) include mother's health in danger, fetal distress, mother's pelvis too narrow for a vaginal delivery, baby's abnormal position, and previous cesareans (Smith, 2000). Medical reasoning is that a cesarean section will likely produce a healthier baby than prolonged labor and a difficult birth. However, the procedure also involves certain risks, such as increased chance of infection for the mother, increased anxiety for parents, longer hospital stays, and longer recovery time associated with the surgery. The success rate for a vaginal delivery after having had a cesarean ranges from 60% to 80%.

A cesarean section is considered major surgery and is not recommended unless necessary. There has been a gradual increase in cesarean births in the United States. The rate is currently at 29%, which means more than 1 million births this year, compared to only 5% as recently as 40 years ago (Bakalar, 2005). Some doctors tend to be conservative when they suspect a risky delivery and therefore recommend a C-section. Some doctors may recommend C-sections, largely because of concern about lawsuits related to vaginal deliveries that have increased in recent

years. There has also been a growing trend of women who request cesarean sections because it provides them with some control over factors such as the baby's delivery date, pain, and stress on the babies' and their own bodies. Fortunately, what was once a surgical procedure used most often as an emergency measure has become less likely to cause problems for the mother and baby than in the past.

Complications and Interventions

The birth process, as complex as it may be, proceeds normally with manageable levels of pain for most women. However, complications arise for women across all cultures, geographic locations, and socioeconomic levels. In industrialized societies, particularly in North America, use of medical monitoring and intervention occurs in an extremely high proportion of cases. Advances in medical technologies (such as assisted fertilization) allow for multiple births and high-risk deliveries to occur, but the chance of complications and use of interventions increase. The following are a few of the more common complications that sometimes occur and the interventions that have been designed to avoid or address them.

BREECH BIRTH

During the last month of pregnancy, most babies "turn" or move into a head-down position. Most babies who don't turn during this time are in the **breech birth** position (see Figure 4.2). It's almost as if the baby is sitting in the uterus, head up and feet down. Breech babies must be carefully guided through the birth

cesarean section Surgery performed to deliver the baby through the abdomen if the baby cannot come through the birth canal.

breech birth Birth in which the baby is born feet first, buttocks first, or in a crosswise position (transverse presentation).

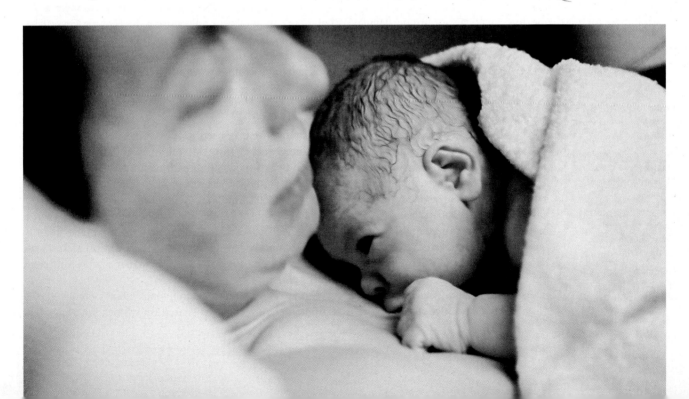

FIGURE 4.2

Fetus in Breech Presentation

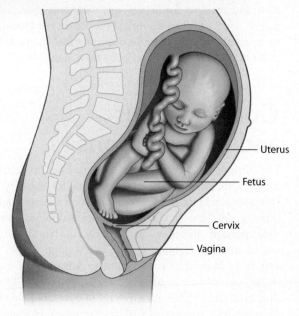

- Uterus
- Fetus
- Cervix
- Vagina

canal feet first, buttocks first, or in a crosswise position, but most are born healthy.

Breech births cause concern and often require a cesarean section because a baby's position in the uterus is not conducive to an optimal delivery. The major concern is with the size of babies' heads in proportion to the rest of their bodies. Several conditions can contribute to a breech presentation: more than one fetus in the uterus, an abnormally shaped uterus, a placenta covering all or part of the uterine opening, and prematurity.

FETAL MONITORING

When a woman enters the first stage of labor, it is not uncommon for her to be fitted with an electronic device called a **fetal monitor** to register the baby's heartbeat and inform medical staff as to any distress or irregularities the baby may be experiencing. This information will affect decisions about delivery proceedings, such as specific techniques, medications, and instruments that will be needed.

Two kinds of fetal monitors are used in hospitals and birthing centers—external and internal monitors. The most common device is external and worn like a belt across the mother's belly during labor. While this is not an invasive device, it can be somewhat uncomfortable for the mother and can hinder some movement during labor. Another type of monitor is inserted through the

fetal monitor Electronic device used to monitor the baby's heartbeat throughout labor.

forceps Metal clamps placed around the baby's head to pull the baby through the birth canal.

vacuum extractor Plastic cup attached to a suction device that pulls the baby through the birth canal.

induced labor Labor initiated by doctors through use of medication and by breaking the amniotic sac

woman's cervix and rests directly on the baby's scalp. This internal monitor is more comfortable for the mother and is also highly sensitive, registering information about the baby as well as the mother's contractions. Both types of monitors are safe, and the medical use of fetal monitoring has resulted in a higher number of safe deliveries in high-risk situations. Even though the use of monitors is not necessary in all cases, doctors in the United States often use them to ensure that they have taken every possible step to facilitate a healthy delivery for mother and newborn.

USE OF INSTRUMENTS

If doctors determine that the baby is in jeopardy, they may opt for the use of special instruments to assist in the delivery of the newborn. Two kinds of instruments are typically used in most cases: forceps and vacuum extractor. This type of assistance has been practiced for centuries when there is sufficient cause for concern over need for a speedier delivery. In the United States, forceps tend to be the preferred tool, whereas vacuum extractors are more frequently used in Europe. **Forceps** are metal clamps that are gently placed around a baby's head to pull the baby through the birth canal. More recently, vacuum extractors are chosen for much the same reason as forceps. A **vacuum extractor** consists of a plastic cup attached to a suction device that pulls the baby through the birth canal. Concern about the use of these instruments is warranted, as forceps use greatly increases the risk of brain injury to the baby as well as damage to the baby's or mother's body. Vacuum extractors can cause bleeding on or beneath the baby's scalp, or create a conelike shape to the baby's head that may last for many months in a small number of cases. However, vacuum extractors are less likely than forceps to injure the mother's body. The baby's scalp is at risk of injury when either instrument is used.

The use of forceps and vacuum extractors has declined in recent years, due to an increased number of cesarean sections and efforts to reduce risk of brain damage to the baby. As complications arise during the birth process, these instruments do continue to be used by doctors in a small percentage of births. Figure 4.3 compares the use of forceps and the vacuum extractor in delivery.

INDUCED LABOR

One strategy that is used to hasten the delivery of a baby is induced labor. **Induced labor** is initiated by doctors through use of medication and occurs before the mother's own body initiates the birth process. Doctors induce labor when they determine that there is significant risk to either mother or child if a pregnancy continues, such as when a baby is well past the due date and growing bigger than is safe for a mother to deliver, or if there are problems with the placenta and the baby is no longer receiving sufficient nutrition.

Some suggestions for inducing labor without medical intervention are often shared by women who have had

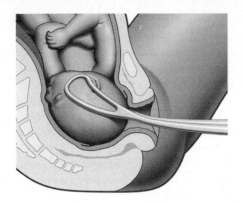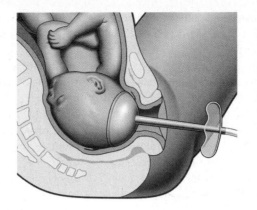

FIGURE 4.3

Forceps vs. Vacuum Extractor in Delivery

babies, and are commonly found in magazines, books, or on the Internet. For example, riding in a car down a bumpy road, being pushed on a park swing, and eating spicy food close to the delivery date are common suggestions. The success of these methods has not been scientifically tested, and yet many women place much confidence in them. The most reliable way to induce labor, however, is for a doctor to break the amniotic sac, which signals the body to go into labor. Coupled with medication, this typically stimulates contractions. For example, oxytocin (Pitocin), a contraction-causing hormone naturally produced by a woman's body during labor, is often given by injection or through an IV to speed up labor.

As a result of induced labor, a woman may experience more intense contractions that occur closer together than with a noninduced labor. This can compromise the baby's oxygen supply and the mother's ability to maintain control using prepared childbirth techniques, such as breathing exercises. The use of medication and instruments becomes greater in these instances. If efforts at an induced labor do not succeed, a cesarean section will likely be the next course of action. In fact, the rate of cesarean sections is much higher for induced labors than for natural labors.

OXYGEN DEPRIVATION

If anything interrupts the flow of oxygen to the fetus during birth, brain damage or death can result. **Anoxia** is the term used for lack of sufficient oxygen supply during labor and delivery. It also can be the result of insufficient blood supply from the mother. A substantial need for oxygen exists during birth because pressure on the fetal head can cause some rupturing of the blood vessels in the brain. Failure to receive oxygen can cause brain damage or death. It is difficult to predict whether the damage is permanent (Carlson, 2004).

Complications with the umbilical cord, placenta, or lungs can also cause anoxia. Before a baby is born, if the umbilical cord is squeezed or otherwise impaired, a baby may suffer oxygen deprivation. Immediately after birth, once the umbilical cord is cut, a delay in lung breathing is also dangerous. Inside the womb, if the mother's placenta separates before the baby is born (placenta abruptio), or

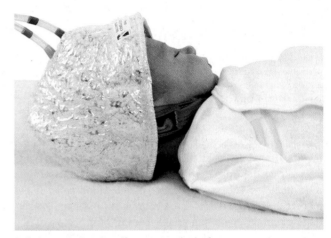

A Cool-cap greatly reduces brain injury and risk of death for infants who experience anoxia.

develops in a position that covers the opening of a woman's cervix (placenta previa) and therefore detaches, an emergency cesarean may need to be performed. A baby's lung development is linked to anoxia, either because the baby experienced prenatal damage to the respiratory system or because the baby's lungs are not able to function well enough for him or her to breathe successfully. When an infant's lungs are in a serious condition, the air sacs may collapse and the infant may need to be supported by medical interventions, such as respirators.

If a baby does experience anoxia and subsequent brain injury, additional brain damage can result even hours after delivery. Researchers have found that cooling an infant's head in a specially designed FDA-approved apparatus (Cool-cap), or placing the infant on a cooling blanket, significantly reduces brain injury and infant death (Shankaran et al., 2005).

Children who have experienced anoxia display impaired cognitive abilities, such as language skills, in early and middle childhood, but these impairments sometimes improve as children age. Milder cases of anoxia tend to result in milder impairment. One condition that results in brain damage before or

anoxia Insufficient oxygen supply during labor and delivery, which can cause fetal brain damage or death.

cerebral palsy A condition resulting from an inability of the brain to control the body; result of brain damage before, during, or after delivery.

Rh factor Involves possible incompatibility between the blood types of mother and child. If the mother is Rh-negative and the child Rh-positive, miscarriage or even infant death can result.

premature birth Early birth; occurs at or before 37 weeks after conception and is defined by low birth weight and immaturity.

small for date Term used for babies born or assessed as underweight for the length of the pregnancy.

isolette Specially designed bed for premature infants that is temperature-controlled and enclosed in clear plastic; often referred to as an incubator.

during labor and delivery, or shortly after birth is **cerebral palsy,** a condition resulting from an inability of the brain to control the body. The disorder is classified into four types: difficult or rigid movement, lack of balance and depth perception, involuntary movements, or a combination of the other types. Approximately 500,000 people in the United States are diagnosed with cerebral palsy, and another 4,500 children are diagnosed annually. About 10% of children diagnosed with cerebral palsy experienced anoxia before or during labor, or after delivery.

THE RH FACTOR

As much as every mother wishes to protect her baby from harm, there are some instances when unintentional damage may occur unless screening measures identify potential risks. In some cases, there is a possible incompatibility between the blood types of mother and baby. This is referred to as the **Rh factor.** The Rh factor is a type of protein located on the surface of red blood cells. If the mother is Rh-negative and the baby is Rh-positive, miscarriage or infant death can result. During birth, some of the baby's blood inevitably enters the mother's bloodstream. The mother then develops antibodies to defend against the Rh factor and is said to be "sensitized" to the Rh factor. The antibodies created by the mother's body can attack the blood cells of an Rh-positive baby, thereby causing the baby to become anemic. In many cases, a woman's first baby may not experience any harm. During later pregnancies, however, these antibodies may pass into the fetus's blood and start to destroy the red blood cells of an Rh-positive baby.

Routine screening during pregnancy, which involves a simple blood test, can provide medical staff and mothers with critical information. This screening is often suggested during the middle stage of a woman's pregnancy. A blood test will indicate whether the Rh factor is positive (present) or negative (absent) in the mother's blood. The majority of women are Rh-positive. An unsensitized Rh-negative mother can be treated with injections of a blood product called Rh immune globulin (RhIg) to prevent sensitization.

PREMATURE BIRTH

Another complication that sometimes occurs despite a mother's best attempts at a

healthy pregnancy is **premature birth.** The average duration of a healthy pregnancy is 40 weeks. Babies who are born early—at or before 37 weeks after conception—are referred to as preterm, or premature, and are often called "preemies." Babies whose birth weight is less than 5½ pounds are also considered preemies. Birth weight has been shown to be the best indicator of a preemie's likelihood of health challenges or successful development. For example, preemies born weighing less than 3½ pounds often struggle with developmental challenges that eventually become impossible to overcome. Even when a preemie succeeds in conquering initial challenges, other problems persist for decades, such as high susceptibility to illness, impaired motor control, emotional and behavioral issues, and learning disabilities. Recent statistics from the Children's Defense Fund estimate the number of uninsured pregnant women in the United States at around 800,000 (CDF, 2009). Lack of insurance may be directly linked to mothers seeking or receiving less prenatal care and the incidence of low-birth-weight babies.

Additional statistics estimate that 2–9% of newborns require care in a neonatal intensive care unit (NICU) (Goldberg & DiVitto, 2002). These babies once had high mortality rates, but today's sophisticated technology greatly increases their chances of survival (Feldman et al., 2002). Mothers who are carrying multiple babies are considered at higher risk for complications for the main reason that there is limited space in the uterus, and at some point there simply isn't enough room for the babies to reach full term in a space that typically holds one baby.

Some babies are identified as **small for date** at the time of delivery, or close to the expected due date. In simple terms, this means that a baby has not grown as large as expected for the length of the pregnancy, and the baby may indeed be full term. A small-for-date baby who weighs 5.8 pounds is considered at low birth weight; a weight of 3.5 pounds or less is considered very low birth weight.

Pregnant mothers' health practices have been linked to the incidence of small-for-date babies, including smoking, poor nutrition, and drug use. Small-for-date babies are typically smaller and weigh less than their peers throughout their lifetimes; they also experience more difficulties than preemies, are at greater risk for infection and brain damage, and are likely to have later childhood learning challenges.

Interventions for premature infants include medical and social procedures and processes. Medical practices involve the use of a specially designed bed called an **isolette.** An isolette provides the preemie with a warm, temperature-controlled environment because the bed is enclosed in clear plastic. Isolettes help preemies who cannot regulate their own body heat and

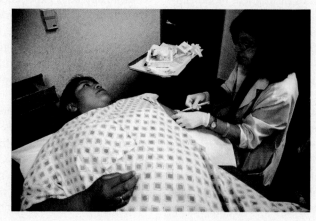

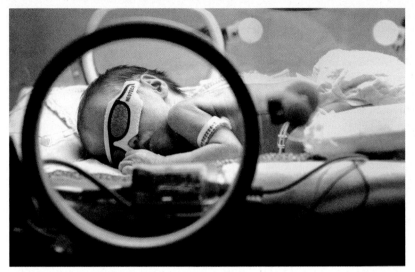

An isolette provides a safe environment for preemies.

on the extreme nature of low birth weight, difficulties vary from one preemie to another. The graph in Figure 4.4 depicts percentages of low-birth-weight babies.

Unfortunately, negative stereotypes exist and impact people's perceptions about preemies and their abilities, temperaments, and overall competence. Preemies are often viewed as vulnerable, fragile, and less competent, even *after* they have caught up with babies who experienced a full-term pregnancy and healthy birth weight. In one study, observers were told that a healthy-looking 9-month-old infant had been premature. These observers subsequently described the baby as "weaker, less physically mature, less sociable, and less cognitively competent" than full-term infants, a tendency called "prematurity stereotyping." Fortunately, studies indicate that by 12 to 18 months, most parents and their preterm babies have established a relationship quite similar to that of full-term infants and their parents (Goldberg & DiVitto, 2002).

protect them from cool drafts of air that could stimulate infection. Air is filtered for the infant, and physical needs relating to feeding and receiving medication can all be done within the isolette through the use of tubes and an intravenous needle, or IV.

Although premature infants may differ from full-term babies in the early days of their development, most reach developmental levels similar to those of full-term babies, although a little more slowly than usual. For example, motor development may develop more slowly for preemies. In a study conducted by Jeng and associates (2000), very low birth weight infants began walking a few months later than infants born full term at healthy weights. Depending

RESILIENCE AND PREMATURITY

The relationships between premature infants and family members are significantly aided when training and support are readily available. Parents who are fairly stable financially and have a strong social network tend to have less stress associated with premature births. They can accommodate the stresses that present themselves with the arrival

FIGURE 4.4

Percentages of Low-Birth-Weight Babies

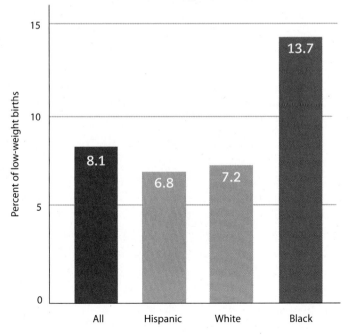

Percent of low-weight births

- All: 8.1
- Hispanic: 6.8
- White: 7.2
- Black: 13.7

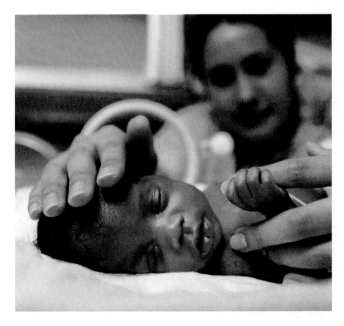

of preemies. When a premature infant is born into a situation that is already compromised because of factors that may have contributed to the prematurity in the first place (such as poverty, drug or alcohol abuse), the stress is compounded for all family members. Parents who live in high-stress, low-income environments greatly benefit from long-term interventions, such as professionals who coach parents in coping with and responding to the needs of their newborns. Parents are not able to hold preemies in the same way they would full-term infants, and preemies do not appear as cute and cuddly as babies parents typically imagine in their minds, which impacts how caregivers and preemies bond in the early months after delivery. Many mothers of preemies report feelings of guilt and low self-esteem and admit to feeling like failures (Bugental & Happaney, 2004).

> *Once we believe in*
> **ourselves,** *we can*
> *risk curiosity, wonder,*
> **spontaneous** *delight,*
> *or any experience that reveals*
> *the* **human spirit.**
>
> **E.E. CUMMINGS**

Whereas it was once considered unwise and unsafe for preemies to be stimulated in their postuterine environment, it is now known to be beneficial for preemies to receive regular forms of stimulation, whether it is music being played in their rooms, parents showing toys to infants and pointing out characteristics such as color and texture, or skin-to-skin contact such as massage or a practice called kangaroo care. **Kangaroo care** involves the baby spending some amount of time every day lying in a vertical position, either on the mother's chest (typically placed between the breasts) or on the father's chest, under clothing so that the baby's skin and caregiver's skin touch for specific periods of time, sometimes several hours at a time.

There are benefits of kangaroo care for both caregiver and infant. The caregiver's body responds to the needs of the infant's body, and it regulates the infant's body temperature more easily than can be done in an isolette. Mother's milk adjusts accordingly, and the baby sleeps more soundly and gains weight more rapidly than when solely in an isolette. Perhaps one of the greatest benefits for caregivers is the confidence they develop with daily experience caring for their newborn. Caregivers are able to gain an appreciation for their new roles as well as their infant's abilities. They also

kangaroo care Practice of skin-to-skin contact, positioning baby against caregiver's bare chest.

neonate An infant in the first days and weeks after birth.

experience the joys of daily gains in physical, cognitive, and social development.

Recall the Werner and Smith longitudinal study described in Chapter 1, in which data were collected on children from their prenatal days through their early 30s. Some of the infants were considered at risk for developmental challenges because of difficult births. What might have been some significant factors that contributed to their resilience? Relationships with family members constitute one possible influence. Individual characteristics—many noticeable at birth—are other possible factors.

Characteristics of Neonates

From the moment of birth until about 1 month, the newborn infant is called a **neonate.** Even as recently as 50 years ago, most people assumed that neonates cannot do much other than lie down, eat, cry, and wait for others to tend to their needs. Today, however, we know that neonates begin to use their abilities to adapt to, and exercise some control over, their environment immediately after birth. Although they are not able to walk or talk, newborn babies display competence that contributes to their survival and elicits attention from others who will provide them with basic care. For example, neonates have the ability to imitate almost immediately after birth. Infants' imitation of tongue movements is well established in babies as young as a few hours (Gopnik, Meltzoff, & Kuhl, 1999; Jones, 1996).

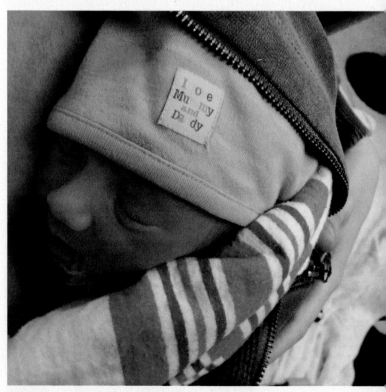

Kangaroo care involves a baby spending time in a verticle position, chest to chest with a caregiver, with their skin touching.

Imitative Behavior of Infants.
....
Courtesy of Dr. Tiffany Field and Science. From Field et al., model and infant expressions from "Discrimination and Imitation of Facial Express by Neonates" in Science, *Fig. 2, Vol. 218, pp. 179–181, October 8, 1982. Reprinted by permission of the American Association for the Advancement of Science.*

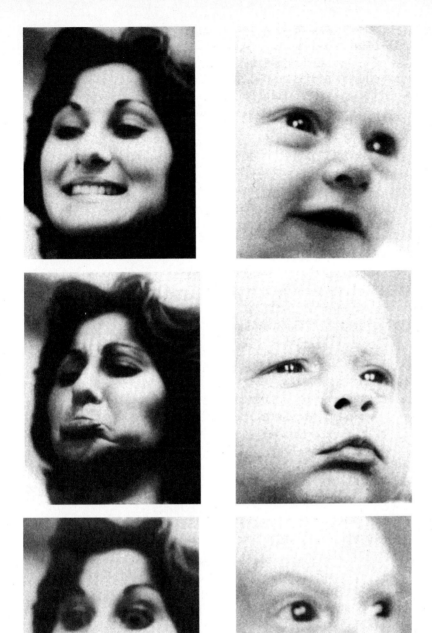

SENSORY COMPETENCE

Neonates are active seekers of stimulation. They want and need people, sounds, and physical contact to stimulate their cognitive development and to give them a feeling of security in their world. Although infants spend much time trying to gain some control and regulate bodily functions such as eating, breathing, and heart rate, for brief moments, sometimes 15 to 20 seconds, they stop these efforts and pay close attention to the environment in search of stimulation.

Vision

There is often some misperception about neonates' abilities to see at birth. They are indeed able to see, yet their visual abilities are the least developed of all the sensory abilities at birth. For example, they are nearsighted, meaning that they can see objects better at close distances (less than a foot from their faces) than farther away. If a neonate's attention is drawn to an object (such as a small, red rubber ball held at about 10 inches from the face), she will track it as the object is moved slowly from side to side.

Neonates do not possess the level of eye-muscle control and eye–brain communication at birth that they will develop rapidly over the next few months. For example, the muscles that control the lens of the eyes are not strong enough to allow neonates to focus on and discriminate images at different distances. Neonates will focus on objects with consistent sharpness or acuity—more accurately, lack of acuity—across a range of distances. Between 2 and 4 months of age, infants generally react to bright colors, and depth perception appears at about 4 to 5 months (Brazelton & Nugent, 1995). The coordination of vision with other senses, such as smell, allows repetitive exposure to certain images to create meaningful preferences for the images, such as a mother's face. As seen on the previous page, infants are able to imitate facial expressions with great accuracy.

Smell

Neonates' ability to distinguish smells is most evident in their reactions to breast milk. Infants show a preference for the scent of human milk, even if it is not their own mother's, over formula in their first days of life (Marlier & Schaal, 2005). Neonates tend to orient themselves toward the smell of their mothers' bodies and have been shown to prefer the smell of their mothers' chests, nipples, and underarm scents to those of other women.

The powerful draw of a mother's scent likely has survival value, for a baby is more likely to survive if she is able to find food and receive care and protection from a stronger, able caregiver. Furthermore, preferences for pleasant odors (such as chocolate) over unpleasant odors (such as vinegar) elicit different facial expressions that provide evidence of neonates' specific tastes. Similar facial expressions are elicited when neonates experience different tastes, because taste is closely associated with smell.

Taste

Neonates tend to make certain faces when they taste sweet flavors (relaxed lips) and quite different faces when they taste sour and bitter flavors (open or arched mouth). As with smell preferences, neonates prefer the taste of human milk, which likely has survival value, ensuring that a neonate remains close to the caregiver. As infants' tastes develop over their first year, they acquire a liking for saltier flavors, which likely facilitates their move from a liquid diet to solid foods.

Hearing

Infants can hear at birth and can perceive the direction of sound. In a famous yet simple experiment, Michael Wertheimer (1962) sounded a clicker from different sides of a delivery room only 10 minutes after an infant's birth. The infant not only reacted to the noise but also attempted to turn in the direction of the sound, indicating that babies immediately tune in to their environment. Although neonates have less developed ear–brain communication at birth than in subsequent months, they are sensitive to a variety of sounds.

Neonates pay closer attention to human speech, regardless of specific language, than sounds constructed in a pattern distinctly different from human sounds. They are able to recognize sound patterns, distinguish between two- and three-syllable sounds, and respond to tone of voice that would indicate a specific mood (e.g., happy versus angry tone). When adults speak to neonates in soft, low tones, for example, they are more able to soothe infants. The connection between sound and feelings associated with comfort and care promotes the bond between neonates and their caregivers.

Touch

You have already learned how the simple act of skin-to-skin contact in kangaroo care can benefit preemies. The same is true for all neonates. Sense of touch plays an important role in how infants gain information about the world around them and stimulates their physical, cognitive, and emotional growth. Certain techniques, such as swaddling an infant, developed as cultures around the world recognized the soothing effect that a warm, tightly wrapped blanket has on an infant's behavior. Infants may learn to respond to swaddling because of the subsequent comfort they feel, or it may be that swaddling and other touch sensations are connected to reflexes that are biologically based, prewired into every human being.

NEONATAL REFLEXES

Unlike the environment, which a baby is born into, a **reflex** is an inborn, automatic response to certain stimuli. Popular examples include the eye blink and the knee jerk. Critical reflexes needed to survive are present at birth (breathing, sucking, swallowing, and elimination) and require no learning to execute. For example, reflexes associated with feeding include sucking and swallowing during the prenatal period and infancy. Infants demonstrate the **rooting reflex** when a nipple or finger is gently placed on their cheek or near their lips. An infant will turn toward the stimulation and attempt to get the nipple or finger into her mouth. The neonate's sucking reflex grows stronger as the infant grows, and eventually the reflex becomes voluntary. Neonates also adjust their breathing accordingly when feeding. Their ability to breathe comfortably while feeding is critical to their survival. They also demonstrate developing breathing control when crying and reacting to new stimuli in their world (Rose, 2005). Breathing patterns are not fully established at birth, and it is common for infants to stop breathing for brief periods (lasting 2-5 seconds) called **apnea.**

The **Moro reflex** is also known as the *startling reflex,* because the neonate's physical movements appear as if the infant is startled. The arms and legs flail out and back in toward the chest quickly, and the back arches. This reflex typically occurs when the neonate experiences a sensation like falling or loss of support—if the infant's head or neck is released suddenly or the infant's crib or stroller is

reflex An inborn, automatic response to certain stimuli.

rooting reflex Automatic response in which an infant turns toward a finger or nipple placed gently on her cheek, attempting to get it into her mouth.

apnea Brief periods when breathing is suspended.

Moro reflex Infant's automatic response to sudden change in position or unexpected movement; arms and legs flail out in back in toward chest and back arches.

bumped into. Absence of the Moro reflex can indicate brain damage or immature development.

Neonates exhibit grasping reflexes of the hands and feet. The **grasping reflex** of the hands is seen when neonates instinctively grasp objects placed in the palms of their hands, whether the object is a human finger, a rattle, or the corner of a blanket. Similarly, the **plantar reflex** is seen when neonates curl their toes toward pressure placed on the balls of their feet. Each of these grasping reflexes diminishes during the first several months of life, and babies develop increasing ability to grasp things voluntarily with their hands (and, at times, with their feet!).

Similar, yet slightly different from the plantar grasp, the **Babinski reflex** is demonstrated when the neonate spreads out her toes in response to gentle stroking of the bottom of the foot, from heel to toes. Eventually this reflex changes and the infant curls toes toward the pressure instead of fanning out the toes.

As early as the first days of life, neonates demonstrate movements that appear similar to walking. If an infant is held under her arms so that her feet are touching a tabletop or other flat surface, she demonstrates the **stepping reflex,** in which her feet look like she is trying to walk, placing one foot down and then the other. Preemies often step in a "tiptoe" manner, whereas full-term babies step heel to toe, in the manner that humans eventually do walk.

When a neonate is placed on her back, and she turns her head to one side, the **tonic-neck reflex** is apparent. The infant extends her arm and leg on the side that corresponds to the direction she's looking, while flexing the arm and leg on the other side. This reflex, also known as the *fencing reflex,* diminishes in frequency over the first few months of life.

Pediatricians are able to assess a neonate's overall neurological functioning by assessing the various reflexes. Many of these reflexes diminish after a few months and are substituted with other, voluntary actions. Other reflexes disappear altogether. The photos below illustrate neonatal reflexes.

grasping reflex Automatic response in which an infant's fingers curl toward palm of hand when object or finger is placed in palm.

plantar reflex Automatic response in which an infant's toes curl inward when pressure is placed on balls of feet.

Babinski reflex Automatic response in which an infant's toes spread out in response to stroking the sole of the foot from heel to toes.

stepping reflex Automatic response in which the neonate, held under the arms with feet touching a flat surface, makes stepping movements similar to actual walking.

tonic-neck reflex Automatic response in which an infant extends arm and leg on same side as the direction in which she is looking, while flexing other arm and leg.

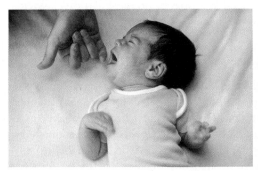

The rooting reflex.

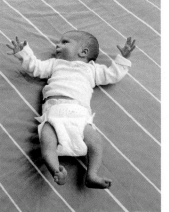

The Moro reflex.

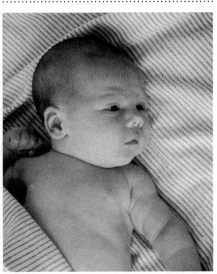

The grasping reflex.

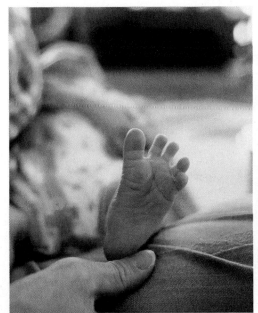

The Babinski Reflex.

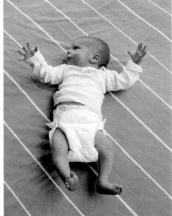

The stepping reflex.

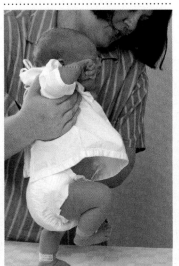

The tonic-neck reflex.

NEONATAL ASSESSMENT TECHNIQUES

Although all infants are born with these reflexes and abilities, they possess them to varying degrees. For example, some neonates demonstrate weaker reflex action than others, which affects their chances of surviving. Links to neurological functioning also influence doctors' desires to gain accurate information about each neonate. Efforts to develop reliable measures of early behavior, called *neonatal assessment,* have therefore increased over time. Three basic neonatal tests used to assess overall health of the infant are the Apgar scale, neurological assessment, and behavioral assessment.

The **Apgar scale,** shown in Figure 4.5, is administered twice—1 minute and 5 minutes after birth—to evaluate a newborn's basic life signs. Using five life signs (heart rate, respiratory rate, muscle tone, reflex irritability, and skin color) an observer evaluates the infant on a 3-point scale. Each life sign receives a 0, 1, or 2, with 0 indicating severe problems and 2 suggesting an absence of major difficulties. A total of 8 or more points indicates a successful transition to life outside the womb (Arenson & Drake, 2007).

Neurological assessment is used for:

- identification of any neurological problem,
- constant monitoring of a neurological problem, and
- prognosis about some neurological problem.

Each of these purposes requires testing the infant's reflexes, which is critical for neurological evaluation and basic for

Apgar scale A test to evaluate a newborn's basic life signs administered at 1 minute and 5 minutes after birth.

neurological assessment A neonatal test that identifies any neurological problem, suggests means of monitoring the problem, and offers a prognosis about the problem.

Brazelton Neonatal Behavioral Assessment Scale Device to assess an infant's behavior; examines both neurological and psychological responses.

postpartum period Period lasting approximately 6 weeks after birth as mother adjusts physically and psychologically.

all infant tests. There are different neurological assessment tools specifically designed for newborns, but they all aim to identify potential problems for the neonates.

The **Brazelton Neonatal Behavioral Assessment Scale** has become a significant worldwide tool for infant behavioral assessment. It focuses on a neonate's reflexes, responses to stimuli (e.g., sounds, light, and touch), attention, how the neonate orients to face and voice, ability to be soothed, motor coordination, and transitions from one emotional state to another. Brazelton and Nugent (1995) believe that the baby's state of consciousness (sleepy, drowsy, alert, or fussy) is the single most important element in the examination. The assessment is administered when the neonate is 3 days old and again a few days later to strive for accuracy. This assessment is intended to measure various aspects of a neonate's behavior, so important for survival.

Postpartum Adjustment

With so much attention placed on the neonate, it is important to focus some attention on the impact that birth has on the mother and other family members. Immediately after birth and continuing for about 6 weeks, women enter the **postpartum period,** a time of physical and psychological adjustment to pregnancy and birth.

DEPRESSION

Hormonal changes after birth, a sense of anticlimax after completing something anticipated for so many months, sheer fatigue, and tension about care of the baby (especially after a first birth) may cause feelings of sadness or a "letdown" in the new mother. Anywhere from 25% to 85% of women have feelings described as "the blues" for a few days postpartum. Such feelings are usually temporary and wane during the first week or two after delivery. However,

FIGURE 4.5
The Apgar Scale

Score	0	1	2
Heart rate	Absent	Slow—less than 100 beats per minute	Fast—100–140 beats per minute
Respiratory rate	No breathing for more than one minute	Irregular and slow	Good breathing with normal crying
Muscle tone	Limp and flaccid	Weak, inactive, but some flexion of extremities	Strong, active motion
Body color	Blue and pale	Body pink, but extremities blue	Entire body pink
Reflex irritability	No response	Grimace	Coughing, sneezing and crying

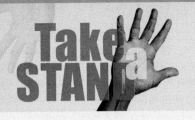

How Much Information Is Too Much?

There is no question that families and medical professionals know more today than they did years ago about neonates' abilities. Technology provides people with access to information before conception, during pregnancy, at the moment of birth, and after. Some people argue that the wealth of available information contributes to a growing anxiety about birth and a neonate's abilities. It is not uncommon for a mother to worry if her newborn does not respond well to sounds at 3 days old—does that mean the child is at risk for future cognitive impairment?

How can people balance the medical benefits of various tests with the emotional effects of anticipation and processing the information provided as a result of the assessments?

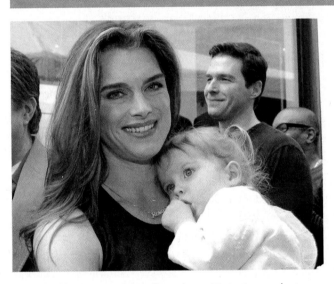

Brooke Shields is a strong advocate for mothers, raising awareness about postpartum experiences and the need for greater awareness and sensitivity.

if these feelings persist longer than 2 or 3 weeks, professional help may be needed. Approximately 7–17% of women who have these feelings are diagnosed with **postpartum depression.** Women with a history of mental illness are at higher risk for experiencing postpartum depression. While it is clearly a difficult experience for the mother, it also seriously impacts her parenting, which has a significant impact on the neonate's development (see Figure 4.6).

Actress and model Brooke Shields has shared her personal experience with postpartum depression, citing feelings of helplessness and shame. She had worked hard to achieve pregnancy, using assisted fertilization techniques, and the letdown after delivery rendered her despondent. She successfully came back from her postpartum depression, after medical and psychological treatment, and is now a strong advocate for mothers and their postdelivery support.

Methods of treating postpartum depression often involve medication and contact with others, such as a parent support group. Most women respond well to brief treatment with antidepressant medication. Because patients are leaving hospitals earlier after delivery than in decades past—due to medical advances and requirements of health insurance—the challenges of motherhood are experienced differently. Mothers are thrust into their new roles and relationships with the privilege and uncertainty attached to navigating uncharted territory.

> **postpartum depression** Feelings of sadness and emotional withdrawal that continue for many weeks or months after delivery.
>
> **bonding** The formation of a close connection between newborn and caregiver, typically parents.

FIGURE 4.6

Postpartum Symptoms Among U.S. Women

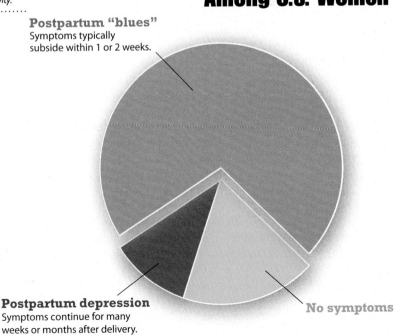

Postpartum "blues"
Symptoms typically subside within 1 or 2 weeks.

Postpartum depression
Symptoms continue for many weeks or months after delivery.

No symptoms

BONDING

Bonding refers to the formation of a close connection, or attachment, between the newborn and caregiver, typically parents. The connection begins as a physical connection but evolves into a psychological and emotional one that is considered crucial for a child's well-being. Hospital practices reflect the importance of bonding, as seen in the increased practice of keeping neonates in their mother's hospital room as much as possible. Mothers are more readily able to hold and feed their babies and begin adjusting to their new role. Still under the care of medical professionals who are concerned for the mother's well-being as well as that of the newborn, mothers can opt for some time alone in the room if they wish.

It is important to note that extended time together immediately after birth does not guarantee a healthy and harmonious parent–child relationship in later years, and lack of time together shortly after birth does not mean that bonding will not occur. For instance, adoptive parents and their adopted children experience deep and rewarding bonding equal to that of biological parents and their children. It may be argued that quality, not quantity (number of hours), of time together more significantly influences the connection.

SINGLE-PARENT FAMILIES

The percentage of babies in the United States born to single (unmarried) mothers is approximately 40% (Martin et al., 2009). The number of births to single mothers has increased by more than 20% since 2002, and in 2006 the highest number of births to single mothers in U.S. history was recorded—1.6 million babies. (See Figure 4.7.) There is no question that support is needed to help these mothers, but it is important to note that to identify a mother as unmarried does not necessarily mean that she is alone or without a loving family or other support network.

Nonetheless, the fact remains that the majority of births to single mothers occur for women who are in their 20s, at a low income level, and without significant social and financial support. The absence of social and financial support can compound feelings of insecurity for women and can negatively impact a child's development for his or her entire lifetime. Interventions, such as counseling, support groups, and home visits by professional social workers or early-intervention specialists, greatly assist mothers and other family members with the transitions associated with welcoming the neonate into the world.

FAMILY DYNAMICS

In many cases, the birth of a baby creates new expectations for family members. For example, it is common that some of the more stereotypical gender-associated activities

fall to the mother. Feeding the neonate is a natural task for mothers, especially if they are nursing their babies. Fathers can feed babies the mother's breast milk in a bottle, which greatly helps the mother with feeding responsibilities. Because all relationships with partners or spouses require cooperation, negotiation, and distribution of labor, the birth of a child often brings these issues to the forefront, regardless of any discussion or agreements that occurred before delivery.

When couples wait until they are older and more established in their chosen careers to become parents, the transition to parenthood is somewhat easier. Fathers tend to be more comfortable with their parenting role if they feel

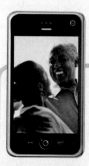

TECH TRENDS

Not Your Mother's Cranial Stimulator

Brooke Shields's sharing of her personal experience with postpartum depression and medical treatment prompted comments from many people who frown upon medical intervention for psychological problems. A new form of treatment that does not rely on medication—the Fisher Wallace Cranial Stimulator—has been approved by the Food and Drug Administration as a safe and effective way to reduce the stress that leads to depression and other psychological problems.

The device consists of a headband, two sponge applicators, and the base unit. The sponges are moistened and held in place with the headband. When the base unit is turned on, it sends mild radio waves to stimulate production of serotonin and dopamine in the brain—two neurotransmitters (chemicals in the brain) associated with mood. Acquiring the device requires a prescription in the United States, but the effects on brain activity have been argued to be a healthy alternative to prescription medication for postpartum and other kinds of depression.

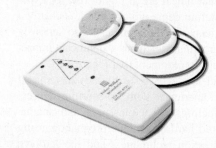

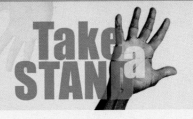

In many workplaces, a woman who delivers a baby is entitled to paid time off (amounts of time off and pay vary by institution) thanks to the Family and Medical Leave Act (see http://www.dol.gov/whd/fmla/index .htm), which allows eligible employees (women and men) to take time off up to 12 workweeks in any 12-month period for the birth or adoption of a child. Because a woman is, in most cases, under the care of a physician during and briefly after pregnancy, many institutions provide benefits to female employees through the short-term disability policies they have in effect in that particular workplace.

Do you agree with the term **short-term disability** as the category under which a woman who is pregnant should receive work-related benefits and compensation? Why or why not?

FIGURE 4.7

Births to Unmarried Women

This graph shows the number of births, birthrate, and percentage of births to unmarried women in the United States, 1940–2007.

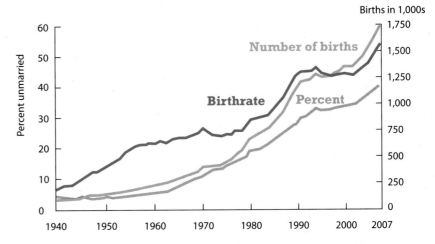

Source: CDC-NCHS, National Vital Statistics System.

more secure financially. Also, a father is more inclined to pitch in with household responsibilities while a mother is regaining strength and establishing routines. All families in whatever form they take, including adoptive families, families with gay or lesbian parents, blended families, and single-parent families, must make an adjustment when the neonate arrives. As the newborn grows into infancy, the strategies used and lessons learned will shift once again.

CONCLUSIONS & SUMMARY

This chapter provides information about the complex birth process as well as many challenges and interventions that impact the experience for mother, child, family members, and the professionals involved in the process. Today, thanks to technological advances, preemies have a much greater chance of survival and of healthy physical and psychological development. As the neonate transitions into the world, assessments highlight strengths and challenges from his or her very first moments and provide information that serves as a baseline for future development. The family's adjustment to the newborn involves multiple factors, including physical, financial, social, and emotional elements.

What is the typical sequence of the birth process?

- Birth occurs as a series of stages that bring the baby from the uterine environment into their new world.
- Complications such as breech presentations, anoxia, and the Rh factor are among the difficulties that can develop during the birth process.

What are some methods of childbirth?

- Childbirth methods are constantly evolving that are designed to ease the transition from womb to world. These include breathing techniques, relaxation, and other methods to alleviate pain and anxiety.

What are some challenges that can arise in childbirth?

- Today, the outlook for premature infants is much more optimistic than in previous times.

What are some characteristics of newborns?

- Neonates exhibit their competence through their sensory abilities and reflexes. Neonatal assessment focuses on neurological functioning and other behaviors to gain information about the neonate's abilities.

How do people adjust after the birth of a newborn?

- Families must adjust to the birth of a new child, which impacts people in different ways, according to expectations and family dynamics. About 10% of women experience postpartum depression, which is related to the physical and emotional letdown following delivery. Medical and other interventions are available to help mothers with this condition.

KEY TERMS

afterbirth 82

analgesics 84

anesthetics 84

anoxia 87

Apgar scale 94

apnea 92

Babinski reflex 93

bonding 95

Braxton-Hicks contractions 80

Brazelton Neonatal Behavioral Assessment Scale 94

breech birth 85

cerebral palsy 88

cesarean section 85

dilation 81

doula 84

episiotomy 81

expulsion 81

fetal monitor 86

forceps 86

grasping reflex 93

induced labor 86

isolette 88

kangaroo care 90

Lamaze method 83

midwife 84

Moro reflex 92

natural childbirth (or prepared childbirth) 83

neonate 90

neurological assessment 94

oxytocin 80

plantar reflex 93

postpartum depression 95

postpartum period 94

premature birth 88

reflex 92

Rh factor 88

rooting reflex 92

small for date 88

stepping reflex 93

tonic-neck reflex 93

vacuum extractor 86

1. Adults typically interact with newborns quite differently than with older children and adults. Is our behavior influenced by what we learn about appropriate means of interacting with neonates, or might some of our behavior be innate?

2. Various forms of neonatal assessment exist to provide information to parents and medical professionals. How many assessments are necessary to gain a clear picture of a neonate's abilities?

3. What is important to know about the postpartum period? What physical and emotional adjustments does a woman make after delivery?

Chapter Review Test

1. When a baby is positioned inside the mother's uterus in a head-down orientation, this is known as a _____ position.
   a. topsy-turvy
   b. upside-down
   c. breech
   d. organic

2. False labor pains are marked by a woman experiencing _____ contractions.
   a. Braxton-Hicks
   b. Brazelton
   c. tight
   d. Moro reflex

3. A woman trained as a caregiver to provide ongoing support to pregnant women in all stages of pregnancy and delivery is a certified
   a. pregnancy mentor.
   b. doula.
   c. nurse-practitioner.
   d. Lamaze coach.

4. The frequency of deliveries by _____ has increased over the years, even though it is considered major surgery.
   a. cesarean section
   b. water birth
   c. induced labor
   d. surrogate delivery

5. A(n) _____ is an electronic device that provides important information about the baby's and mother's conditions during labor.
   a. episiotomy
   b. epidural
   c. spinal block
   d. fetal monitor

6. _____ is the term used to describe a muscle condition caused by brain damage before, during, and after delivery.
   a. Braxton-Hicks
   b. Cerebral palsy
   c. Locus of control
   d. Episiotomy

7. Babies who are born more than 3 weeks before full term and weigh less than 5 1/2 pounds at birth are considered
   a. premature.
   b. slow to warm up.
   c. breech.
   d. complex deliverables.

8. The practice of skin-to-skin contact that is recommended for preemies and their caregivers is known as
   a. swaddling.
   b. attachment.
   c. kangaroo care.
   d. Babinski reflex.

9. The _____ reflex is sometimes called the startling reflex because the neonate flails her arms and legs out and back in toward her chest and arches her back.
   a. grasping
   b. rooting
   c. plantar
   d. Moro

10. Women who experience lingering feelings of sadness and withdrawal after delivery may suffer from postpartum
    a. anoxia.
    b. hypertension.
    c. depression.
    d. anxiety.

INFANCY

As You READ

After reading this chapter, you should be able to answer the following questions:

- What are the major physical accomplishments of the infancy period?

- How do infants acquire information about their world?

- What are the differences between Piaget's view of cognitive development in infancy and that of information processing?

- How do infants acquire their language?

- What is the role of relationships in psychosocial development?

- How do children develop and control their emotions?

- How would you assess the importance of attachment in psychosocial development?

- How does temperament affect the relationship between parents and their children?

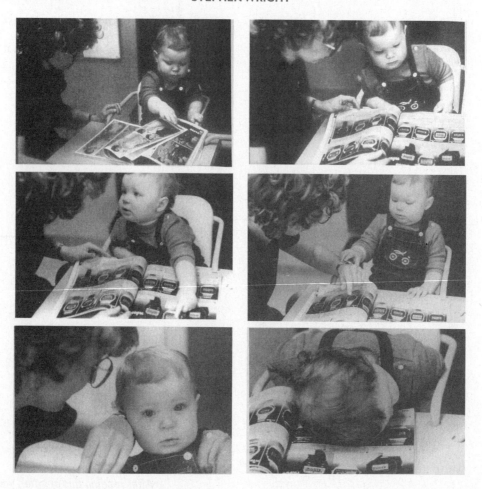

Infants are more than cute and cuddly, drooling and squirming milk-guzzlers. Between birth and the age of 2, children master an incredible array of physical, cognitive, and emotional skills and tasks. Because they are so dependent on their caregivers, however, infants are often completely underestimated in their abilities. Theorists in the field of lifespan development have viewed infants along a range of competencies, from small sponges waiting for something to absorb (Skinner), to active constructors of their own world (Piaget). Beliefs about what infants are capable of have powerful impact—on parents' views of their children, on educators' views of how infant/toddler care should be designed, and on policymakers' views of how money and resources should be allocated.

One of the most influential approaches to infant/toddler and preschool education is widely recognized in the work of educators in Reggio Emilia, Italy, who are known for their innovative approach to early education. One principle of the Reggio Emilia philosophy is that even the youngest infants exercise some control over the direction of their learning. One feature that distinguishes the municipal infant/toddler centers and preschools in Reggio Emilia is their systematic use of

documentation to inform and extend the learning experiences of the children as well as the educators and families.

The images of Laura above speak to the curiosity and competency of young children and have been recorded, analyzed, and revisited by people around the world. Notice how she and the teacher are looking at a catalog, at a picture of a watch. The teacher, seeing Laura's interest in the watch, shows Laura her own wristwatch and lets Laura listen to the ticking sound the watch makes. Laura, using the new knowledge she's just acquired, puts her ear to the catalog to see if the watch in the photo also makes a ticking sound. Not even 1 year old, Laura has taken her new learning, generated a hypothesis (all watches make a ticking sound), and tested her hypothesis (if I listen to the photo of a watch, will it tick?). At the heart of the Reggio Emilia approach, exemplified in these images, is a celebration of relationships—between child and teacher, child and environment, teacher and caregiver(s), and all combinations of these participants in children's learning and development.

This chapter will help you to understand how development in infancy is viewed today. First, infants' physical development is presented, followed by specific domains of infant

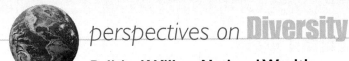
A CNN.com report (Green, 2006) stated that "almost all newborn and maternal deaths take place in developing nations—99 percent and 98 percent, respectively." Countries that have a history of war and other conflicts, such as Liberia, Afghanistan, Iraq, and Angola, have especially high infant mortality rates. There also seems to be a direct link between mothers and their status (health, education, and support) and infant mortality. But while we might assume that the problem lies in the wealth of a nation, Green argues that the political priorities of the country make more of a difference.

Countries that rank as rather poor countries on a global scale, such as Colombia, Mexico, and Vietnam, rank higher than many other countries in terms of infant mortality. Perhaps political and cultural factors that provide for mothers ultimately serve to protect infants as well.

development: motor, perception, cognitive, language, and social and emotional. Themes relating to biopsychosocial interactions are woven throughout the material, and you'll notice how virtually every aspect of development is affected by multiple influences. For example, early interactions between a parent and an infant are very powerful and are affected by factors such as cultural traditions, birth order, the parent's health, and the infant's temperament. Many factors influence the interactions between parent and infant; they also set the stage for interactions that will evolve over a lifetime.

Physical Development in Infancy

Infancy is a time of rapid physical development—nature's way to ensure an infant's survival and attempts to cope with the world. A typical newborn weighs about 7½ pounds and is about 20 inches long. In the year after birth, an infant's length increases by one half and its weight almost triples. While infancy is a time of rapid growth and increasing physical ability, it is also a time of extreme vulnerability. The infant morality rate is the number of deaths that occur in the first year of life for 1,000 live births. The National Center for Health Statistics reported that the U.S. infant mortality rate in 2006 was 6.3, which is 3 times higher than the infant death rate in Japan and 2.5 times higher than in Finland, Norway, and Iceland. Figure 5.1 shows the changes in infant mortality rankings from 1960 to 2009 for various countries around the world. Although infant death in the United States is often due to babies being born too small or too early, there is a link to poor mothers with less education being at a higher risk of early delivery.

DEVELOPMENTAL MILESTONES OF INFANCY

Growing children experience rapid changes in body shape and composition, distribution of tissues, and in motor skills. For example, the infant's head at birth is about a quarter of the body's total length, but in the adult it is about one sev-

FIGURE 5.1

Infant Mortality Rates

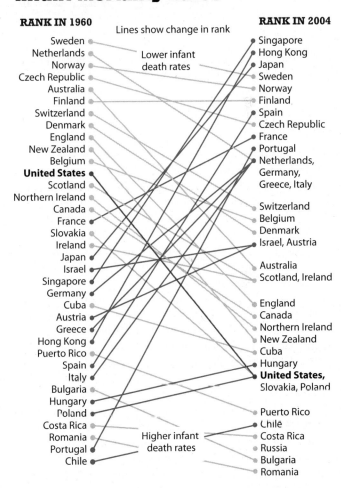

In 1960, only 11 countries could boast a lower infant mortality rate than the United States. In 2004, 28 countries surpassed the U.S. for lower infant mortality rate.

Source: Copyright 2009 The New York Times Company.

enth of body length. The head becomes noticeably smaller compared to the rest of the body as we develop. (See Figure 5.2.) Total growth represents a complex series of changes

FIGURE 5.2
Changes in Proportions of the Human Body

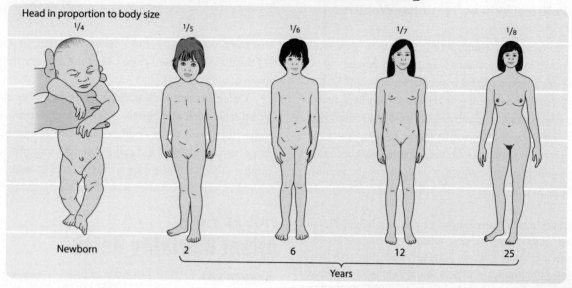

Head in proportion to body size

| ¼ | ⅕ | ⅙ | ⅐ | ⅛ |

| Newborn | 2 | 6 | 12 | 25 |

Years

that occur in developmental sequence. Underlying this rapidly unfolding and complex process is, of course, proper nutrition.

NUTRITION

Good nutrition is critical for a healthy baby, and ideally all infants would receive a balance of necessary nutrients. Yet infants' nutritional needs are quite different from adults'. Meeting ideal needs can be difficult because of an infant's small stomach and an immature digestive system (Ball & Bindler, 2006). Fortunately, until infants' bodies develop the mechanisms needed to chew, swallow, store, and digest solid food, their nutritional needs can be taken care of through liquid nutrition in the form of breast milk or formula. Just as babies do not choose the families they are born into, they also do not choose whether or not their caregivers follow a healthy diet or whether they are breast- or formula-fed. The decision to breast-feed is one that is often influenced by pressure from family and society.

Breast-Feeding Versus Bottle-Feeding

Most doctors, nurses, and mothers agree that human milk is the ideal food for infants up to six months (Leifer, 2003), and yet this belief wasn't always the dominant viewpoint. Throughout much of the 20th century, women were discouraged from breast-feeding as some medical experts believed that babies could get better nutrition through formulas. Doctors and family often actively discouraged breast-feeding, which was frowned upon in public places and banned in some of them.

Breast-feeding has definite advantages over formula-feeding. First is protection against disease. Breast-fed babies tend to experience less illness than formula-fed babies. Second, breast-fed babies are less at risk for aller-

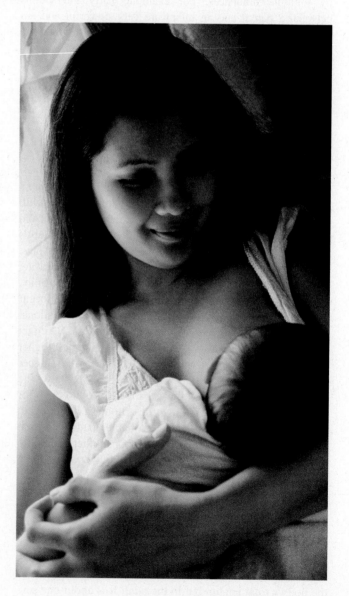

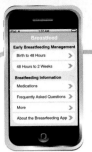
Podcasts for Nursing Mothers

In case mothers aren't multitasking enough, the following application for iPhone or iTouch (available via iTunes) offers free information about breast-feeding that interested women can access while exercising, driving, working...or nursing! Called Breastfeeding Management, this app was designed to help clinicians identify and treat common breast-feeding problems. This app has a link to the LactMed database and news about medications, which most mothers might find interesting but not use as often as other key features—frequently asked questions and links to highly respected resources, such as the World Health Organization.

gic reactions than are formula-fed babies. Other findings from research indicate that breast-fed babies have stronger bones, more advanced cognitive development, easier transitions to solid food, and lower risk for obesity than those who are formula-fed. The American Academy of Pediatrics recommends that babies have breast milk exclusively for the first six months of life and that nursing should continue for at least a year. The number of mothers who choose to nurse has dramatically increased since the 1970s.

There are specific situations, however, when a woman should not breast-feed her baby. If a woman is infected with AIDS or another infectious disease, has active tuberculosis, or is currently taking medication that could be harmful to the child, then she should not breast-feed her child.

The availability of formula is an important factor in the decision of feeding an infant. One of the advantages of formula feeding is that others, including fathers, can feed the baby. This is a relief to some mothers who, despite their wishes to breast-feed, are not able to physically. Although breast feeding is best for babies' health and development, some mothers will need or want to bottle-feed and can be reassured that the nutrition of most formulas is sufficient. Assuming that the formula is appropriate, nutritional problems should not arise.

In the course of one year, infants progress from either breast- or bottle-feeding to eating a variety of solid foods. As infants develop, tremendous brain growth occurs that helps make advances in feeding possible, and the more diverse range of foods, in turn, fuels the brain for more growth. The motor skills needed to pick up small pieces of food, the chewing and swallowing required to digest the food, and the language skills that emerge as a child learns to ask for "more!" are all connected to the brain.

BRAIN DEVELOPMENT

infantile amnesia The inability to remember events from early in life.

Scientists have reexamined their ideas about babies' brains. Rather than an empty vessel waiting to be filled, the baby's brain is actually more active than an adult's brain, taking in large amounts of information in short periods of time. What once had been viewed as a deficit, such as infants' undeveloped language ability or short attention span, is now considered essential to the learning process (Lehrer, 2009). Nature has taken amazing steps to ensure that a baby will be able to adapt to its challenging environment, and daily discoveries about the structure of the brain inform decisions that impact human development. Figure 5.3 illustrates the various areas of the brain.

Because babies aren't able to tell us what they're thinking or feeling, and we all experience the phenomenon called **infantile amnesia**—the inability to remember events from early in life—brain researchers rely heavily on tests that provide results they can then compare to results from an adult brain. Any conclusions that researchers make about infant brains are therefore speculative, and supported with stronger or weaker data from various techniques:

- *Electroencephalogram.* Electrodes are placed on the scalp to (1) measure neuron/nerve activity that registers as electrical signals and (2) identify different behavioral states, such as deep sleep.

- *Computed tomography (CT).* An advanced version of X-ray techniques, the commonly used CT scan presents three-dimensional pictures of the brain.

FIGURE 5.3

The Human Brain

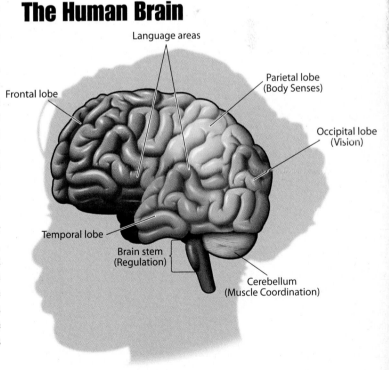

- *Positron emission tomography (PET).* PET scans measure the amount of blood flow associated with brain activity. Tiny radioactive elements (about the same amount of radioactivity you would receive from a chest X-ray) are injected into the bloodstream and become tracers that the PET scan can detect.

- *Magnetic resonance imaging (MRI).* The popular MRI depends on the magnetic quality of blood to measure internal structures.

EEGs are most often used with infants, because radiation poses a risk to their health and they won't stay still for an MRI. Findings from EEGs have noted bursts of activity that may correspond to bursts in cognitive and language development, and they have also been used as predictors of behavior problems in toddlers.

During infancy, the baby's brain is about one fourth of its adult weight and contains billions of nerve cells, called **neurons.** Neurons transmit information by electrochemical signals, and at this age connections between neurons increase to as many as 100 to 1,000 connections for each of the billions of neurons. The brain grows from ½ pound at birth to about 1½ pounds at the end of the first year. By age 5, the brain weighs about 3 pounds and is adult size (Eliot, 2000). Because infants' neck muscles are not well developed and provide little support for their heads, any violent movement thrusts the brain back and forth in the skull and puts infants at risk for brain trauma. In

neurons Nerve cells that transmit information with electrochemical signals.

axons Branchlike ends of neurons that send electrochemical signals between cells.

dendrites Branchlike ends of neurons that receive and conduct the electrochemical signals between the cells.

synapse A small gap between neurons.

myelin Sheath of insulation around axons that facilitates communication between neurons.

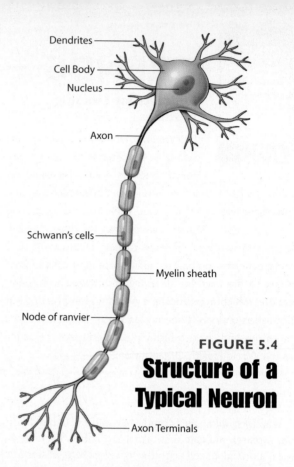

Dendrites
Cell Body
Nucleus
Axon
Schwann's cells
Myelin sheath
Node of ranvier
Axon Terminals

FIGURE 5.4

Structure of a Typical Neuron

the injury known as *shaken baby syndrome,* frustrated caregivers shake babies so hard that brain damage occurs, resulting in a baby's loss of control over such vital functions as heart rate, respiration, blood pressure, and temperature. The National Center on Shaken Baby Syndrome puts the number of SBS babies at about 1,300 per year.

Thanks to research, we know that infants shape their brains through their experience with the outside world. An infant translates information from the outside world into brain action in the following way:

- Electrical nerve impulses travel along **neurons** (see Figure 5.4), forming connections between **axons** and the **dendrites** of other neurons along their pathways. The axons send the signals from one neuron to another, and dendrites catch and conduct the electrochemical signals between the cells.

- The small gaps between neurons are called **synapses.** Each synapse allows communication between neurons to occur.

- The process is made quicker because of a sheath (coating) on the axons called **myelin,** which is like insulation around the axon that is critical for brain function. Myelination, the formation of a myelin sheath around axons, is rapid during the first 2 years of life and allows for quicker communication among axons by improving the efficiency of the signal transmission.

As infants process information from stimuli, the brain works to form connections that shape learning and develop-

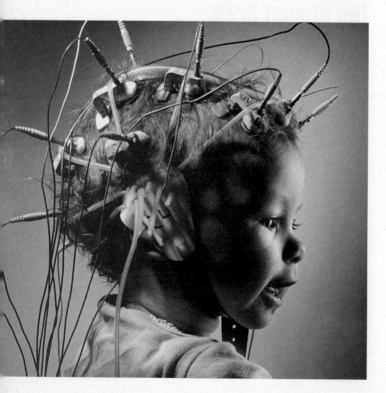

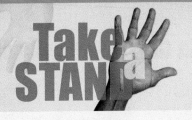
Creeping and Crawling, or Just Plain Creepy?

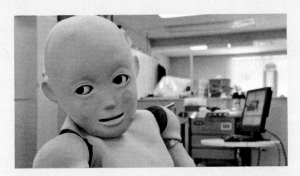

An example of startling new breakthroughs in the applications of brain research is the work of Japanese scientists who have designed a robot that mimics infants' learning. Called the CB2, this robot is designed to develop abilities in the same manner that a human infant would, including cognitive and physical development. The research team, led by Minoru Asada and based at Osaka University, consists of engineers, brain specialists, psychologists, and experts in other fields.

CB2 can "breathe" with rhythmic movements, record images with internal processors and lump input into categories that relate to emotional states, such as happy or sad, and can recognize human touch with sensors under its "skin." The robot can even pair emotional expressions with physical movements or sensations.

The benefits of developing a "robo species" range from the altruistic (providing companions to the elderly) to the practical (a robot secretary) to sheer entertainment (creating a football team to win the World Cup Championship by 2050). While skeptics argue that a robot can never have the same emotional capacity of humans, Japanese cultural beliefs in *animism* (the belief that things in nature have souls or consciousness) may contribute to wider acceptance of a robo species.

Do you think it's possible for **artificial intelligence** (human intelligence simulated by machines) to replicate or replace human capabilities? What boundaries, if any, should be placed on such research? Do you think funding could be better aimed at human conditions—why or why not?

---

ment. The brain cells that receive new or familiar information survive; those that don't, die. It's as simple as that. Activity is critical to sustaining brain function in an infant's environment.

Environmental stimulation—teachers, parents, and other people and events—affect all parts of the brain. The infant's brain awaits sensory stimulation and experiences that will guide brain development. As the brain is stimulated, neurons continue to form connections, resulting in an increase in synapses. More synapses, in turn, increases communication systems in the brain that foster development of more complex skills. Neurons that are not stimulated lose their synapses in a pruning process, thereby allowing those neurons to be utilized in other synaptic connections. The warmer and more supportive the baby's environment is, the more connections in the brain the baby makes relating to emotions and relationships. The role of environment on physical and cognitive brain growth underscores the biopsychosocial model of development and implications for life experiences.

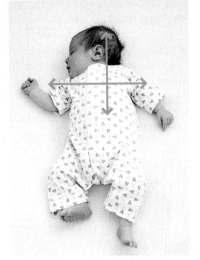

MOTOR DEVELOPMENT

Parents are fascinated by their child's motor development: Is he holding up his head? Shouldn't she be crawling by now? When will he walk? Motor development occurs in two directions—from head to feet (cephalocaudal) and from the center of the body to the arms and legs (proximodistal). In the early years, most growth occurs from the head to feet, with brain development leading the way. For example, a baby can see things and communicate about them before he can grab them or crawl to them. Likewise, a baby can control her midsection and core muscles enough to sit up before she can control her fingers. Although there is a typical

> **artificial intelligence**
> Human intelligence simulated by machines; a specific field of computer science.

FIGURE 5.5

Milestones in Gross Motor Development

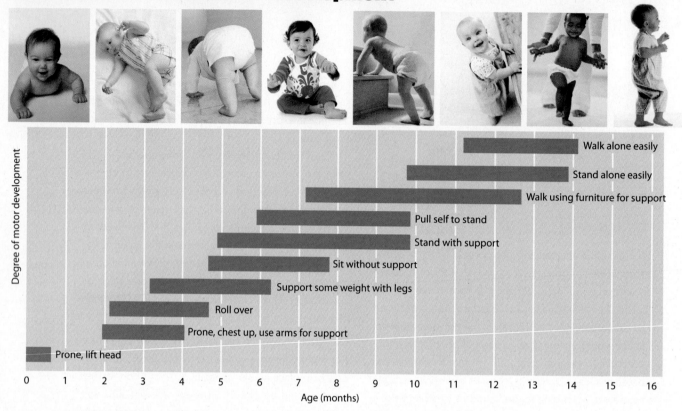

progression, as shown in Figure 5.5, there is always variation among individual babies.

Important characteristics of motor control include head and body movement.

Head Control

A baby's most obvious initial head movements are from side to side, although a 1-month-old infant can occasionally lift his head when lying face down. Four-month-old infants can hold their heads steady while sitting and will lift their head and shoulders to a 90-degree angle when on their stomachs. By the age of 6 months, most babies can balance their heads quite well.

creeping Movement whereby the infant's abdomen touches the floor and the weight of the head and shoulders rests on the elbows.

crawling Movement on hands and knees; the trunk does not touch the ground.

Creeping and Crawling

Creeping and crawling are two distinct developmental phases. In **creeping,** the infant's abdomen touches the floor, and the elbows support the weight of the head and shoulders. Movement occurs mainly by arm action. The legs usually drag, although some youngsters push with their legs. Most youngsters can creep after age 7 months. **Crawling** is more advanced than creeping, because movement is on hands and knees and the middle of the body does not touch the ground. After age 9 months, most youngsters can crawl.

The typical progression is from movement on the abdomen to quick movements on hands and knees, but the sequence varies. Babies display an amusing array of positions and movements that can only be loosely grouped together.

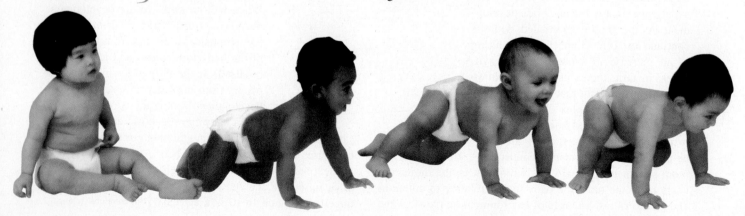

Standing and Walking

After about age 7 to 9 months, babies, when held, support most of their weight on their legs. Coordination of arm and leg movements enables babies to pull themselves up and gain control of leg movements. First steps are clumsy waddles, with each step down heavy and deliberate. Gradually a smooth, confident step emerges. The world now belongs to the infant.

Once babies begin to walk, their attention darts from one thing to another, thus sharpening their perception. Tremendous energy and mobility, coupled with innate curiosity, drive infants to explore their world. It is an exciting time, but a watchful time for caregivers, who must draw the line between encouraging curiosity and initiative, and protecting the child from injury. The task is not easy. It is, however, a tension found in all stages of development between giving reasonable freedom and showing unreasonable restraint. All infants experience bumps and bruises, but some infants enter the world with specific challenges.

Neonatal Problems

Occasionally the typical developmental sequence does not progress smoothly. The most common newborn problems include failure to thrive, sudden infant death syndrome, sleeping disorders, and respiratory distress syndrome.

FAILURE TO THRIVE

Failure to thrive (FTT) is a condition that occurs when an infant does not grow at the expected rate. The weight and height of failure-to-thrive infants is consistently far below average. Such infants are estimated to be in the bottom 3% of height and weight measures.

There are two types of FTT: organic and nonorganic. Organic FTT accounts for 30% of FTT cases, and the problem is usually some gastrointestinal disease and occasionally a problem with the nervous system. Nonorganic FTT, much more difficult to diagnose and treat, lacks a physical cause. Researchers have identified environmental causes such as poverty, neglect, abuse, and ignorance of good parenting practices (Block et al., 2005). The seriousness of this problem is evident from the outlook for FTT infants: Almost half of these infants continue to experience physical, cognitive, and behavioral problems for several years. A follow-up study of FTT children at age 8 (Black et al., 2007) indicated that FTT negatively affected height, math performance, and study habits.

SUDDEN INFANT DEATH SYNDROME (SIDS)

One of the most devastating and perplexing problems facing parents and researchers is **sudden infant death syndrome (SIDS),** a condition in which an infant dies suddenly, usually during the night, without an apparent cause. An estimated 2,500 infants from 2 to 4 months old die each year from SIDS, and it is the primary cause of death for infants under 1 year in industrialized nations. There is little warning, although many cases are preceded by mild cold symptoms and are later connected to early physical problems such as low birth weight, weak muscle tone, irregular heartbeat, and respiratory issues. Most cases usually occur in late winter or early spring (American SIDS Institute, 2009), which is likely linked to the fact that many infants who have died from SIDS are discovered wrapped in blankets and warm clothing.

Other theories about the cause of SIDS involve impaired brain functioning, which can result in infants being unable to change their positions or turn their heads if their breathing is hindered by clothing, bedding, or spit-up. Environmental factors, such as cigarette smoking and drug abuse during and after pregnancy, increase the risk of SIDS. It is particularly devastating for parents because of the lack of warning. You can imagine the effect this has on caregivers, particularly the feelings of guilt they have. Today, special services have been established to counsel grieving families.

Although no definite answers to the SIDS dilemma have yet been found, current research encourages caregivers to put babies to sleep on their backs rather than on their stomachs or sides and to eliminate soft bedding, which could interfere with babies' breathing. Campaigns have been established, urging caregivers to be mindful of their children's sleeping and breathing. These practices have contributed to a decrease in SIDS mortality (Malloy & Freeman, 2000).

> People who say they
> sleep *like a* **baby**
> usually don't have one.
> _____
> **LEO J. BURKE**

SLEEPING DISORDERS

Although less serious than FTT or SIDS, some infant sleeping problems negatively affect development. Sleep specialist Richard Ferber (2006) explains that parents often have a child between the ages of 5 months and 4 years who does not sleep readily at night and wakes repeatedly. Parents therefore become tired, frustrated, and angry and the relationship between parents becomes tense. Most often a sleeping disorder has nothing to do with parenting, and nothing is wrong with the child—physically or mentally. Yet some sleep problems do exist because of physical or psychological influences, such as a bladder infection or night terrors.

Most parents would agree that sleep becomes a precious commodity once babies arrive. Sleep patterns in infants

failure to thrive (FTT) Medical term for infants whose weight gain and physical growth fall far below average during the first years of life.

sudden infant death syndrome (SIDS) Unexpected death of an apparently healthy infant, usually between 2 and 4 months of age.

REM (rapid eye-movement) sleep A period of deep sleep marked by eye movements; when vivid dreams occur.

FIGURE 5.6

Sleep Patterns Across the Lifespan

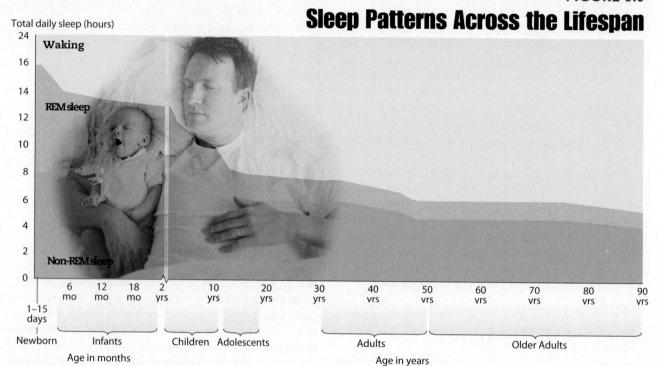

Total daily sleep (hours)

Waking

REM sleep

Non-REM sleep

| 1–15 days | 6 mo | 12 mo | 18 mo | 2 yrs | 10 yrs | 20 yrs | 30 yrs | 40 yrs | 50 yrs | 60 yrs | 70 yrs | 80 yrs | 90 yrs |

Newborn   Infants   Children   Adolescents   Adults   Older Adults

Age in months   Age in years

respiratory distress syndrome (RDS) Problem common with premature babies; caused by lack of a substance that keeps air sacs in the lungs open.

perception The process of obtaining and interpreting information from stimuli.

range from about 16 to 17 hours in the first week to 13 hours at age 2, with most deep-sleep periods lasting about 20 minutes. **REM (rapid eye-movement) sleep** refers to a period of deep sleep marked by eye movements and is known to be the time when vivid dreams occur. Infants tend to spend 80% of sleep in REM sleep (compared to 20–25% in adults), and brain activity during REM sleep is similar to that when infants are awake. Perhaps the large amount of REM sleep provides infants with the extra stimulation they need to promote healthy brain development. As infants grow into toddlerhood and later childhood, the patterns of sleep change, as do patterns of brain development. Figure 5.6 shows sleep patterns from newborn to older adulthood.

Some adults choose to bring their babies into their own beds so that they can get some sleep and their children can also fall asleep feeling safe and loved in the parents' bed, but parents need to exercise caution when they take children into their own beds (called *shared sleeping* or *cosleeping*). Agreement between parents, safety considerations for the child, and a decision about when to stop cosleeping must be considered (Ferber, 2006).

RESPIRATORY DISTRESS SYNDROME

Although most common with premature infants, **respiratory distress syndrome** may strike full-term infants whose lungs are particularly immature. RDS is caused by the lack of a

substance that keeps air sacs in the lungs open. When the air sacs close up, the lungs can collapse, causing severe breathing problems. Because most babies do not produce sufficient substance until the 35th prenatal week, it is a serious problem for premature infants. Full-term newborns whose mothers are diabetic and babies who have undergone a difficult birth also seem vulnerable to RDS. The good news is that today 90% of these youngsters survive, and early detection and treatment make their outlook excellent.

Perceptual Development

If you stop reading for a moment and look around, you'll see some things that you recognize immediately: this book, a lamp, shoes, paper, cell phone, and such. But you may also notice something that seems new or unfamiliar, such as a new student in class or a flyer announcing an upcoming concert. Our ability to recognize the familiar and to realize what we don't know depends on perception.

Perception is defined as the process of obtaining and interpreting information from stimuli. It is the key to our experiences in the world. It is also the basis for growth of thought, regulation of emotions, social interactions, and progress in almost all aspects of development.

Infants are quite clever at obtaining information from stimuli around them. During infancy the capacity to take in information through the major sensory channels, make sense of the environment, and assign meaning to information improves dramatically (Bornstein, 2002). In the first

A Global Look at the Rush to Toilet Train (or Not)

While sleep issues can drive caregivers crazy and create stress in the household, toilet training is another major source of stress for families. In the United States and most Western societies the "norm" for toilet training is to start training when a child is about 18 months old. This assumes that up until that age children aren't able to regulate their own body functions (bladder, anus) and control when and where they pee or poop.

Cultural belief systems influence the timing of toilet training. In traditionally Eastern countries such as China, toileting routines with infants are begun much earlier, even as early as 1 month old. Cultural practices typically emphasize interdependence between adult and infant, and an adult is readily available to hold an infant over the toilet. Open-crotch garments facilitate the process. Economic realities also play a role. In a small affluent family that can

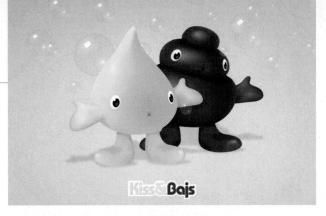

Swedish children's characters, Kiss and Bajs (Pee and Poo).

afford disposable diapers, the need to get children toilet trained is not urgent. A large family with less disposable income might be more motivated to get children toilet trained as early as possible.

Despite "expert" opinions on the benefits of toilet training at a certain age, families have been operating for thousands of years with varying toileting practices. Cultural and individual preferences, as well as health conditions, should be the primary considerations for when a baby is ready for the potty.

---

year of life, infants discern patterns, depth, orientation, location, movement, and color. During infancy, babies also discover what they can do with objects, which furthers their perceptual development.

Infants are born ready to attend to changes in physical stimulation. Stimuli presented often cause **habituation,** a decrease in an infant's attention. If the stimuli are altered, the infant again pays attention, showing awareness of the difference. For example, if you show an infant an engaging picture, he or she is first fascinated, but then becomes bored; the infant has habituated. If you change the picture, you can regain the infant's attention.

Perception depends on both learning and maturation. An infant's perceptual system undergoes much development following birth, as she becomes familiar with objects and events in the world and continues to grow. Most research on infant perceptual development has emphasized vision and hearing because of their importance and rapid development.

VISUAL PERCEPTION

Infants are born able to see and quickly exhibit a preference for patterns. They tend to show definite preferences based on as much complexity as they can handle (Gibson & Pick, 2000). Robert Fantz's (1965) classic work on visual preferences revealed that children look at different things for different amounts of time. He designed a "looking chamber" so that an experimenter could see which of two images an infant looked at longer. The knowledge about babies' visual preferences is apparent today—a stroll through the newborn section of any toy store will lead you past many black,

white, and red toys, and you'll also see many checkerboard, striped, and polka-dotted items. Human faces, which are remarkably complex, also capture babies' attention on mobiles and other items.

> **habituation** A decrease in an infant's attention.

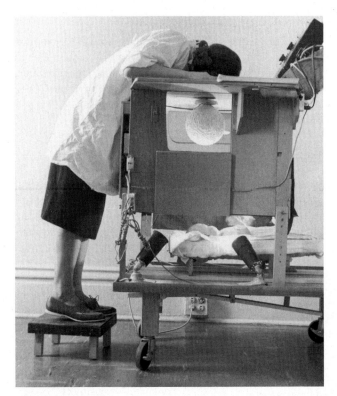

Fantz's "looking chamber"

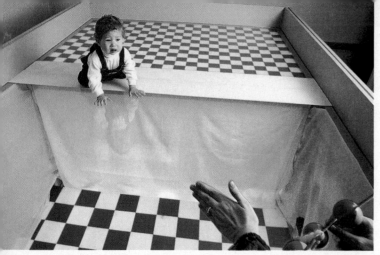
The visual cliff

DEPTH PERCEPTION

The study of visual development sparks questions about how visual skills help infants to adjust to their environment. In their famous visual cliff experiment, Gibson and Walk (1960) reasoned that infants would use visual stimuli to gauge both depth and distance. The visual cliff consisted of a board dividing a large sheet of heavy glass. A checkerboard pattern was attached to one half of the bottom of the glass, giving the impression of solidity. The investigators then placed a similar sheet on the floor under the other half, creating a sense of depth—the visual cliff. Thirty-six infants from ages 6 to 14 months were tested. After each infant was placed on the center board, the mother called the child from the shallow side and then the cliff side. Twenty-seven of the youngsters moved onto the shallow side toward the mother. When called from the cliff side, only three infants ventured over the depth. The experiment suggests that infants discriminate depth when they begin crawling.

By 2 to 4 months of age, infant perception is fairly sophisticated. Infants perceive figures as organized wholes, react to the relationship among elements rather than single elements, perceive color, and are fascinated by complex patterns. They scan the environment, pick up information, then encode and process information (Gibson & Pick, 2000).

AUDITORY PERCEPTION

Infants display notable auditory abilities in the uterus and at birth. Hearing and auditory discrimination are well developed since sounds are carried to the fetus through the amniotic fluid as a series of vibrations. Infants display sensitivity to differences in the quality of sounds. For example, some babies may prefer music to other sounds, they can discriminate their mothers' voices from those of other women, and they can locate the direction of a sound.

Infants pay special attention to speechlike sounds (Siegler & Alibali, 2005). Although significant in itself, this perceptual sensitivity underscores the importance of auditory perception in language development. For example, infants begin to differentiate the sounds of their language and tune in to the speech they hear around them (Bjorklund, 2005). It's as if nature has determined that infants must immediately attend to important information in their aural environment.

egocentrism Piaget's term for the child's focus on self in early phases of cognitive development.

sensorimotor period The first 2 years of life.

circular reactions Piaget's term for infants' motor activity that is repeated in developing stages.

Cognitive Development

The biological basis of cognition plays a role in human behavior, such as genetic influences on behavior, the role of the brain in processing music, and biological insights into language development. The study of cognitive development must therefore examine both the brain's role and the sociocultural basis of cognitive development (Bjorklund, 2005).

PIAGET'S SENSORIMOTOR PERIOD

As you will recall from Chapter 2, the work of Jean Piaget embodies the interaction between biological, psychological, and social factors. Did you ever wonder what infants are thinking? How their interactions with their environment shape their thinking, which, in turn, shapes the structure of the brain? These are questions that Piaget addressed, and his research made a lasting impression on studies of cognitive development.

Piaget believed that the first few years of life are marked by extraordinary mental growth and influence the entire course of development. It is through the senses that an infant begins to make sense of the world. Initially, everything centers on them, and they see the world only from their point of view. **Egocentrism** describes this initial relationship of children to their world. Unlike an egocentric adult who knows that other viewpoints exist, but disregards them, the egocentric child is simply unaware of any other viewpoint.

The remarkable changes of the **sensorimotor period** (about the first 2 years of life) occur within a sequence of six stages that involve **circular reactions.** An infant experiences something through her own motor activity, even by pure chance, and tries to repeat the experience. Finally, she adds the action to a growing body of knowledge about the world and the way things work.

Stage 1

During the first stage, simple reflexes, children do little more than exercise their inborn reflexes. For example, Piaget (1952b) stated that the sucking reflex is hereditary and functions from birth. At first, infants suck anything that touches their lips, then they suck when nothing touches their lips, and then they actively search for the nipple. This involves steady development of the coordination of the eye, mouth, arm, and hand. Through these activities, patterns form in the brain—physically through neuron connections and emotionally through memory and learning—that build a foundation for forming cognitive structures.

Stage 2

Piaget referred to stage 2 (from about 1 to 4 months) as the stage of **primary circular reactions.** During stage 2, first habits emerge as infants tend to repeat actions involving their bodies, even if the actions are accidental. For example, they have learned that they are fed when hungry, and they have mastered the sucking reflex so that it can now be done voluntarily, even when nothing is present. Infants seem to have no external goals behind these actions other than the pleasure of self-exploration, but they are learning something about their own bodies.

Stage 3

Secondary circular reactions emerge during the third stage, which extends from about 4 to 8 months. During this stage, infants direct their activities toward objects and events outside themselves. For example, a baby may accidentally swat a mobile with one hand while squirming in the crib, and the mobile makes a jingling sound and moves. The infant will try again to swat the mobile. Secondary circular reactions produce results in the environment, and not, as with the primary circular reactions, on the child's own body.

Stage 4

From about 8 to 12 months of age, infants engage in **coordination of secondary schemes** to form new kinds of behavior (Piaget & Inhelder, 1969). The baby first decides on a goal, such as finding an object that is hidden under a small blanket. Then the infant attempts to move the blanket to reach the object. In stage 4, the infant coordinates previously learned actions to carry out the desired goal. Infants use multiple senses in the process of coordinating their actions and learning about materials. They often look at and feel items, or shake and listen to items. Here we see the first signs of intentional behavior.

Stage 5

Tertiary circular reactions appear from 12 to 18 months of age. In the tertiary circular reaction, repetition occurs again, but now with variation. The infant is exploring the world's possibilities. Piaget thought that the infant purposefully attempts to provoke new results instead of merely reproducing activities. Tertiary circular reactions indicate experimentation and an interest in novelty for its own sake.

Have you ever seen a baby standing in a crib, dropping everything on the floor? Through Piaget's lens you could watch how the baby drops things, from different locations and different heights. Does it sound the same when it hits the floor as when it hits the rug? Is it as loud dropped from here or higher? Each repetition is actually a chance to learn.

Stage 6

During stage 6 (between 18 and 24 months), the last stage of the sensorimotor period, children develop a basic kind of **internalization of schemes.** They begin to use symbols (internalized representation of an event) to think about real events without actually experiencing them. For example, a budding toddler has seen her father using a leaf blower outside their house many times. She picks up a discarded paper-towel tube and moves her arm in a side-to-side motion, making a "Brrrrrrrr . . ." sound, mimicking the sound of the leaf blower.

Progress through the sensorimotor period leads to four major accomplishments:

- **Object permanence:** Children realize that objects continue to exist even when out of sight. Out of sight does not mean not gone forever. This is significant because it signals that babies have a sense that objects are separate from them.

- Sense of space: Children realize objects in the environment have a spatial relationship.

- Causality: Children realize the relationship between actions and their consequences.

- Time sequences: Children realize that one thing comes after another.

By the end of the sensorimotor period, children move from purely sensory and motor functioning to symbolic kinds of activity, in which the child takes a real-life event and re-creates it according to her own ideas. This is seen as children develop their make-believe play and represent happenings from their own world in play settings.

EVALUATION OF PIAGET

Although Piaget left a major legacy, his ideas have not gone unchallenged. Piaget proposed a theory of development as a sequence of distinct stages, each of which entails important changes in the way a child thinks, feels, and behaves. However, acquiring cognitive structures may be gradual rather than abrupt and may not be a matter of all or nothing. For some theorists, a child's level of cognitive development depends more on the nature of the task than on a rigid classification system.

In one of the first important challenges to Piaget, Gelman and Baillargeon (1983) found that children can accomplish specific tasks at earlier ages than Piaget believed. Criticism that Piaget underestimated infants' abilities has led to a closer examination of the times during which children acquire certain cognitive abilities. For example, Piaget believed that infants will retrieve an object that is hidden from them (in stage 4) beginning at about 8 to 12 months. Before this age, if a blanket is thrown over a toy the infant is looking at, the child stops reaching for it as if it doesn't exist. More recent research has argued that infants can see objects as separate from themselves as early as age 3 to 4 months.

primary circular reactions Infants' actions that are focused on their own bodies and reflexes.

secondary circular reactions Piaget's term for infants' activities that are directed toward objects and events outside themselves.

coordination of secondary schemes Piaget's term for when infants combine secondary schemes to obtain a goal.

tertiary circular reaction Piaget's term for repetition with variation; the infant is exploring the world's possibilities.

internalization of schemes Children's use of symbols to think about real events without actually experiencing them.

object permanence Refers to children gradually realizing that there are permanent objects around them, even when these objects are out of sight.

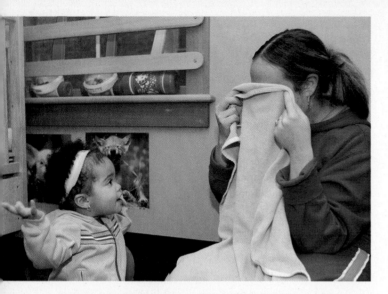

INFORMATION PROCESSING IN INFANCY

Information-processing theorists propose that cognitive development occurs through the gradual refining of such cognitive processes as attention and memory. Information processing theorists share three assumptions (Munakata, 2006):

- The first assumption relates to limited capacity—we can process only so much information at any one time.

- The second assumption refers to the belief that all thinking is information processing—making sense of external stimuli. The major focus of these theories is on such functions as attention and memory, not on stages of development.

- The third assumption is that most children devise a wide variety of thinking strategies and select what they think is the most appropriate strategy. Strategies that produce successful solutions increase in frequency, whereas those that do not decrease in frequency.

The sequence of information processing is shown in Figure 5.7.

Infants and Attention

Attention strategies enable children to decide what is important, what is needed, or what is dangerous. They also help infants gradually ignore everything else. Infants attend to different stimuli for a variety of reasons: intensity, complexity of the stimuli, visual ability, and novelty. They enjoy human faces, voices, and movements.

The brain is the biological basis of attention, and when infants attend to something, a series of brain activities is activated. For example, auditory receptors pick up the sound of the mother's voice, and a structure in the brain stem brings the baby to a higher state of alertness. An inner-brain system now swings into action, which involves memory and emotion. Finally, cortical areas interpret what was said and how it was said. Was it directed at something? Was it soothing? Was it pleasant?

In terms of psychology, the following describes what attention means for the developing infant:

- *Their attention is selective*—infants can't attend to everything.

- *Their attention involves cognitive processing*—infants don't just passively accept stimuli, they actively process incoming information.

- *Their attention is limited*—infants can attend only to a limited number of things at the same time.

Adults must assume some responsibility for monitoring the sights and sounds that their infants experience to shield them from overly intense stimulation. Many caregivers intuitively read their babies' signals and react appropriately, which reflects sensitive responsiveness to a child's needs.

Infants and Memory

Four important discoveries should frame your thinking about infant memory:

1. The brain as a whole is involved in memory; memories don't reside in one particular location.

2. Memories are retrieved in the same manner as they were formed.

3. Memories are stored in the brain's synapses, which are the connections between neurons.

4. These synaptic connections can be strengthened through use, and learning can form new synaptic processes.

Obviously, infants must have some ability to remember, or they could never learn about their world. They love to repeat actions that bring them pleasure. Infants demonstrate one type of memory (habituation) after the first few months following birth. By the end of the second year, an infant's memory more closely resembles that of older children, and they can recall sounds that, when strung together, elicit responses from others and a mutual understanding based on a shared language.

FIGURE 5.7

Information-Processing Model

| Stimuli from the environment (hearing, seeing, etc.) | → | Sensory registers | → | Short-term memory (briefly holds information from the environment) | → | Long-term memory (our permanent storage base) |

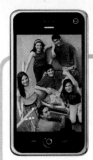
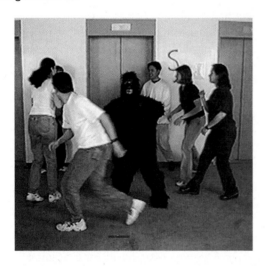
It's my **belief** *we developed language because of our deep inner need to* **complain.**

LILY TOMLIN

Language Development

One of the most amazing accomplishments in infancy is the beginning of speech. With no formal training—in fact, often exposed to dramatically faulty language models—children learn words and meanings, and how to combine them in a logical, purposeful manner. Because all children acquire their own language in a similar manner, it's important to consider this drive toward language.

Children in all parts of the world go through a process whereby they first emit sounds, then single words, two words, and then complex sentences (see Table 5.1). By the time they are about 5 years old, they have acquired the basics of their language—a huge accomplishment.

THE PACE OF LANGUAGE ACQUISITION

How does this uniquely human achievement occur? First, children learn the rules of their language, which they then apply in a wide variety of situations. Then, by the end of the second year, children learn to apply a label to an object without anyone telling them. Even when children don't understand a word, they acquire information about it from the surrounding context, a phenomenon called **fast mapping** (Bjorklund, 2005).

The process of acquiring language goes on at a fast pace until the fundamentals have been acquired, around age 5 for most children. By the time children enter elementary school, they are remarkably sophisticated language users. Then it becomes a matter of expanding and refining language skills, a task that can often define success or failure in a formal education setting.

VYGOTSKY'S STAGES OF LANGUAGE DEVELOPMENT

Psychologist Lev Vygotsky emphasized the role of context in language development. He argued that language begins as preintellectual speech and develops into a sophisticated form of what he called *inner speech*. The use of speech propels cognitive development as we literally talk ourselves through a task. In *Thought and Language* (1962), Vygotsky clearly presented his views about the four stages of language development.

> **fast mapping** Children's use of surrounding context to understand words' meaning.

TABLE 5.1

Language Development During Infancy

Language	Age
Crying	From birth
Cooing	2–5 months
Babbling	5–7 months
Single words	12 months
Two words	18 months
Phrases	2 years

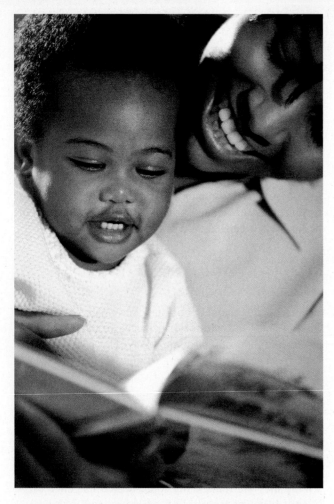

1. The first stage, which he called **preintellectual speech,** refers to such early processes as crying, cooing, babbling, and bodily movements that gradually develop into sophisticated forms of speech and behavior. Although human beings have an inborn ability to develop language, they must then interact with the environment if language development is to fulfill its potential.

2. Vygotsky referred to the second stage of language development as **naive psychology,** in which children explore the concrete objects in their world. At this stage, children begin to label the objects around them and acquire the grammar of their speech.

3. At about 3 years of age, **egocentric speech** emerges, that form of speech in which children carry on lively conversations, whether or not anyone is present or listening to them.

Career Apps

As a speech therapist, how could you help families recognize children's early sounds as serious attempts at communication?

4. Finally, speech turns inward (**inner speech**) and serves an important function in guiding and planning behavior. Inner speech often accompanies physical movements, guiding behavior. What begins as talking aloud to herself, eventually turns inward. For difficult tasks, inner speech is used to plan as well as guide behavior. For example, a child working on a jigsaw puzzle might remind herself to look for the flat-edged pieces so that she can form the border to frame the puzzle.

In many cases, children who aren't permitted these vocalizations struggle to accomplish a task. In fact, the more complex the task, the greater is the need for egocentric and inner speech.

KEY MILESTONES OF LANGUAGE DEVELOPMENT

During the first 2 months, babies develop sounds associated with breathing, feeding, and crying. **Cooing** (gurgling, vowel-like) appears during the second month. Between 5 and 7 months, babies play with the sounds they can make, and this output begins to take on the sounds of consonants and syllables, the beginning of **babbling.** Babbling probably appears initially because of biological maturation. At 7 and 8 months, sounds like syllables appear—da-da-da, ba-ba-ba, a pattern that continues for the remainder of the first year (Pinker, 1994). This is a phenomenon that occurs in all languages.

First Words

Around their first birthday, babies produce single words, about half of which are for objects (food, clothing, toys). Throughout the world, children's first words express similar meanings. These words refer to people, animals, toys, vehicles, and other objects that fascinate children. Children quickly learn the sounds of their language (**phonology**), the meanings of words (**semantics**), how to construct sentences (**syntax**), and how to communicate (**pragmatics**).

At 18 months, children acquire words at the rate of 40 per week (Woodward & Markman, 1998). This rapid increase in vocabulary lasts until about 3 years of age and is frequently referred to as the **word spurt.** Vocabulary constantly expands, but estimating the extent of a child's vocabulary is difficult because youngsters know more words than they articulate. Estimates are that a 1-year-old child may use from two to six words, and a 2-year-old has a vocabulary ranging from 50 to 250 words. Children at this stage also begin to combine two words (Pinker, 1994). By first grade, children may understand 10,000 words, and by fifth grade they understand about 40,000 words (Woodward & Markman, 1998). These first words, or **holophrases,** are usually nouns, adjectives, or self-inventive words and often contain multiple meanings. The single word "ball" may mean not only the ball itself but also "Throw the ball to me."

Two-Word Sentences

At about 18 to 24 months of age, children's vocabularies begin to expand rapidly, and a form of communication

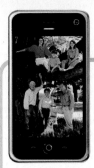

TECH TRENDS

Sound Design

For the Disney movie *WALL-E,* sound designer Ben Burtt used sounds from real-life things to create the language for the machines featured in the film. By putting pieces of sounds together to form new sounds, he and his design team re-created the process that infants use to make language. The team recorded thousands of sounds—motors, generators, and even an old crank from a 1930s bi-plane. Burtt said the technique goes back to the early days of Disney cartoons, when wind machines and blowing machines were used to make sounds that are recognizable to the human ear, but in a different context the sounds take on a new life and a new meaning.

Some examples from the film are the sounds WALL-E makes when he is surprised by something: his eyebrows make the sounds of a Nikon camera shutter and his arms are the sound of a motor on a tank.

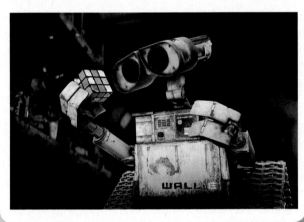

called **telegraphic speech** appears. Telegraphic speech consists of simple two-word sentences without conjunctions, articles, and (often) verbs. For example, the phrase "Mommy milk" might stand for "Mommy, I would like to have a glass of milk."

When the two-word stage appears (any time from 18 to 24 months), children initially struggle to convey tense (past and present) and number (singular and plural). They also experience difficulty with grammar. Children usually employ word order ("me go") for meaning, only gradually mastering inflection (how language handles plurals, tenses, possessives, gender, and so on) as they begin to form three-word sentences. They use nouns and verbs initially ("doggie sleep," "mama kiss"), and their sentences demonstrate grammatical structure like that of adults.

Children begin to use multiple words to refer to the things that they previously named with single words. Rather than learning rules of word combination to express new ideas, children learn to use new word forms. Combining words in phrases and sentences suggests that children are learning the structure of their language.

Word order and inflection become increasingly important. During the first stages of language acquisition, word order is paramount. At first, children combine words without concern for inflections, and word order provides clues as to their level of syntactic (grammatical) development. Once two-word sentences are used, inflection soon appears, usually with three-word sentences ("Where *ball* go?"). The appearance of inflections seems to follow a pattern: first the plural of nouns, then tense and person of verbs, and then possessives.

The biopsychosocial model of development is evident as various phases of development converge in a child's use of language (see Table 5.2). Motor development is visible when a child runs excitedly toward her mother. Language development is visible when the child lifts her arms upon reaching her mother, saying, "Mommy, UP!" Cognitive development is visible in terms of the attachment the child displays to her mother. The integration of these developmental forces is linked to social and emotional factors that shape the infant's life.

preintellectual speech Vygotsky's category for cooing, crying, babbling, and bodily movements that develop into more sophisticated forms of speech.

naive psychology Vygotsky's stage in which children explore objects and label objects as they acquire the grammar of their speech.

egocentric speech The form of speech in which children carry on lively conversations with themselves or others.

inner speech Internal speech that often accompanies physical movements, guiding behavior.

cooing Early language sounds that resemble vowels.

babbling Infants' production of sounds approximating speech between 5 and 7 months.

phonology Sounds of a language.

semantics Meaning of words and sentences.

syntax The way in which words are put together to construct sentences.

pragmatics Ability to communicate with others.

word spurt Rapid increase of vocabulary from 18 months to 3 years.

holophrases One word that can communicate many meanings and ideas.

telegraphic speech Initial multiple-word utterances, usually two or three words.

Social and Emotional Development

Think back to the example of Laura at the beginning of this chapter and the importance of relationships in a child's development. Relationships can be considered as patterns of interactions between people over time. A baby's relationships involve many aspects of development, such as playing (physical and social), talking and communicating (language), understanding self and others (cognitive), and attachment (emotional). In other words, a relationship is a good example of the importance of biopsychosocial interactions.

TABLE 5.2

Developmental Characteristics of Infancy

Age (months)	Height (inches)	Weight (pounds)	Language Development	Motor Development	Cognitive (Piaget)
3	24	13–14	Cooing	Supports head in prone position	Primary circular reactions
6	26	17–18	Babbling: single syllable sounds	Sits erect when supported	Secondary circular reactions
9	26	20–22	Repetition of sounds signals emotions	Stands with support	Coordination of secondary schemes
12	29.5	22–24	Single words: mama, dada	Walks when held by hand	Same
18	32	25–26	3–50 words	Grasps objects accurately, walks steadily	Tertiary circular reaction
24	34	27–29	50–250 words, 2–3-word sentences	Walks and runs up and down stairs	Representation

FIGURE 5.8

The Brain and Language

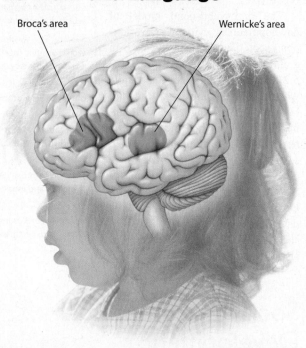

Broca's area

Wernicke's area

Specific areas of the brain have been identified for their role in language production and comprehension. Debate exists over whether the acquisition of these skills is innate or learned.

CHILDREN'S DEVELOPING RELATIONSHIPS

reciprocal interactions
Interactions that shape relationships with others.

Infants interact with their environments and begin to structure their own relationships according to their individual temperaments. The interactions occurring among family members—parent–parent, parent–siblings, sibling–sibling—produce a ripple effect that colors the parent–child relationship. Thus, the nature of the relationships between parents and their children emerges from the temperament and characteristics of each and from the interactions that occur among them (Rubin, Bukowski, & Parker, 2006).

Infants quickly focus on their mothers as sources of relief and satisfaction. Mothers, in turn, rapidly discriminate between their infants' cries: for hunger, discomfort, or fear. Thus, a pattern of interactions is established. Relationships can usually be labeled using adjectives such as warm, cold, rejecting, and hostile. Any relationship may be marked by seemingly contradictory interactions. A mother may have a warm relationship with her child as shown by hugging and kissing, but she may also yell when yelling might be needed to protect the child from harm. To understand the relationship, we must understand the interactions.

THE ROLE OF RECIPROCAL INTERACTIONS

From the moment children are born, they immediately seek stimulation from their environment and instantly interpret and react to how they are being treated—a process called **reciprocal interactions.** Not only do infants attempt to make sense of their world as they develop cognitively, they also "tune in to" the social and emotional atmosphere surrounding them and immediately begin to shape their relationships with others.

Infants are not merely passive, but also exercise some control over the interactions. Adults respond to infants partly because of the way that infants respond to adults.

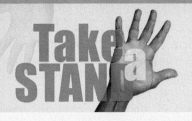

There has been ongoing debate about whether language is a biological, innate ability that all humans possess or learned through interactions in the environment. Noam Chomsky (1957) argued that humans are born prewired with the ability to acquire the rules of language, detect and re-create sounds, and receive and express meaning. He called this inborn ability a *language acquisition device (LAD),* and while not situated in a specific region of the brain (such as Broca's area, involved in producing words, or Wernicke's area, involved in comprehension), there is evidence that people in all different parts of the world develop language in the same sequence.

Behaviorists believe that environment and reinforcement are at the heart of language development.

They believe that infants exposed to a certain language acquire the language based on the responses that caregivers give them. Currently, people who argue for the influence of environment on language development find that context plays a large role. For instance, a child who grows up exposed to many books and printed materials will be more likely to acquire language skills than a child who does not grow up in a print-rich environment.

Do you think biology or environment plays a bigger role in language development? What examples can you think of to support your argument? What implications does this have on children's early education?

An infant's staring, cooing, smiling, and kicking can all be used to maintain interactions. Early interactions establish the nature of the relationship between parent and child, giving it a particular tone or style.

Parents bring some preconceived ideas about the role they should play in their relationships with their children. How they exercise their power and how their children react to their suggestions and encouragements, their demands and commands, ultimately determine the success of the relationship. In an ideal world, their ideas, expectations, and sense of their roles as parents should mesh perfectly with their child's personality and abilities.

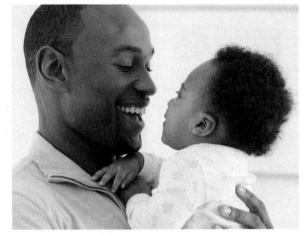

ROLE OF EMOTIONS IN DEVELOPMENT

It's easy to see how a child's life is affected by the impact of attachment and early relationships. Healthy emotional development helps children to define their individuality. During infancy, emotions generate adaptive functions that help to define the meaning of a child's experiences. How can we define emotions? According to pediatrician, psychiatrist, and author Daniel Siegel, "Emotions represent

dynamic processes created within the socially influenced, value-appraising processes of the brain" (p. 123). For example, infants' emotions motivate them to either approach or withdraw from situations and to either communicate or not communicate their needs to those around them. When others respond, infants learn about social exchanges, which furthers their social development. These emotional interchanges help to explain why emotions are often referred to as the language of infancy (Emde, 1998).

Appropriate emotions and behavior are heavily influenced by cultural values. For example, in a study of Asian and American children, Cole, Bruschi, and Tamang (2002) found notable differences in emotional expression. Children from the United States expressed their anger more openly than did the children from the other cultures. Asian children demonstrated that one can feel differently than one reveals.

When we think about various emotions, we must remember that *different* responses may be made to any *one* emotion. A smile, for example, may signal joy, nervousness, or some other emotion. Also, different theorists may suggest slightly different schedules for the appearance of various emotions, but the basic explanation of *how* they develop is identical. Emotional development occurs as the result of an infant's dispositional tendencies combined with a complex interaction between growing cognitive skills and social interactions (see Table 5.3).

In the first year of life, infants gradually develop the ability to stop or reduce the duration and intensity of emotional reactions. Two processes seem to be involved—one related to the appearance of emotions and one involving the management of emotions. Any psychological explanation of child development must recognize the importance of emotions as motivators. Emotions can help infants analyze situations and prepare themselves to act.

ANALYZING EMOTIONAL EXPRESSIONS

One of the first signs of emotion is a baby's smile, which most parents immediately interpret as a sign of happiness. Yet newborns' smiles don't indicate pleasure in the sense that the smiles of older infants do. By the baby's third week, the human female voice elicits a brief, real smile, and by the sixth week the beginnings of the true social smile appear, especially in response to the human face.

Two-month-old infants are often described as "smilers," whereas frequent and socially significant smiles emerge around 3 months (Kagan & Fox, 2006). Babies smile instinctively at faces—real or drawn—and this probably

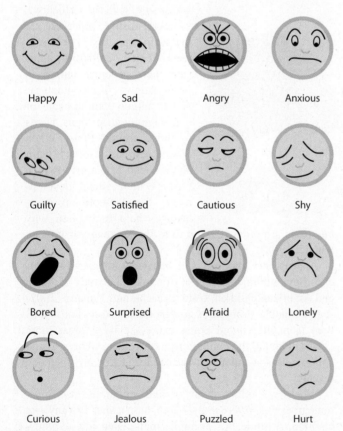

Happy	Sad	Angry	Anxious
Guilty	Satisfied	Cautious	Shy
Bored	Surprised	Afraid	Lonely
Curious	Jealous	Puzzled	Hurt

Children and adults recognize the various emotions that they display with each other in everyday interactions.

TABLE 5.3
Timetable of Emotional Development

Age	Emotion	Features
Birth–3 months	Pleasure, distress, disgust	A range of emerging emotions from happiness to anger
3–6 months	Delight, wariness, anger	More specific responses to specific stimulation
6–9 months	Fear, anxiety, shyness, pleasure	Emotions slowly becoming differentiated with increasing cognitive development
9–12 months	Stranger anxiety, separation anxiety	Concentrated focus on main caregiver
12–18 months	Elation, security	Feelings of security and well-being encourage exploration of environment
18–24 months	Shame, defiance	Integration of emotional and cognitive features

reflects the human tendency to attend to patterns. Infants gradually learn that familiar faces usually mean pleasure, and smiling becomes a key element in securing positive reinforcement from those around the infant.

Finally, infants smile at any high-contrast stimuli and at the human beings around them, and they discover a relationship between their behavior and events in the external world. When infants smile, they elicit attention from those around them and begin to associate the human face with pleasure. Current research on emotional development reinforces the biopsychosocial basis for this book: Emotional expression appears immediately after birth, acquires meaning, and expands rapidly because of the socially interactive nature of emotional communication. As children grow, the circumstances that elicit their emotions change; that is, the emotional experiences at different ages vary drastically. The happiness that a 6-month-old child shows when tickled by her mother is far different from a 16-year-old's happiness sharing a funny story with a friend. We may label both "happiness," but is the emotion the same?

Emotional development seems to move from the general (positive versus negative emotions) to the specific—general positive states morph into such emotions as joy and interest; general negative states morph into fear, disgust, or anger. These primary emotions emerge during the first 6 months. Sometime after 18 months of age, secondary emotions appear that are associated with a child's growing cognitive capacity for self-awareness. As early as 2 or 3 years of age, children begin to display complex emotions, such as shame, guilt, and jealousy (Volling, McElwain, & Miller, 2002). These new emotions emerge from a child's increasing cognitive maturity, and they have a strong influence on self-

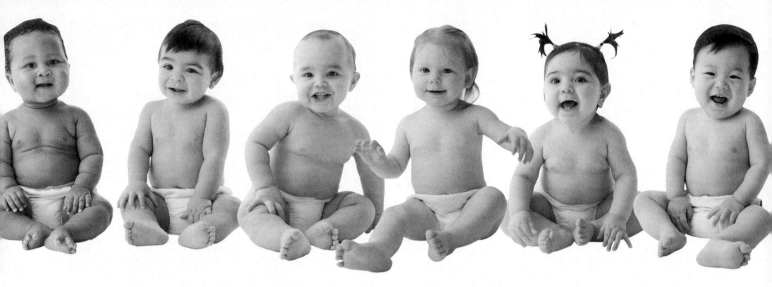

esteem. For example, embarrassment or shame at spilling a cup of water may weaken a child's sense of competence. For emotions such as embarrassment to appear, children must have developed a sense of self.

Attachment

How significant is the mother–infant relationship in the first days and weeks after birth? Infants who develop a secure **attachment** to their mothers have the willingness and confidence to seek out future relationships. Attachment figures are secure bases that encourage infants to explore their environments but remain reliable retreats when stress and uncertainty appear. Among the first researchers to stress the significance of relationships in an infant's life were John Bowlby and Mary Salter Ainsworth.

EXAMINING ATTACHMENT

Using concepts from psychology and **ethology,** a field that stresses behavior is strongly influenced by biology, John Bowlby formulated his basic premise: A warm, intimate relationship between mother and infant is essential to mental health, because a child's need for its mother's presence is as great as its need for food. A mother's continued

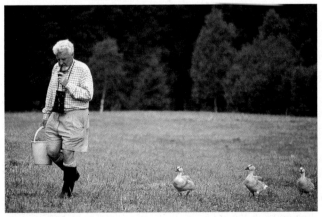

Konrad Lorenz

absence can generate a sense of loss and feelings of anger. Even though most attachment research tends to focus on mothers' relationships with children, Bowlby stated that an infant's principal attachment figure can be someone other than the biological mother. Further, Bowlby noted that attachment patterns between fathers and children closely resemble those between mothers and their children. This is reminiscent of the work of ethologist Konrad Lorenz (1965), who determined that newborn ducks and geese would follow the first object they saw after hatching. In a now-famous experiment, the first thing these young geese saw after hatching was Lorenz!

Bowlby and his colleagues initiated a series of studies in which children were separated from their parents. A predictable sequence of behaviors was observed: (1) *Protest* begins almost immediately and lasts up to 1 week, with loud crying, extreme restlessness, and rejection of all adult figures; (2) *despair* is typified by a growing hopelessness, with monotonous crying, inactivity, and steady withdrawal; and (3) *detachment* appears when an infant displays renewed interest in its surroundings—but a remote, distant kind of interest. Bowlby described the behavior of this final phase as apathetic, even if the mother reappeared. Bowlby also believed that although attachment is most obvious in infancy and early childhood, it can be observed throughout the life cycle.

To assess the quality of attachment, Mary Salter Ainsworth (1973, 1979; Ainsworth & Bowlby, 1991), designed an experiment known as the **strange situation.** In her experimental scenario, Ainsworth had a mother and an infant taken to an observation room. The child was placed on the floor and allowed to play with toys. A stranger (female) then entered the room and began to talk to the mother. Observers watched to see how the infant reacted to the stranger and to what extent the child used the mother as a secure base. The mother then left the child alone in the room with the stranger; observers then noted how distressed

attachment Behavior intended to keep a child (or adult) in close proximity to a significant other.

ethology Scientific field that stresses behavior is strongly influenced by biology and is linked to evolution.

strange situation Measure designed to assess the quality of attachment.

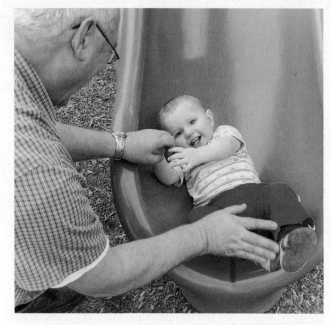

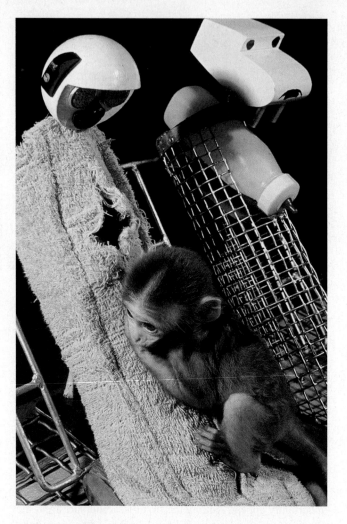

the child became. The mother returned and the quality of the child's reaction to the mother's return was assessed. Next, the infant was left completely alone, followed by the stranger's entrance and then that of the mother. The behavior exhibited by children in the strange situation is used to categorize children as follows:

- *Securely attached children,* who use their mothers as a base from which to explore. Separation intensifies their attachment behavior; they exhibit considerable distress, stop their explorations, and seek contact with their mothers at reunions.

- *Avoidantly attached children,* who rarely cry during separation and avoid their mothers at reunion. The mothers of these babies seem to dislike or are indifferent to physical contact.

- *Ambivalently attached children,* who manifest anxiety before separation and who are intensely distressed by the separation. Yet on reunion, they display ambivalent behavior toward their mothers; they seek contact but simultaneously seem to resist it.

- *Disorganized/disoriented children,* who show a confused sort of behavior at reunion. For example, they may look at the mother and then look away, showing little emotion.

Ainsworth reported other studies, conducted in Baltimore, Washington, D.C., Scotland, and Uganda, noting that cultural influences may affect the ways in which different attachment behaviors develop. Nevertheless, geographic location did not affect the existence of attachment behaviors.

ATTACHMENT CHALLENGES

Obstacles to successful attachment exist in many forms, such as child maltreatment and neglect. In a classic study, the Harlows (1971) studied rhesus monkeys that were caged without real mothers but, instead, with substitute "mothers"

temperament Individual differences; unique and stable styles of behaving.

constructed out of wire or terry-cloth towels. The Harlows found that the monkeys placed in cages with the softer surrogate mothers fared better than those monkeys caged with the cold, hard stand-ins, but in each case the monkeys exhibited clear effects from being deprived of maternal affection. For example, as the monkeys grew older, they tended to avoid other monkeys and cowered in the corner when confronted or attacked, rocking themselves back and forth. Later studies placed the socially deprived monkeys in cages with younger monkeys, and researchers found that deprived monkeys would eventually interact playfully with others.

Clearly, ethical and moral parameters would prevent such a study with children, but there is strong evidence of the impact that neglect and abuse have on children raised in neglectful orphanages and other institutions. Receiving little to no attention, children in such settings display signs of depression and impaired emotional regulation, even if their physical needs are met in terms of minimal food, shelter, and clothing. In the United States, children across the country live in settings that do not promote healthy attachments and developmental benefits such as emotional and intellectual growth. Organizations such as the Children's Defense Fund (http://www.childrens defense.org) and the U.S. Department of Health and Human Services (http://www.hhs.gov) work to ensure that children receive the care they deserve as citizens and unique individuals.

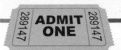

Temperament

Simply put, **temperament** refers to individual differences—our unique and stable styles of behaving. Temperament is a critical personality trait, especially in the first days and weeks after birth, and is persistent. Temperaments provide clues to why infants behave in the ways they do and the manner in which they interact with others.

THE DIMENSIONS OF TEMPERAMENT

Throughout life, a child's family, the social environment, socioeconomic status, and cultural influences contribute to the shaping of a child's temperament. Examining this developmentally interactive process, Thompson (1999) concluded:

- A child's temperament may or may not mesh well with the demands of the social setting. This **goodness of fit** between temperament and environment has a major impact on personality and adjustment. Yet a child's environment changes dramatically through the years, and these changes have powerful effects on development and adjustment.

- Temperament influences how a child selects and responds to different aspects of the environment. This affects how people respond to the child.

- Temperament impacts how a child perceives and thinks about the environment.

Based in biology, temperament is an evolving feature of behavior that is influenced by other factors.

KAGAN'S BIOLOGICAL INTERPRETATION

Harvard professor and developmental psychologist Jerome Kagan has proposed that biology, especially the brain, is a major contributor to temperament. He proposed that most temperamental biases are due to inherited variations in neurochemistry or anatomy, although some may be due to unknown prenatal events. And yet, because our development is based on the critical role of reciprocal interactions, we can't overlook the interactions between biology and the environment. Kagan describes temperament as an inherited physiology that is preferentially linked to an envelope of emotions and behaviors. The interaction of biology and other forces has been examined by other researchers from different perspectives.

CHESS AND THOMAS'S CLASSIFICATION OF TEMPERAMENT

Two child psychiatrists, Stella Chess and Alexander Thomas (1987, 1999), were struck by the behaviors of their own children in the days immediately following birth—differences that could not be attributed solely to the environment. Intrigued, they devised the **New York Longitudinal Study** of 141 children. Chess and Thomas discovered that even with children as young as 2 or 3 months of age, they could identify and categorize three types of temperament:

- *Easy,* characterized by regularity of bodily functions, low or moderate intensity of reactions, and acceptance of, rather than withdrawal from, new situations (40% of the children).

- *Difficult,* characterized by irregularity in bodily functions, intense reactions, and withdrawal from new stimuli (10% of the children).

- *Slow to warm up,* characterized by a low intensity of reactions and a somewhat negative mood (15% of the children).

Note that a significant number of children (35%) could not be classified into any of the categories. If parents recognize similar characteristics in their children—the need for sleep at a certain time; a unique manner of reacting to strangers or the unknown, the intensity of concentration on a

goodness of fit Concept coined by Chess and Thomas (1977) that describes the match between a child's temperament and his/her environment.

New York Longitudinal Study Long-term study by Chess and Thomas of the personality characteristics of children.

task—they can use their knowledge of such characteristics to build a goodness-of-fit relationship. Table 5.4 summarizes the behaviors of children in three categories of temperament.

The importance of parents' and children's temperaments in establishing a goodness-of-fit relationship has shown the significance of **sensitive responsiveness.** An example of sensitive responsiveness would be that although most infants like to be held, some dislike physical contact. How does a mother respond to an infant who stiffens and pulls away, especially if her older children liked being held when they were young? Infants instantly tune in to their environment. They give clues to their personalities so that a mother's and father's responses to their child's signals must be appropriate for *that* child; that is, greater parental sensitivity produces more responsive infants.

sensitive responsiveness
The ability to recognize the meaning of a child's behavior.

TABLE 5.4

Categories of Temperament

Behaviors	Easy Children	Difficult Children	Slow-to-Warm-Up Children
Activity level	Varies	Low to moderate	Varies
Approach or withdrawal	Positive approach	Withdrawal	Initial withdrawal
Adaptability	Very adaptable	Slowly adaptable	Adaptable
Quality of mood	Positive	Negative	Slightly negative

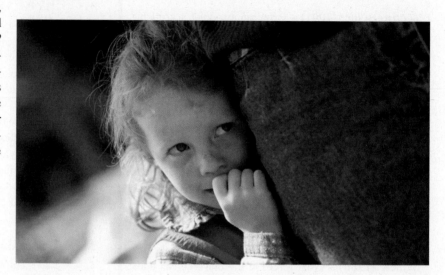

CONCLUSIONS & SUMMARY

Our view of an infant today is of an individual with enormous potential, one whose activity and competence are much greater than originally believed. It is as if a newborn enters the world with all systems ready to function and eager for growth. What happens during the first two years has important implications for future development. Setbacks—physical and psychological—will occur, but need not cause permanent damage. Human infants show remarkable resiliency.

What are the major physical accomplishments of the infancy period?

- Newborns display clear signs of their competence: movement, seeing, hearing, interacting.
- Infants' physical and motor abilities influence all aspects of development.
- Motor development follows a well-documented schedule.

How do infants acquire information about their world?

- Infants are capable of acquiring and interpreting information from their immediate surroundings.
- From birth, infants show preferences for certain types of stimuli.

What are the differences between Piaget's view of cognitive development in infancy and that of information processing?

- Infants, even at this early age, attempt to answer questions about their world, questions that will continue to occupy them in more complex and sophisticated forms throughout their lives.
- One of the first tasks that infants must master is an understanding of the objects around them.
- A key element in understanding an infant's cognitive development is the role of memory.

How do infants acquire their language?

- Infants show rapid growth in their language development.
- Language acquisition follows a definite sequence.

The role of relationships in development has achieved a prominent place in our attempts to understand children's growth. From the initial contacts with the mother to the ever-expanding network of siblings and peers at all ages, children's relationships exert a powerful and continuing influence on the direction of development.

How do children develop and control their emotions?

- The brain plays a major role in the development and appearance of emotions.
- As emotional development occurs, children acquire a necessary degree of emotional regulation.

What is the role of relationships in psychosocial development?

- Relationships involve almost all aspects of development.
- Infants, as active partners in their development, help to shape their relationships.
- To understand relationships, we must analyze and understand the reciprocal interactions involved.

How would you assess the importance of attachment in psychosocial development?

- Bowlby and his colleagues, studying the separation of children from their parents, identified attachment as an important part of psychosocial development.
- Ainsworth's strange situation technique is designed to assess the security of an infant's attachment.
- Attachment is a cross-cultural phenomenon that offers clues to psychosocial development.

How does temperament affect the relationship between parents and their children?

- Temperament refers to a child's unique way of interacting with the environment.
- An infant's temperament immediately affects interactions with adults.
- To maintain goodness of fit, parents must constantly adapt their parenting style to match the developmental changes in their children.

KEY TERMS

artificial intelligence *107*

attachment *121*

axons *106*

babbling *116*

circular reactions *112*

cooing *116*

coordination of secondary schemes *113*

crawling *108*

creeping *108*

dendrites *106*

egocentric speech *116*

egocentrism *112*

ethology *121*

failure to thrive (FTT) *109*

fast mapping *115*

goodness of fit *123*

habituation *111*

holophrases *116*

infantile amnesia *105*

inner speech *116*

internalization of schemes *113*

myelin *106*

naive psychology *116*

neurons *106*

New York Longitudinal Study *123*

object permanence *113*

perception *110*

phonology *116*

pragmatics *116*

preintellectual speech *116*

primary circular reactions *112*

reciprocal interactions *118*

REM (rapid eye-movement) sleep *110*

respiratory distress syndrome (RDS) *110*

secondary circular reactions *113*

semantics *116*

sensitive responsiveness *124*

sensorimotor period *112*

strange situation *121*

sudden infant death syndrome (SIDS) *109*

synapse *106*

syntax *116*

telegraphic speech *117*

temperament *123*

tertiary circular reaction *113*

word spurt *116*

1. The shift from considering an infant as nothing more than a passive sponge to seeing infants as amazingly competent carries with it certain responsibilities. What are some rights that babies have, as our youngest citizens, that deserve attention and advocacy efforts? How does the environment impact the rights of infants?

2. Testing infants has grown in popularity during the past two decades. What are some cautions that the public should be aware of when gaining and interpreting data from infant assessments?

3. After reading this chapter on infancy, how do you feel about this stage of life as one in which seeds for the future are planted? Select one phase of development (for example, cognitive development) and show how a stimulating environment can help to lay the foundation for future cognitive growth.

Chapter Review Test

1. Which of the following is *not* a reflex?
   a. breathing
   b. sucking
   c. swallowing
   d. laughing

2. Piaget noted that _____ are a critical feature of the sensorimotor stage.
   a. circular reactions
   b. rootings
   c. babblings
   d. habits

3. The famous experiment conducted by the Harlows examined social deprivation in
   a. monkeys.
   b. kittens.
   c. infants.
   d. rats.

4. The final area of the brain to develop is the
   a. sensory region.
   b. motor area.
   c. visual area.
   d. auditory area.

5. When infants demonstrate a decrease in attention, this is called
   a. repression.
   b. habituation.
   c. egocentrism.
   d. permanence.

6. What parents see as their ___ affects parent–child relationships.
   a. interactions
   b. function
   c. background
   d. role

7. Children's _____ contribute(s) significantly to their interactions with their environments.
   a. ages
   b. gender
   c. temperaments
   d. culture

8. Chess and Thomas described a child with a low intensity of reactions and a somewhat negative attitude as
   a. slow to warm up.
   b. difficult.
   c. easy.
   d. depressed.

9. Biologically based individual differences are known as
   a. interactions.
   b. attachments.
   c. temperament.
   d. parental signposts.

10. The author of the strange situation test is
    a. Ainsworth.
    b. Bowlby.
    c. Brazelton.
    d. Kagan.

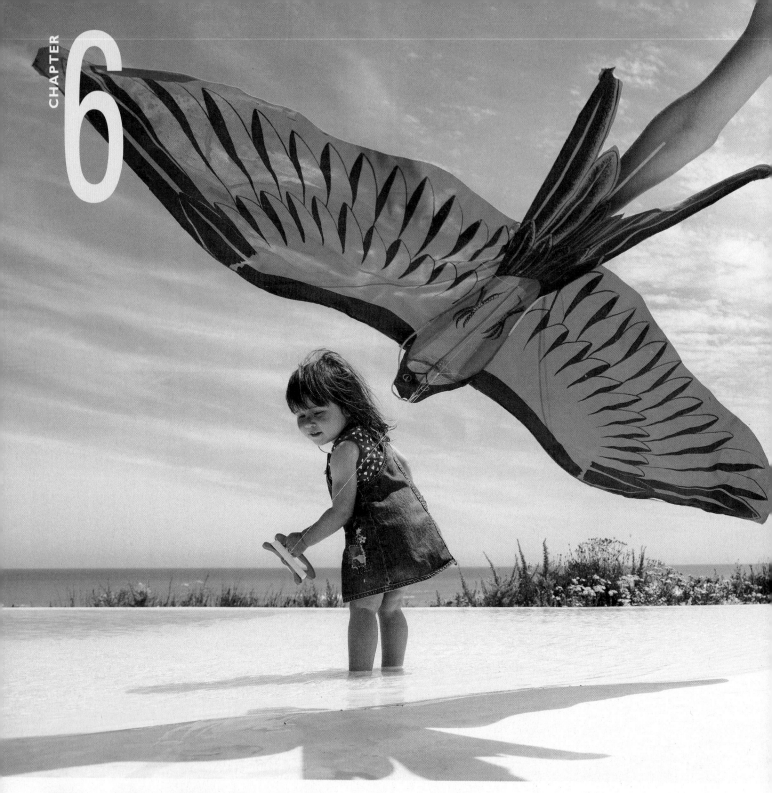

EARLY CHILDHOOD

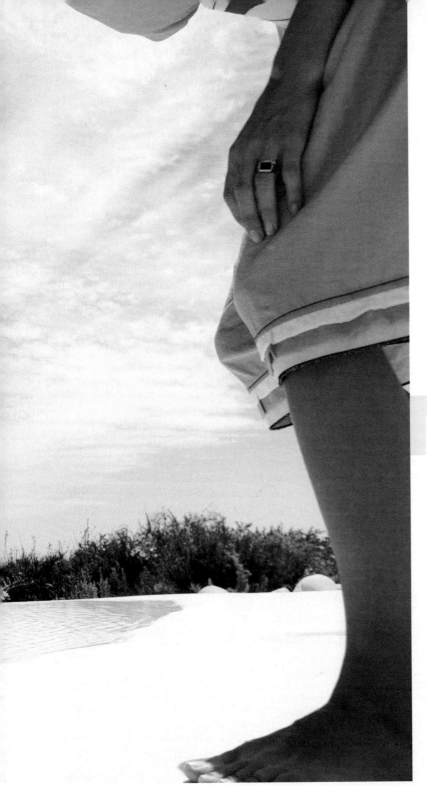

As You READ

After reading this chapter, you should be able to answer the following questions:

- What are the major physical and motor accomplishments of the early childhood years?

- How do Piaget's views on cognitive development differ from those of information-processing theorists?

- What types of early childhood education seem most promising?

- How does children's language acquisition proceed during these years?

- What role does family play in development during these early childhood years?

- How do children of this age acquire a sense of self?

- How do children come to understand the meaning of gender?

- What is the value of play for children's development and learning?

129

> These are "magic" years because children in their early years are magicians—in the psychological sense. Their earliest conceptions of the world are magical ones; they **believe** that their actions and thoughts can bring about events. Later, they extend this magic system and find human attributes in natural phenomena and see human or **suprahuman** causes for natural events or for ordinary occurrences in their lives.
>
> SELMA FRAIBERG, *THE MAGIC YEARS* (1959), P. IX

In one of the great classics describing early childhood, Selma Fraiberg immortalized ages two to six as *The Magic Years*. She describes how children perceive and interpret events through the use of "magical thought," the idea that children believe their thoughts can bring about the events they witness. Wonderful at times, such as when magical thought enables children to see themselves as the heroic firefighter saving others, magical thought can also be upsetting, such as when children blame themselves for their parents' divorce. The early childhood years are exciting, rewarding, and challenging—for both children and those who care for them. The goal of this chapter is to help you better understand the magical world of early childhood.

Boundless energy, constant curiosity, and growing mental maturity all characterize children from 2 to 6 years of age. Children's developmental changes combine with feelings of confidence—"I can do it myself!" Cognitively, the preschool years correspond to the second stage in Piaget's theory of development, the preoperational period, when children begin to use symbols such as language to represent objects. During this time, many young children also experience some form of preschool education, which contributes to their cognitive and social growth on many complex, interconnected levels. As children's own mental structures interact with messages and values in their environment, they increasingly make sense of their world. While the demands of this period of life are many, healthy children have abundant energy required to tackle these challenges.

Physical and Motor Development

Growth in early childhood proceeds at a slower pace than in infancy, yet is quite complex (see Figure 6.1). Some changes are obvious—during the years 2 to 6, children grow about 12 inches and continue to gain weight at the rate of about 5 pounds a year. Boys and girls show about the same rate of growth during these years, and although there is a predictable pattern for growth in most parts of the body, growth varies from child to child. Other changes are not visible, but critically important—rapid growth in the brain's frontal lobe impacts planning and organizing of thought and actions.

FEATURES OF PHYSICAL DEVELOPMENT

We know that different cells, tissues, and organs grow at different rates. In early childhood, children tend to slim down as their trunks lengthen and body fat declines. While girls tend to be a bit shorter and less heavy than boys, girls' bodies tend to have more fatty tissue than boys' bodies, which have more muscle tissue. As children begin to notice obvious differences in physical appearance and growth,

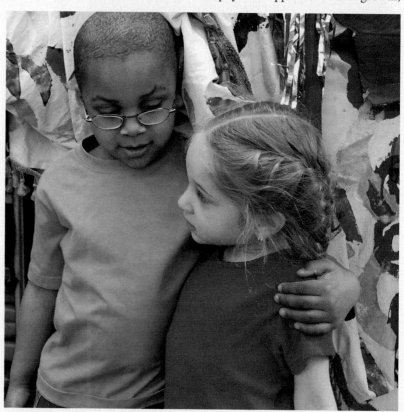

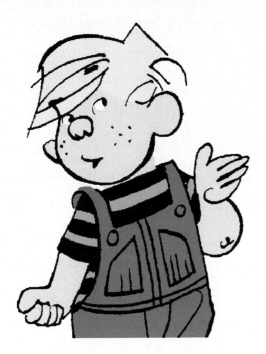

they enjoy comparing their body parts to learn about themselves and others. For example, children are happily aware of loose and missing teeth as "baby" teeth fall out to make way for "grown-up" teeth.

BRAIN DEVELOPMENT

As young children compare themselves to others, their brain development allows them to construct new understandings. Although the brain does not grow as much in early childhood as it did during infancy, the number of patterns in specific parts of the brain, such as the frontal lobe, increase tremendously. The patterns that form in the brain promote connections in the form of neural pathways (nerve impulses that travel along axons and connect with dendrites of other neurons along the way) and connections between children and their environment, as an increasing number of cognitive abilities enable them to participate in richer experiences and interactions. Young children are exposed to tremendous amounts of information in their world that they take in through their five senses. The patterns in the specific part of the frontal lobe known as the *prefrontal cortex* (see Figure 6.2) allow young children to organize their attention and actions.

Over time, this organized information helps children plan their activities and use resources efficiently. At times this organization occurs automatically, as brain matter grows to accommodate the growing number of pathways that are formed and other areas pare down unused brain cells. In Chapter 5, the process by which nerve impulses travel along axons was introduced. Recall that myelin refers to the layer of fat cells that insulate the axons. The presence of myelin speeds up the rate that information travels throughout the nervous system in a process called **myelination,** which continues throughout childhood. Myelination has been shown to influence visible skills, such as hand-eye coordination, as well as skills that are harder to detect, such as a child's ability to focus attention.

The ability to organize information is also impacted by behavior, such as children's preference in handedness. Although the brain's two hemispheres seem to be almost

> **myelination** Process by which speed of information traveling through nervous system increases, due to a fatty layer of cells on nerve cells in the brain.

FIGURE 6.1
Growth Curves for Boys and Girls

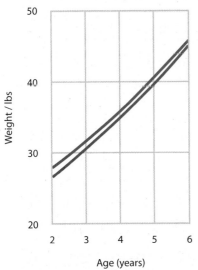

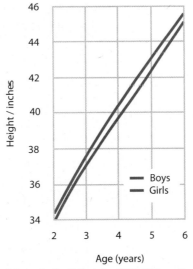

Source: Centers for Disease Control and Prevention, National Center for Health Statistics. (2000). CDC growth charts: United States. http://www.cdc.gov/growthcharts.

FIGURE 6.2
Prefrontal Cortex

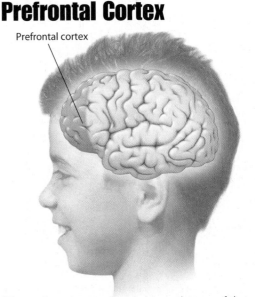

The prefrontal cortex in relation to the rest of the brain.

identical, there are important differences between the two halves of the brain that are linked to specific functions, a concept called *lateralization*. More people around the world are right-handed than left-handed, and for decades parents and teachers forced children to write with their right hand, even when they showed a clear preference for their left hand. The reasons for this include superstitions as well as the reality that much of the world is geared toward right-handedness (consider scissors, musical instruments, and notebook bindings). Today, most adults allow children to pursue the handedness to which they naturally gravitate, and many brain functions have been recognized as being linked to both hemispheres. In fact, a person's ability to utilize both hemispheres of the brain and coordinate function between them is tied to increased performance in several areas, such as creativity and language processing, production, and recall (see Figure 6.3).

GROWING MOTOR SKILLS

It's easy to take the physical accomplishments of 6-year-olds for granted, but a great deal of neuromuscular develop-

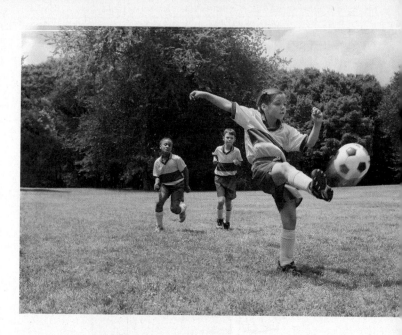

ment must occur before the motor skills involved in actions such as kicking, cutting, throwing, zipping, and tying shoes become effortless.

These actions fall into two types of motor skills: **gross motor skills** (using the large muscles) and **fine motor skills** (using the small muscles of the hands and fingers). Gross motor skills are visible as young children enjoy a wider variety of movement, from running to dancing to hopping and climbing. As their abilities increase, children are more prone to taking some risks in their physical play, such as climbing a structure on the playground that once seemed unconquerable. Fine motor skills, such as picking up objects using finger and thumb (pincer grip), develop greatly during early childhood and are evident in children's play with puzzles and building blocks, as well as in their evolving writing and drawing. Table 6.1 gives examples of gross and fine motor skills at ages 2 to 6 years.

FIGURE 6.3

Lateralization and Handedness

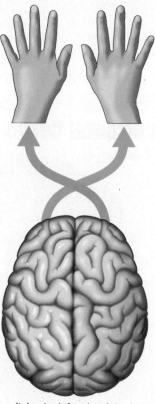

Lateralization links the left side of the brain with right-handedness and the right side of the brain with left-handedness.

TABLE 6.1

The Emergence of Motor Skills

Age	Gross Motor Skills	Fine Motor Skills
2 years	Runs, climbs stairs, jumps from object (both feet)	Throws ball, kicks ball, turns page, begins to scribble
3 years	Hops, climb stairs with alternating feet, jumps from bottom step	Copies circle, opposes thumb to finger, scribbling continues to improve
4 years	Runs well, jumps skillfully, begins to skip, pedals tricycle	Holds pencil, copies square, walks balance beam
5 years	Hops about 50 feet, balances on one foot, can catch large ball, good skipping	Colors within lines, forms letters, dresses and undresses self with help, eats more neatly
6 years	Carries bundles, begins to ride bicycle, jumps rope, chins self, can catch tennis ball	Ties shoes, uses scissors, uses knife and fork, washes self with help

BIOPSYCHOSOCIAL INFLUENCES ON PHYSICAL DEVELOPMENT

Physical development impacts all aspects of children's lives, but the interplay between biological, psychological, and social forces plays a huge role in developmental outcomes. Some major forces that interact to influence physical development are as follows:

- *Genetic elements.* Genes, which we inherit from our parents, control growth to some degree. The genetic growth plan is created at conception and functions throughout the lifespan.

- *Nutrition.* Active preschoolers need a well-balanced diet. Healthy eating habits established in early childhood last a lifetime.

- *Disease.* Short-term illnesses do not permanently impede growth rate, although if the child's diet is consistently weak, problems can occur. Major disease usually causes a slowing of growth, followed by a catch-up period if the situation improves.

- *Psychological issues.* Stress and anxiety are associated with a predisposition to physical and mental disorders (Rutter & Taylor, 2002), but they certainly impact ordinary experiences, such as transition to school and relationships with new adults. For some children, seemingly simple experiences can feel traumatic.

- *Socioeconomic status.* Children from different socioeconomic backgrounds differ in average body size at all ages. A consistent pattern appears in research studies, indicating that children in more favorable circumstances develop differently than those growing up under less favorable economic conditions, perhaps due to factors including nutrition, sleep, and recreation (Graham, 2005).

The forces described above illustrate the influence of biopsychosocial interactions. It's impossible to argue that physical growth is determined solely by heredity or the environment. The neuroscientist Lise Eliot (2000) summarizes this reality when she notes that while genes direct the formation of the organs of the nervous system, experience ultimately determines the extent of children's brain development. An array of factors combine to explain skills acquired throughout development.

Physical changes, while observable and exciting, are not the only significant changes occurring during early childhood. Young children's cognitive abilities develop with their increasing use of ideas and rapid growth in language.

Theories of cognitive development help explain what is happening in the cognitive world of young children.

Cognitive Development

Piaget's theory of cognitive development is perhaps the best-known theory relating to children's thinking, yet other ideas about children's intellect provide additional insights into children's competence in early childhood and the mechanisms that enable them to make sense of the world, such as Vygotsky's consideration of social and cultural influences and information-processing theory.

PIAGET'S PREOPERATIONAL PERIOD

During Piaget's **preoperational period,** young children begin to use symbols to represent objects and events in their environment, and the relationships among them. They remember and talk about their memories, which signals growing symbolic ability and language acquisition. They gradually acquire the basics of their language, a feat of such magnitude that its secret still eludes scholars.

In early childhood, children become more comfortable with symbols, such as reading and understanding what they read. They continue to explore and learn about their environment through their play. Yet their mental ability during these years remains limited. For Piaget, *preoperational* refers to children who cannot take two things into consideration at the same time (a flower is both red and a tulip), who cannot return to the beginning of a thought sequence (how to reverse the action of $3 + 2 = 5$), and who cannot believe that the properties of substances remain the same even if you change their shape or arrangement. These children are at a level of thinking that precedes operational thought (thinking marked by reversible mental actions).

Features of the Preoperational Period

For Piaget, the great accomplishment of the preoperational period is a growing ability to represent, which is how we record or express information. For example, the word "car" is a **representation,** because it stands for the idea of something with wheels that people drive. Pointing an index finger at a playmate and saying "Stick 'em up" is also an example of representation, because it refers to a specific type of play with guns and "bad guys."

Other activities typical of preoperational children reflect their use of internal representation and include the following:

- **Animism** Young children tend to believe that inanimate objects have thoughts and feelings like they do. At the preoperational stage, children attribute actions and abilities to objects and animals. You'll

preoperational period Piaget's second stage of cognitive development, extending from about 2 to 7 years.

representation A child's application of abstract thinking during the preoperational period.

animism Children's preoperational activity in which they consider inanimate objects to possess human thought, feelings, and actions.

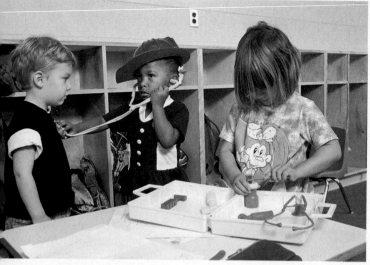

Imitative and symbolic play

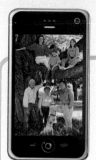
notice that most children's literature features animals as the main characters, which supports this kind of thinking.

- **Deferred imitation** Preoperational children can imitate some action or event they previously witnessed; for example, they walk like an animal they saw at the zoo earlier in the day.

- **Symbolic play** Children enjoy pretending that they are someone or something else. Piaget argued eloquently for recognizing the importance of play in a youngster's life. As children adapt to social and physical worlds that they only slightly understand and appreciate, they must have some outlet that permits them to assimilate reality to themselves. Children find this possible through play, using the tools characteristic of symbolic play.

deferred imitation Children's preoperational behavior that continues after they witnessed the original action or event.

symbolic play Children's mental representation of an object or event and reenactment of it in their play; one object may represent a different object in the play scenario.

egocentrism Piaget's term for the child's focus on self in early phases of cognitive development.

centration Feature of preoperational thought; the centering of attention on one aspect of an object and the neglecting of any other features.

Limitations of Preoperational Thought

Although we see the steady development of thought during this period, preoperational thought has several limitations. In the period of preoperational thought, children cannot assume the role of another person or recognize that other viewpoints exist, a state called **egocentrism.** In Piaget's classic experiment, illustrated in Figure 6.4, a child is shown a display of three mountains varying in height and color. The child stands on one side of the table, looking at the mountains; a doll is then placed at various spots around the mountains. The child is next shown several pictures of the mountains and asked to pick the one that shows what

FIGURE 6.4

Piaget's Mountains Task

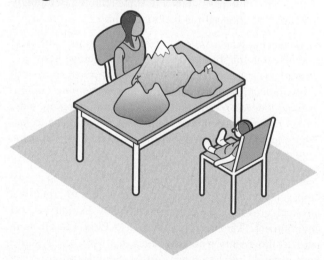

part of the mountains the doll saw. Egocentric children pick the photo that shows the mountains as they saw them.

Another striking feature of preoperational thought is **centration,** the centering of attention on one aspect of an object and the neglecting of any other features. Preoperational children are unable to notice features that would give balance to their reasoning. A good example of this is

FIGURE 6.5

Piaget's Conservation Task

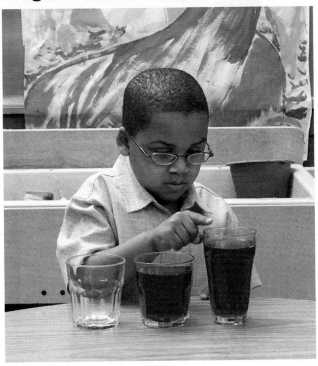

the process of **classification.** Piaget and Inhelder (1969) provide a fascinating example of the limitations of classification at this age. If there are 8 roses and 4 daisies, preoperational youngsters can differentiate between the roses and the daisies. But when asked if there are more flowers or more roses, preoperational children will generally say there are more roses than flowers. The understanding that subclasses can be part of a larger class does not appear until about age 8.

Another limitation of the period is the lack of **conservation,** the understanding that an object retains certain properties no matter how its form changes. The most popular illustration is to show a young child two identical glasses, each half-filled with water, as shown in Figure 6.5. The child agrees that each glass contains an equal amount. But if you then pour the water from one of the glasses into a taller, thinner glass, the preoperational child now says that the new glass contains more liquid because the water level is now higher. Children consider only the appearance of the liquid and ignore what happened. They also do not perceive the reversibility of the transformation—if they pour the water back into the original glass, the amounts of water will be equal.

Reversibility is a cognitive act in which a child recognizes that she can use stages of reasoning to solve a problem and then proceed in reverse, tracing the steps back to the original question or premise. The preoperational child's thought is irreversible, and although the child is able to rationalize her thinking and actions, the adults see the contradictions in the child's logic.

Evaluation of Piaget

Piaget's theory has been tested, retested, challenged, and refuted in many respects. Training studies have repeatedly shown that young children possess more cognitive competence than Piaget believed. For example, 4-year-olds can be taught conservation (Bjorklund, 2000). (See the conservation task illustrated in Figure 6.6). Other theories complement Piaget's theory and fill some of the gaps that critics identify as weaknesses in understanding children's cognitive development.

> **classification** Ability to group objects with some similarities within a larger category.
>
> **conservation** The understanding that an object retains certain properties even though surface features change.
>
> **reversibility** A cognitive act in which a child recognizes that she can use stages of reasoning to solve a problem and then trace the steps back to the original question or premise.

FIGURE 6.6

Conservation Tasks

Type of Conservation	Initial Presentation	Manipulation	Preoperational Child's Answer
Number	Two identical rows of objects are shown to the child, who agrees they have the same number.	One row is lengthened and the child is asked whether one row now has more objects.	Yes, the longer row.
Matter	Two identical balls of clay are shown to the child. The child agrees that they are equal.	The experimenter changes the shape of one of the balls and asks the child whether they still contain equal amounts of clay.	No, the longer one has more.
Length	Two sticks are aligned in front of the child. The child agrees that they are the same length.	The experimenter moves one stick to the right, then asks the child if they are equal in length.	No, the one on the top is longer.

VYGOTSKY'S THEORY

Recognizing that children do not develop in isolation, Vygotsky stressed the role of social interactions and learning contexts, two areas less emphasized by Piaget but deserving much attention. Both Vygotsky and Piaget believed learning to be an active process, known as **constructivism** in the fields of education and psychology, but Vygotsky's attention to social influences gave rise to the term **social constructivism.**

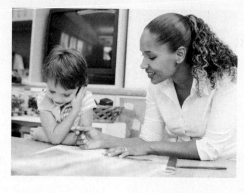

One of the social influences that Vygotsky stressed as important to children's learning is instruction, which may be formal, such as teacher–child instruction in the classroom, or informal, such as parent–child interaction at the dinner table. Vygotsky developed the term **zone of proximal development (ZPD)** to refer to the range of ability that a child has when faced with a task. The range includes what a child can do alone and what a child can do with guidance from adults or older children, and it reflects the dynamic nature of children's cognitive abilities at a given point in time. With practice or assistance from others, children's zones of proximal development can improve greatly.

The concept of **scaffolding** is linked to the ZPD and refers to the systematic support that a child receives from a parent or teacher to help him get from one point to the next in a given task. For example, a first-grade teacher wouldn't expect a 6-year-old to know how to write a journal entry on the first day of school. By the end of the year, when the child has had direct instruction and practice writing, editing, and "publishing," he will have a well-formed idea of what is involved in writing a journal entry. Just as we notice scaffolding on the outside of buildings under construction, children's thinking is supported through smaller, structured tasks on the way to completing a larger task.

INFORMATION-PROCESSING THEORY

In early childhood, children process huge amounts of information. Information-processing theory attempts to explain the ways in which children's thinking develops. Rather than being attributed to one individual theorist, such as Piaget or Vygotsky, information-processing theory provides a broad theory of children's cognitive development that has been interpreted and adapted by different theorists since the 1960s. The underlying belief is that as children develop strategies to notice and process information, they are better able to retain and recall this information (Munakata, 2006). Major factors in information-processing theory provide both energy and capacity for cognitive mechanisms to function.

Attention involves a lengthy process in which children translate what they know into appropriate actions and then rely on these strategies to gather new information. Selective attention—the ability to focus on specific activities or stimuli—becomes increasingly important as children move through early childhood and become better at concentrating on pertinent information. The selectivity with which children focus their attention on relevant items increases greatly between 3 and 8 years. Much the same holds true for memory.

Memory

Unlike Piaget's or Vygotsky's theories, information-processing theory assumes that our minds, like computers, have a limited space with which to operate efficiently. It is therefore critical that children (1) develop strategies for attending to relevant information to carry out tasks, (2) remember relevant information using rehearsal and organization strategies, and (3) retrieve information relevant to the task.

During the early childhood years, children begin to develop memory strategies, such as rehearsal, organization, and retrieval. **Rehearsal** (repeating target information) allows children to hold on to information for as long as possible, increasing the possibility of storing the information in long-term memory, memory that can last from a few days to decades. Such strategies also impact short-term memory (up to 30 seconds, or longer with rehearsal), as children actively work on tasks in the immediate, present situation.

Organization (discovering or imposing structure on a set of items to guide behavior) allows children to group items in chunks and reduce the number of things they are trying to remember. If a child is shown a list of 20 items to

---

constructivism The belief that children create, organize, and transform knowledge through active engagement in their environment.

social constructivism The belief that children construct knowledge through social interactions.

zone of proximal development (ZPD) The range of ability a child possesses on a given task, from working independently to working with assistance from adults or older children.

scaffolding The systematic use of support to assist a child in his or her performance on a given task.

rehearsal Mnemonic strategy that describes a person repeating target information.

organization Memory strategy that entails discovering and imposing an easy-to-remember structure on items to be memorized.

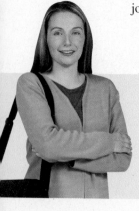

Career Apps

As a day care provider, how might you satisfy the desire of a screaming 3-year-old who wants two cookies at snack time, when his parents explicitly asked you to limit his sugary treats? (Hint: Most cookies break easily.)

Harlem Children's Zone

Harlem Children's Zone (HCZ) is an organization that embodies the notion of social interaction impacting children's thinking and overall development. Under the leadership of president and CEO Geoffrey Canada (who was named to the "Top 50 Power and Influence" list in *The Nonprofit Times* for 2009), HCZ is in its 35th year offering innovative programs designed to address problems such as failing schools, violence, crime, and poor health, and to break the cycle of poverty for more than 17,000 families in Harlem. Classroom support includes volunteers from AmeriCorps participating in the Harlem Peacemakers program, which trains young people to help make neighborhoods safe for children and families; the Harlem Gems preschool program, an all-day pre-kindergarten program that prepares children to enter kindergarten; and the Promise Academy, a public charter school. The impact of the HCZ's programs on families and the larger community helps to ensure that the scaffolding children experience extends beyond the classroom.

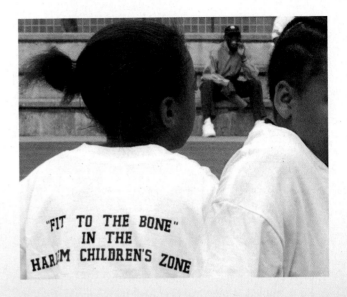

remember, organizing the items into 5 categories relating to function would help the child remember the list. Such strategies allow much information processing to occur in the mind's limited space.

Retrieval (obtaining information from memory) takes two forms: recognition and recall. Most children find recognition tasks fairly simple, but recall offers a challenge.

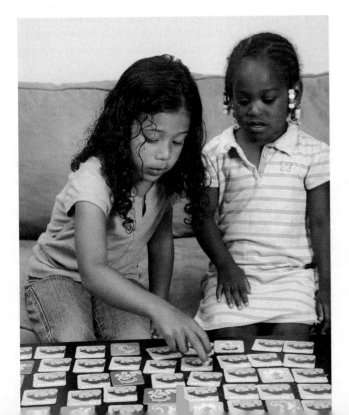

An older child tends to use spontaneous retrieval cues, such as remembering what color shirt she was wearing when she ate a certain flavor of ice cream, more often than a preschooler will.

THEORY OF MIND

As children's cognitive processes develop, they become aware of their own thinking and begin to understand that the thinking of others may be different than their own. Known as **theory of mind** (Flavell, 1999), children's understanding of their own thoughts and mental processes develops throughout childhood. Around ages 2 to 3 years, children begin to understand what it means to desire something, and they also realize that the success or failure to obtain something results in related feelings of happiness, sadness, frustration, and so on. A key development around ages 4 to 5 years is the ability to recognize false beliefs—beliefs that are not true.

One study of false beliefs involved a box of Band-Aids (Jenkins & Astlington, 1996). Children were asked what was inside the box, but when they opened the box to verify their answers, they found pencils inside! The children were then asked what other children might think was inside the box. Three-year-old children often answered, "Pencils," whereas 5-year-old children often answered, "Band-Aids!"

retrieval Memory strategy that enables obtaining information from memory; includes recognition and recall.

theory of mind Children's understanding of their own thoughts and mental processes.

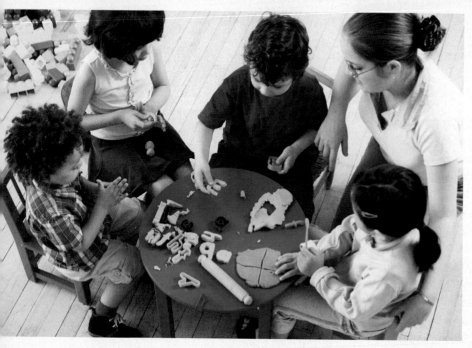

sider when choosing an optimal educational environment?

CONSTRUCTIVIST APPROACHES TO LEARNING

Early childhood programs based on developmental theory rather than behavioral theory reflect constructivism, an approach to learning influenced by Piaget's and Vygotsky's theories. In the **constructivist approach,** children are encouraged to be active participants in constructing knowledge and learn by interacting with their environment. Early childhood programs integrate content so that one cooking activity can meet state standards for math (quantity), science (measuring ingredients, noting changes in temperature), and literacy (reading a recipe). Relationships with others are stressed, including teacher–child, child–child, caregiver–child, and all permutations. The value of social interaction is seen in examples of collaborative activities, such as children working at clusters of desks, rather than sitting at individual desks in rows.

The older children could understand that other children could be fooled as they had been, but the younger children were tied to the reality of what was actually in the box.

Early Childhood Education

Early childhood education refers to classrooms for infants through 8-year-olds, but most people think of preschool and kindergarten when they hear the term *early childhood*. As Howard Gardner (2003) noted, two considerations are critical in any early childhood program: assumptions about the minds of children and our views about the kind of society we desire. Are children's minds empty vessels to be filled, or are children curious and competent? Are children equal citizens in a community, entitled to rights and privileges like adults, or are they not? Classroom expectations and responsibilities will reflect such beliefs in the environment and materials that children encounter. Early childhood education tends to reflect a rich mixture of ideas from educational philosophy and educational and developmental psychology.

An understanding of the complexities of children's thinking at different developmental levels is important as educators design classroom practices that are appropriate for young children. As you read about different approaches to early childhood education in this section, recall the case study of Amshula Khare from Chapter 2, and consider what you know about children's development. Which approach might be best suited for Amshula? What factors in her family context are important to con-

Although Piaget never specified using his developmental theory as part of a constructivist approach to learning, his emphasis on a child's progression through cognitive stages has clear implications for classroom practice, such as use of materials. For example, a 3-year-old might not be able to complete a jigsaw puzzle successfully, whereas a 6-year-old can complete a jigsaw puzzle more easily, as well as describe specific strategies he uses to work with puzzles, such as finding all of the straight-edged pieces first. Piaget's theory stresses children's active interactions with their environment, not the rote memorization of facts. Rather than expecting children to memorize names of animals based on seeing pictures of them, providing colorful plastic or wooden animal figures and a farm area to play with (or taking a field trip to a farm) is a more engaging learning strategy, as children create their own meaning from the experiences.

constructivist approach
Learning approach in which children are encouraged to be active participants in constructing knowledge and learn by interacting with their environment.

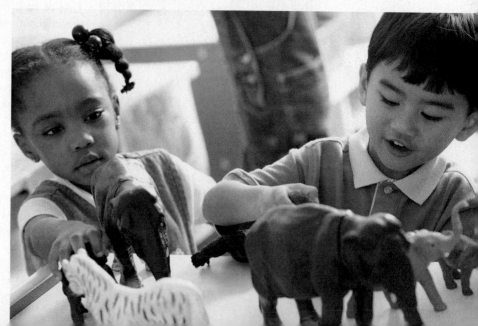

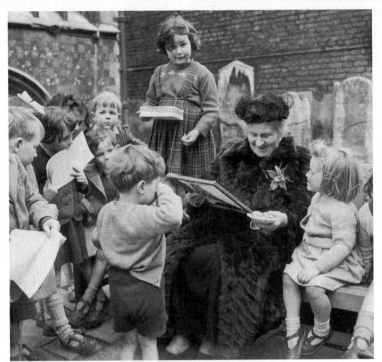

Maria Montessori with her students.

Chapter 5 are a beautiful example of the Reggio Emilia philosophy in action.

In the Reggio Emilia schools, the classroom and school environment are considered another teacher, which means that beauty, nature, and transparency (to foster communication between individuals) are explicitly demonstrated in many ways—from placement of windows in the building to allow ample natural light and views into other classrooms to the array of natural materials from which children create sculptures, collages, and other creations. Many people have the misperception that Reggio Emilia–inspired schools in the United States are for children from wealthy, advantaged families. On the contrary, some of the most inspirational work has been conducted in urban, economically challenged schools, such as the work in the Chicago Commons Reggio Exploration (see www.chicagocommons.org and *We Are All Explorers: Learning and Teaching with Reggio Principles in Urban Settings* by Scheinfeld, Haigh, and Scheinfeld, 2008).

Maria Montessori (1870–1952), an Italian educator, was a vocal proponent of early childhood programs. She believed that developing children pass through different physical and mental growth phases that alternate with periods of transition, suggesting that there are times when a child is especially ready for certain types of learning. These periods—called **sensitive periods**—differ so sharply that Montessori referred to them as a "series of new births."

Another Italian influence in early childhood education comes not from one person, but from an entire community. Recognized in 1991 by *Newsweek* magazine as some of the best preschools in the world, the schools in Reggio Emilia, Italy (also see discussion in Chapter 5), embody an approach to early childhood education that has been widely embraced around the world (Edwards, Gandini, & Forman, 1998).

Following the devastation of World War II, community members in Reggio Emilia began the process of rebuilding schools brick by brick. A young teacher named Loris Malaguzzi visited Reggio Emilia and, inspired by what he observed, became the driving force behind what came to be the first infant–toddler centers and preschools of the community. Viewing children as curious and competent citizens with rights and valuable contributions, educators and families in Reggio Emilia value collaboration and support children's developing interests. Experts in pedagogy and art work with classroom teachers on a daily basis to document and extend the learning that occurs in the classrooms. The pictures of Laura at the beginning of

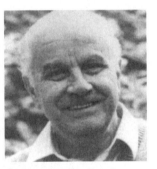

Loris Malaguzzi, founder of the Reggio Emilia approach.

HEAD START

Head Start is a national program to increase school readiness among children by providing educational, health, nutrition, social, and other services to low-income children and their families. It was originally conceived as part of President Lyndon Johnson's War on Poverty in the 1960s and has enrolled more than 24 million preschool-aged children in its programs since its inception in 1965. Early Head Start programs began in 1995 and address prenatal, infant, and toddler-aged children and their families. In 2007, the Office of Head Start had a budget of about $7 billion to provide services to the one million children registered in its almost 20,000 Head Start Centers (Office of Head Start, 2007). Recent funding under the American Recovery and Reinvestment Act (ARRA) has allocated an additional $1 billion in funds and grants to Head Start programs.

Head Start centers feature the characteristics of good preschools: low teacher-child ratio, specially trained teachers, availability of resources, and recognition of children's individual differences. The programs are designed to provide children with age-appropriate, enriching, enjoyable experiences. Although the long-term benefits of Head Start have been debated, research shows that participants in high-quality intervention programs are less likely to cost taxpayers money for subsequent health, educational, and public assistance services.

sensitive periods Montessori's term for periods of children's development marked by sensitivity/readiness to learn.

Head Start Government-supported early childhood program that provides education, health, and parenting education services to low-income families.

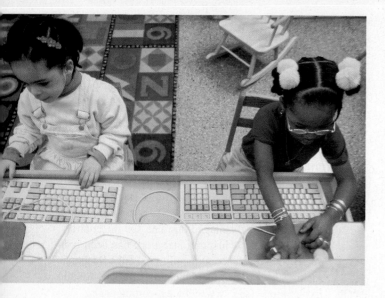

LANGUAGE RULES

As children acquire the basics of their language, they learn the guidelines that make language a powerful tool. For example, by the age of 4 or 5, children know that rules exist for combining sounds into words, that individual words have specific meanings, and that there are rules for combining words into meaningful sentences and participating in a dialogue. These rules help children to detect the meaning of a word with which they are unfamiliar. Rules also provide a foundation from which children create their own expressive vocabulary and become more active participants in their environment.

The rules can be summarized as follows:

- Rules of phonology describe a language's sound system—that is, how to put sounds together to form words. Children notice and imitate sounds in rhymes, songs, and names, even creating their own sounds to represent objects and happenings in their world.

- Rules of syntax determine sentence structure and word order. Children realize that word placement changes with a question or statement, such as when they ask, "Where doggie go?" versus stating "Doggie go home."

- Rules of semantics describe how to interpret the meaning of words. Children gain new vocabulary words at an amazing rate between ages 18 months and 6 years, aiding their understanding of new words in relation to familiar ones.

- Rules of pragmatics describe how language is used in social contexts, how people converse. Children learn to speak about past, present, and future events accordingly, and they tailor their speech to speak to younger children (and animals!), whom older children recognize might not be as advanced in their own speech.

FIGURE 6.7
Head Start Data

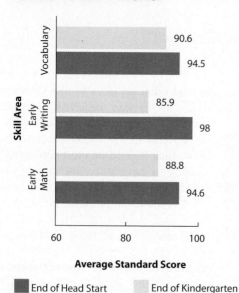

Research has shown that Head Start graduates make further academic progress toward national benchmarks in kindergarten.
Source: FACES, 2000.

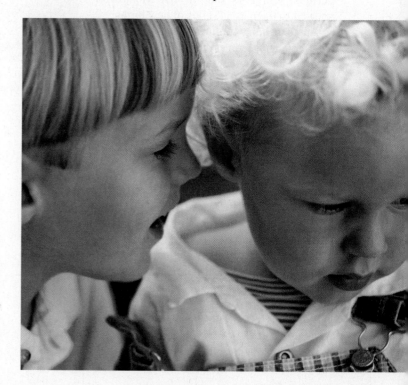

Language Development

Language acquisition is a key milestone in early childhood development. With no formal training, and often exposed to incorrect language models, children learn sounds, combine sounds into words, and—following a complex sequence of grammatical rules—form sentences. The acquisition of language skills is an accomplishment that is often taken for granted, yet by the time children are ready to enter first grade, most have a vocabulary of about 14,000 words; use questions, negative statements, and dependent clauses; and have learned to use language in a variety of social situations. They are relatively sophisticated language users.

As we trace the path of language development in the early childhood years, children clearly show an ability for **receptive language** before they produce language themselves, **expressive language.** They are able to indicate that they understand words before they are able to articulate them themselves.

> *Simply by making noises*
> *with our* mouths, *we can*
> *reliably cause precise new*
> combinations *of ideas*
> *to arise in each other's* minds.

STEVEN PINKER

LANGUAGE IRREGULARITIES

When speech emerges, children tend to use certain language irregularities that are quite normal and to be expected. For example, **overextensions** mark children's beginning words. Assume that a child has learned the name of the house pet, doggy. Think what that label means: an animal with a head, tail, body, and four legs. Now consider what other animals "fit" this label: cats, horses, donkeys, and cows. Consequently, children may briefly apply "doggy" to all four-legged creatures; they quickly eliminate overextensions, however, as they learn about their world.

Overregularization is a similar phenomenon in which children extend regular grammatical rules to irregular words. As youngsters begin to use two- and three-word sentences, they struggle to convey more-precise meanings by mastering the grammatical rules of their language. For example, many English verbs add *-ed* to indicate past tense. Youngsters who do not know that the past tense of *come* is *came* may say "Daddy comed home" instead of "Daddy came home."

During the early childhood years, children begin to display a growing mastery of meaning. As their vocabulary continues to increase dramatically, they begin to combine words to refine their meaning. Yet they also must learn to suggest the correct meaning for the correct word. For example, saying, "Right!" could indicate correctness or direction. Sometimes children's levels of understanding are more advanced than their language ability, so instead of saying, "That dog licked me!" a young child might say, "I got tongued!" Their meaning is still clear.

As children come to the end of the early childhood period, several language milestones have been achieved. At this point, children

- are skillful at building words, adding suffixes such as *-er, -man,* and *-ist* to form nouns (the person who teaches is a *teacher*);

- are comfortable with passive sentences (the glass *was broken* by the rock);

- can pronounce almost all speech sounds accurately;

- have experienced the "language explosion"—vocabulary has grown rapidly; and

- are aware of grammatical correctness.

One of the most noticeable features of children's language development is a child's ability to express herself and communicate ideas and feelings to others. A developing awareness of the self involves a complex interaction between numerous biopsychosocial variables that affect individual children.

The Self Emerges

Young children's cognitive and emotional development paves the way for greater self-awareness in all aspects of development. How do children construct a sense of self—this sense of who they are and what makes them different from everyone else? Children's increasing ability to understand people and happenings in the world provides them with deeper insights into themselves. Children recognize that they are individuals as well as members of a larger group.

THE DEVELOPMENT OF SELF

Initially, in describing themselves, most children tend to focus on physical characteristics—hair color, color of eyes, presence of freckles, and so on—or on tangible things such as food and toys. As children grow, their sense of self isn't limited to their reflections in a mirror, and they have acquired language to tell us what they think of themselves. Their self-judgments reflect their changing cognitive and social maturity. As representational thinking continues to improve and they compare their performances with those of others, more realistic evaluations begin to appear (Harter, 2006).

Erik Erikson categorized early childhood as the stage when children grapple with initiative versus guilt. They experience a tension between their increasing abilities and their developing conscience. Although they may feel proud and confident with their initiative to tackle various challenges, they also feel the effects of judgment from self and others. Examples of this are when a 5-year-old tries to pour herself a bowl of Cheerios and the Cheerios spill all over the table, or when a 6-year-old reads aloud from a favorite book and his older brother corrects his pronunciation of words. Interestingly, the opinions of others become increasingly important as children strive to establish their self-understanding.

Social Development

When we consider the interplay between many variables affecting

receptive language The ability of the child to understand written and spoken language.

expressive language The language children use to express their ideas and needs.

overextensions A language irregularity in which children apply a word in a broad manner to objects that do not fit.

overregularization Children's strict application of language rules they have learned.

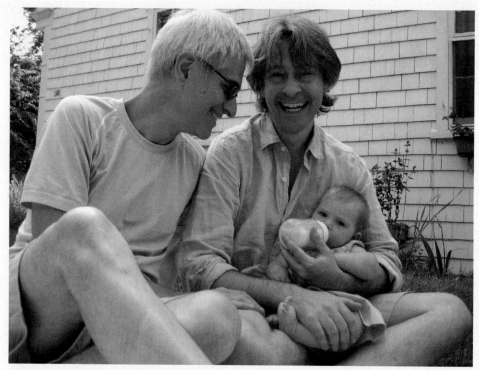

Authors of the children's book And Tango Makes Three, *Justin Richardson and Peter Parnell recently welcomed daughter Gemma into their family.*

and children construct their relationships together, and no one model fits all. Diana Baumrind's (1967, 1971, 1986, 1991a, 1991b) pioneering work on parenting style identified three kinds of parental behavior, and later research (Maccoby & Martin, 1983) suggested a fourth style of parenting that impacts children's development and family relationships.

• **Authoritarian parenting** These parents are demanding, and for them immediate obedience is the most desirable trait in a child. When there is any conflict between these parents and their children, no consideration is given to the child's view or communication. It's a simple case of "Do it my way or else!"

• **Authoritative parenting** These parents respond to their children's needs and wishes. Believing in parental control, they attempt to explain the reasons for it to their children. Authoritative parents expect mature behavior and will enforce rules, but they encourage their children's independence and attempts to reach their potential.

• **Permissive parenting** These parents take a tolerant, accepting view of their children's behavior, including both aggressive and sexual urges. They rarely use punishment or make demands of their children. Children make almost all their own decisions.

• **Uninvolved/neglectful parenting** These parents tend to be quite detached from their children's lives. They place few demands on their children, but are also unresponsive and communicate little, while still tending to their children's basic needs. In the extreme, these parents may reject or neglect their children.

human development, we realize that social relationships influence children both directly and indirectly. Children's developing sense of self, combined with the ability to express themselves and appreciate the perspective of others, is very much influenced by their relationships with family and peers.

THE ROLE OF THE FAMILY

Parenting styles, sibling relationships, and other caregivers can impact children in positive and negative ways. Despite many changes that have occurred in the definition of family over time, the vast majority of individuals live in some type of family, which testifies to the enduring strength of the family as the basic social structure.

PARENTING STYLES

Parents do many things—select clothes, limit television time, and enforce rules—but they alone can't determine the nature of the relationship with their children. Parents

In a longitudinal study from preschool to adolescence, Baumrind (1991c) found that authoritative parenting was associated with positive developmental outcomes. More

The family generally, and **parenting** *specifically, are today in a greater state of flux, question, and redefinition than perhaps ever before. We are witnessing the emergence of striking* **permutations** *on the theme of parenting: blended families, lesbian and gay parents, teen versus 50s first-time moms and dads.*

MARC BORNSTEIN, *HANDBOOK OF PARENTING* **(2002)**

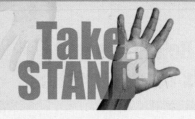

No child is perfect, and most parents are concerned about what to do when their children misbehave. Punishment generally takes one of two paths: Something unpleasant is done to a child (scolding or corporal punishment, i.e., spanking), or something pleasant is withdrawn (temporary loss of a video game).

Most child experts, including pediatricians, oppose the use of corporal punishment for many reasons, mostly because it too often leads to child abuse. New research indicates that corporal punishment can lead to lower IQs in children (Straus & Paschall, 2009). Nonphysical methods, such as positive reinforcement, time-out, or removal of privileges are more desirable. Still, spanking is routinely used by many parents who believe it is the most effective form of punishment (see Figure 6.9).

Do you think that corporal punishment is a valuable way to handle a child who misbehaves? Would you spank your child?

FIGURE 6.8

Effects of Spanking on Cognitive Activity

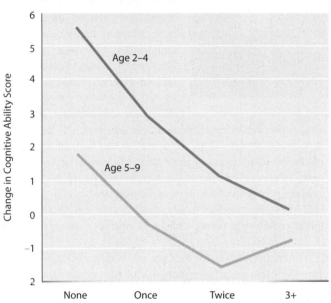

American children who were spanked had a lower cognitive ability 4 years later than those who were not spanked.

dren's characteristics in response to the four types of parental behavior.

THE ROLE OF SIBLINGS

Because of their behavior toward one another, siblings create a unique family environment and play a critical role in socialization. In early childhood, older siblings often act as caregivers for their younger brothers and sisters, which provides opportunities for them to learn about the needs of others (Eisenberg, Fabes, & Spinrad, 2006). Older siblings become models for younger children to imitate. Older siblings often ease the way for younger ones by running interference with parents. In this way, bonds are formed that usually last a lifetime, often longer than those between husband and wife or parent and child.

authoritarian parenting
Baumrind's term for parents who are demanding and want immediate obedience as the most desirable trait in a child.

authoritative parenting
Baumrind's term for parents who respond to their child's needs and wishes; they believe in parental control and attempt to explain the reasons for it to their child.

permissive parenting Baumrind's term for parents who take a tolerant, accepting view of their child's behavior and rarely make demands or use punishment.

uninvolved/neglectful parenting Term for parents who are undemanding and emotionally unsupportive of their child.

recent research suggests that in some ethnic groups authoritarian parenting leads to positive outcomes (Chao, 2001), stressing the role of context in development. It's important to remember that Baumrind's findings don't necessarily indicate a cause-and-effect relationship between the categories and a child's characteristics. A child's temperament also affects how she or he is treated. Table 6.2 lists chil-

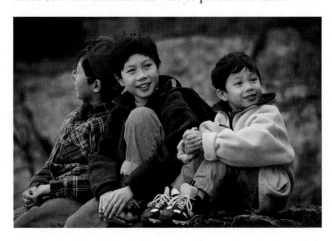

TABLE 6.2

Parental Behaviors and Children's Characteristics

Parental Behaviors			
Authoritarian	*Authoritative*	*Permissive*	*Uninvolved*
Children's Characteristics			
Withdrawn	Self-assertive	Impulsive	Antisocial
Lack of enthusiasm	Independent	Low self-reliance	Low self-regulation
Shy (girls)	Friendly	Low self-control	Low self-control
Hostile (boys)	Cooperative	Low maturity	Low maturity
Low need	High need	Aggressive	High need
Achievement	Achievement	Low achievement	Low achievement
Low competence	High competence	Lack of responsibility	Low competence

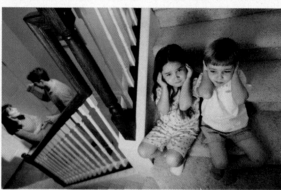

As young children make sense of their world, siblings act as nonthreatening sounding boards for one another. New behaviors, new roles, and new ideas can be tested on siblings, and their reactions, whether positive or negative, lack the doomsday quality of many parental judgments. Siblings also form subsystems that are the basis for the formation of powerful coalitions, often called the **sibling underworld.** Older siblings can warn their younger brothers and sisters about parental moods and prohibitions, thus averting problems. An older sibling can also contribute to a sense of inferiority as the younger child struggles to keep up with the older sibling. There are many complex issues related to sibling relationships, including sibling rivalry, birth order, and only children. Some common perceptions about siblings exist, such as that first-borns tend to be more motivated and academically oriented and that only children tend to interact more comfortably with adults and are highly verbal. Generalizations about birth order and only children must be considered in light of the specific family context and should not become stereotypes, even though many similarities exist between first-borns and between youngest siblings that have attracted attention in research studies. In general, however, research has shown that birth order has a limited ability to predict behavior.

sibling underworld Familial subsystem, or coalition, of brothers and/or sisters.

CHILDREN OF DIVORCE

The changes and stress associated with typical family life are challenging, but children in divorced families experience multiple challenges. Today's divorce rate is still about 50% of all first marriages and about 62% of remarriages; 60% of the divorces in the United States involve children. Examining the current state of children of divorce, Judith Wallerstein and her colleagues note that as a society we have not yet come to terms with a divorce culture (Wallerstein, Lewis, & Blakeslee, 2002). Expectations for relationships have changed, there is fear of commitment, and hesitancy to trust a companion's intentions and to express intimate feelings have impacted the nature of relationships. These have long-term influences on children's understanding of adults' behavior and responsibilities.

Because the conflict that leads to divorce begins long before the divorce itself, young children too often witness displays of hostility, anger, and arguments between their parents. Viewing angry adults is emotionally disturbing for children and may lead to childhood and adolescent problems such as aggression and poor psychological adjustment unless adults also model reconciliation and forgiveness (Friedman & Chase-Lansdale, 2002). Parents' actual separation may not be the major cause of any problem behavior, because too many other possible factors may have intervened, including exposure to conflict, economic decline, and erratic parenting. As families attempt to adjust to life after divorce, overall quality of life and parent–child relationships play an important role in children's long-term well-being.

Although studies of the age at which children most strongly experience the effects of divorce remain inconclusive, suspicion persists that young children are particularly vulnerable. Unable to understand the reasons for the family upset, they are more adversely affected by the divorce than are older children (Hetherington & Stanley-Hagan, 2002). Their ability to engage in abstract thinking is still limited, and they may think that they are responsible for the divorce. During early childhood, children may demonstrate intense separation anxiety and fear of abandonment by both parents (Hetherington & Stanley-Hagan, 1995; Lamb et al., 1999).

Some researchers have explored whether children are better off living in intact families where parents may be fighting or unhappy than in divorced families, and the findings vary. Most agree that children from divorced families show poorer adjustment and are more likely to have social

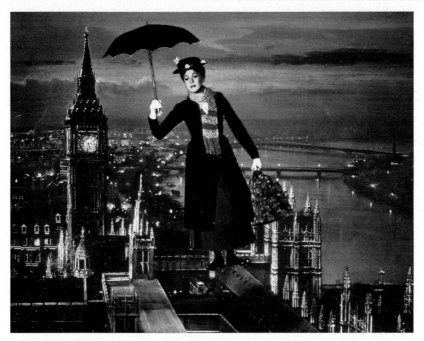

"Mary Poppins, practically perfect in every way."

and academic problems than children who live in intact families where parents are fighting or unhappy (Conger & Chao, 1996; Hetherington, 2005). Yet one study found that an overwhelming majority of adult children of divorce believed their parents' decision to divorce was the right choice (Ahrons, 2004). Ultimately, children's temperament and support from outside caregivers have a significant impact on their overall adjustment.

NONPARENTAL CHILD CARE

In their thoughtful analysis of nonparental child care, Michael Lamb and Lieselotte Ahnert (2006) pose two questions intended to help researchers reshape their evaluation of modern child care:

- What type of and how much care do young children receive from adults other than their parents?

- What effects do such care arrangements have on the children's development?

These questions shape the direction of current research and evaluation, because we now realize that it is useless to ask simply whether child care is good or bad for children. Rather, researchers must examine the nature, extent, quality, and age at onset of child care as well as the characteristics of the children from different backgrounds and needs.

Facts About Day Care

When most people hear the term *caregiver*, they tend to think of day care. **Day care** typically refers to child care outside the home, as opposed to the more general term *child care*. Considering the fact that some children spend more time each day under the care of a day care provider than a parent, the influence of day care is significant because of its impact on children's development. Estimates are that there are over 116,000 licensed day-care centers in the United States and about 254,000 licensed family day-care settings (Children's Foundation, 2003).

The types of child care arrangement vary enormously: One mother may charge another mother several dollars to take care of her child; a relative may care for several family children; businesses may run large operations; some centers may be sponsored by local or state government as an aid to the less affluent; others are run on a pay-as-you-go basis. In 2009 the average annual cost of child care for one child in a day-care center was $4,000 to $11,000, according to the National Association of Child Care Resources and Referral Agencies. Almost everyone agrees that the best centers hire teachers with a background in early childhood education.

Existing research on day care offers the following conclusions:

- In the United States, the majority of children under 5 years of age receive some kind of nonparental day care (Clarke-Stewart & Allhusen, 2005; Harvey, 1999; Zigler & Finn-Stevenson, 1999).

- Attendance in a day-care facility can aid motor development and seems to be associated with increases in height and weight. However, children in day-care centers contract colds, flu, and ear infections earlier than children who do not attend day care. They tend to contract fewer illnesses after they begin school.

- Children who attend day-care programs are more independent of their mothers, but their attachment to their mothers is not threatened (Clarke-Stewart & Allhusen, 2005).

- Enrollment in day-care during early childhood does not aid or impede positive relationships with peers (Lamb & Ahnert, 2006).

- Children who attend day-care programs have advanced cognitive and language development (Clarke-Stewart & Allhusen, 2005).

- Nonparental child care may be associated with increased behavior problems, a result closely linked with the quality of care offered (Lamb & Ahnert, 2006).

- High-quality day care may have a positive effect on children's intellectual development (Clarke-Stewart & Allhusen, 2005).

Table 6.3 lists the characteristics of high-quality day care.

day care Services and care for children provided outside the children's home.

TABLE 6.3
Characteristics of High-Quality Day Care

Site Features	Functional Features
Good staff-child ratio	Concern with personal care
Superior staff education	Supervised motor activities
Good staff training	Attention to language
Higher staff wages	Opportunity for creativity
Attractive, safe environment	Social relationships encouraged

sex Biological maleness or femaleness.

gender Social/psychological aspects of being male or female.

gender identity The conviction that one is either male or female.

gender stereotypes Rigid beliefs about characteristics of males and females.

gender role Culturally defined expectations about how females and males should act.

Gender Development

Although expectations for gender roles are slowly changing, sharp differences of opinion are still evident. Many parents want their children to follow traditional gender roles (sports for boys, dolls for girls), whereas other parents want to break down what they consider to be rigid gender stereotypes. Young children are influenced by social interactions and come to recognize that qualities they notice in others reflect aspects of themselves. A boy who admires a classmate's ability to catch the ball and play "tough" during kickball may wish he was less afraid of getting hurt during a kickball game so that he could also display such bravery and skill.

Developmental psychologists have urged that the terms *sex* and *gender* be used carefully. Therefore, in this discussion, **sex** refers to biological maleness or femaleness (the sex chromosomes) and **gender** refers to the psychosocial aspects of maleness and femaleness.

Within this framework, we can distinguish among gender identity, gender stereotypes, and gender role.

- **Gender identity** is a conviction about being male or female.

- **Gender stereotypes** reflect rigid beliefs about the characteristics associated with being male or female.

- **Gender role** refers to culturally defined expectations about how females and males should act.

THEORIES OF GENDER DEVELOPMENT

Various theorists have seen gender development through a particular lens. The following are the most popular explanations, which have generated most of the research in this area:

- *Biological explanations.* Advocates of biological explanations of gender development have turned to the rapidly growing body of research relating to chromosomes and hormones. At about the sixth prenatal week, embryos start to differentiate into males and females. In male embryos, the Y chromosomes secrete hormones that eventually lead to development of male sex organs. In female embryos, lower levels of certain hormones permit development of female sex organs.

- *Social learning theory explanations.* Social learning theorists believe that parents, as the distributors of reinforcement, reinforce gender-role behaviors. By their choice of toys, by urging "boy" or "girl" behavior, and by reinforcing this behavior, parents encourage their children to engage in gender-specific behavior. Today's social learning theorists have incorporated cognition in their explanations (Bandura, 1997; Eisenberg, Martin, & Fabes, 1996). For example, if parents have a strong relationship with their children, they become models for their children to imitate, encouraging them to acquire additional gender-related behavior. Children also learn appropriate gender behavior from other social influences such as siblings, peers, media, and school (Ruble, Martin, & Berenbaum, 2006).

- *Cognitive development explanations.* The cognitive development perspective posits that children first acquire their sense of gender identity and then display and identify appropriate behaviors (Lips, 2007). In other words, as a result of cognitive development—as children construct their own understandings of the world—children begin to build concepts of maleness and femaleness (Unger & Crawford, 2000). In a home environment, a daughter's understanding of "dinnertime" may lead her to understand that women cook the meals and men watch television. She will likely ask her mom if she can help cooking family meals.

- *Gender schema explanations.* Gender schema theory is related to cognitive development theory. Whereas cognitive development explanations describe behavior that children develop once they've acquired a sense of their own gender, a gender schema explanation is visible when children attempt to organize the flow of information they receive every day. A schema is a mental blueprint for organizing information, and this theory proposes that children develop a schema for gender. Children form a network of mental associations about gender, which they use as a guide to interpret and store information about male and female before they've solidified any identity of their own (Margolis, 2005; Ruble & Martin, 1998; Ruble, Martin, & Berenbaum, 2006).

ACQUIRING GENDER IDENTITY

One of the first categories children form is sex related—there is a neat division in their minds between male and female. For example, children first indicate their ability to label their own sex and the sex of others between 2 and

3 years of age. By 4 years of age, children are aware that sex identity is stable over time. They then come to realize that sex identity remains the same despite any changes in clothing, hairstyle, or activities (Lips, 2007; Ruble, Martin, & Berenbaum, 2006).

Children move from the observable physical differences between the sexes and begin to acquire gender knowledge about the behavior expected of males and females. Depending on the source of this knowledge, gender-role stereotyping has commenced and attitudes toward gender are being shaped. What do we know about the forces influencing this process?

Role of the Family
Evidence clearly suggests that parents typically treat boy and girl babies differently—even before birth— by the toys they supply, the way they decorate the baby's room, and the type of gender behavior they encourage (Ruble, Martin, & Berenbaum, 2006). Adults tend to engage in rougher play with boys, give them stereotypical toys (cars and trucks, dinosaurs and soldiers), and speak differently to them than they do to girls. Parents often reinforce girls for playing with dolls and boys for playing with trucks, reinforce girls for helping their mothers around the house and boys for being brave. Parents are usually unaware of the extent to which they engage in this type of reinforcement.

Because about 80% of children have siblings and spend considerable time with them, sibling relationships also exercise considerable influence on gender identity. An older brother shows a younger brother how to hold a bat, and a younger sister watches her older sister play with dolls. Although same-sex siblings would seem to exercise a greater influence on gender-typed activities by modeling or reinforcing gender-appropriate behavior, the influence of other-sex siblings on gender typing is quite strong.

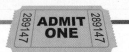

FEATURED MEDIA

Films About Childhood and Gender

***Billy Elliot* (2000)** – How does a boy balance his desire to please his father and follow his own heart to pursue ballet lessons? How can political and emotional issues impact all aspects of a young boy's life?

***Boys Don't Cry* (1999)** – How does a transgender teen find the courage to live life and find love in a society that holds no respect for any visible differences? What protection can society offer teens who find themselves in dangerous situations based on their human needs?

***Ma Vie en Rose (My Life in Pink)* (1997)** – What happens when a French boy's natural inclinations toward stereotypical girl behavior become more than passing fancy? How does the discomfort of others affect his identity?

***Mulan* (1998)** – What lengths would a Chinese girl go to save her father's life and her family's honor, and to risk severe penalties as a result of ignoring cultural expectations for women? How does the film's conclusion fit with implicit and explicit messages of the rest of the film?

Role of Peers
When children form friendships and play, activities often foster and maintain sex-typed play. Depending on the environment, when children engage in nonstereotypical play (boys with dolls, girls with a football), peers may make comments and even isolate them ("sissy," "tomboy"). Although these stereotypes have decreased in recent decades, the tendency to sexually compartmentalize behavior increases with age until most adolescents react to intense demands for conformity to stereotypical gender roles.

During development, youngsters of the same sex tend to play together, a custom called **sex cleavage.** If you think back on your own experiences, remember your friends at this age and recall how imitation, reinforcement, and cognitive development come together to intensify what a boy thinks is masculine and what a girl thinks is feminine.

Role of the Media
Another influence on gender development that carries important messages about what is desirable for males and females is the media, especially television. Television has assumed such a powerful place in the socialization of children, it is safe to say that it is almost as significant as family and peers. What is most disturbing is the stereotypical behavior that it presents as both positive and desirable. The more television children watch, the more stereotypical is their behavior (Lips, 2007).

With this brief examination of the biological and environmental forces that contribute to gender identity and the theories that attempt to explain the process, let's next look at what happens when gender stereotypes are formed.

sex cleavage Youngsters of the same sex tend to play and do things together.

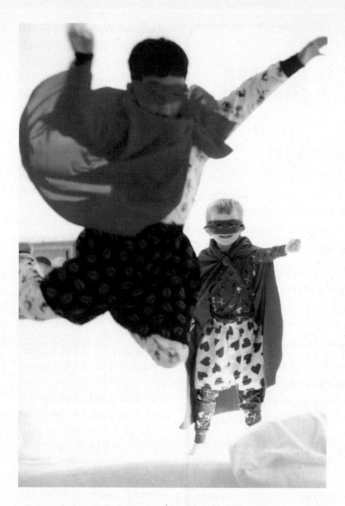

to change the sociopolitical culture in which they live, but play does provide children opportunities to be protagonists in their own physical, cognitive, and social development.

The Importance of Play

One thing that children do effortlessly and without training is to play. **Play** is an activity that children engage in because they enjoy it for its own sake. Some of the benefits of play are that it allows children to explore the environment on their own terms and to take in any meaningful experiences at their own rate and on their own level. Young children also play for the sheer exuberance of it, which enables them to exercise their bodies and improve motor skills. Such uninhibited behavior also permits children to relieve tension and cope with anxiety. When children play, they learn about themselves, others, and their world, and play becomes the medium through which other processes occur.

> *Play may be one of the most* **profound** *expressions of human nature and one of the greatest innate resources for learning and* **invention**.

MARTHA BRONSON, EARLY CHILDHOOD EDUCATOR AND ADVOCATE

Play in early childhood may also influence the learning skills and interests of the future. What children learn as "fun" can become the foundation for intrinsic motivation later. For example, a love of board games that involve counting dice or tallying numerical scores can lend itself to a child's desire to solve math problems. What kind of play did you enjoy as a child? How do you think it contributed to who you are today?

KINDS OF PLAY

In their efforts to understand the role of play in a child's life, scholars have presented several types of classification. One of the earliest and most enduring schemes was proposed in 1932 by Mildred Parten, who suggested categories of play that children tend to progress through as they mature:

- *Unoccupied play,* in which children are seen as observers and not actually engaged in any activity

- *Solitary play,* in which children play by themselves and are not involved with others

- *Onlooker play,* in which children watch others and do not become active themselves, but may call out suggestions or questions

GENDER STEREOTYPING

As mentioned earlier, gender stereotyping refers to beliefs that we have about characteristics and behavior associated with males and females. Recent research (Ruble, Martin, & Berenbaum, 2006) advances that children are aware of gender stereotypes by 2½ years of age and that knowledge of child and adult activities appears between 3 and 5 years peaking at about the time of entrance to first grade.

Video and computer games reflect and underscore gender stereotypes. In one year, the six best-selling computer games for girls were all Barbie games. Popular boys' games take them into virtual worlds where enemies are defeated, aliens are battled, and race cars break speed records. When the characteristics associated with a label create a negative image, problems arise. Even so-called positive images or stereotyping can be problematic, once people start to treat others according to the stereotype. The implications for such stereotyping are great, especially in the classroom context. Although sexual equality is widely accepted today, gender stereotyping is still alive and well. One way that young children can challenge stereotypes and attempt to gain mastery over their observations and ideas is through play. Girls can play the part of "Mommy" but can also be police officers who save the day. Boys can wear a dress and pocketbook in the dramatic play area but still build rocket ships with Lego bricks. It is not up to children

play Activity people engage in because they enjoy it for its own sake.

- *Parallel play,* in which children play beside, but not with, other children
- *Associative play,* in which children play with others but seem more interested in the social interactions than the activity itself
- *Cooperative play,* in which children play with others and are active participants in the goal of the activity

DEVELOPMENTAL ASPECTS OF PLAY

It is clear that play involves developing social skills and awareness of enjoyment, but children's play also impacts other areas of development. In a significant event held in 1989, the United Nations Convention on the Rights of the Child recognized that all children possess certain rights, including "the right of the child to rest and leisure, to engage in play and recreational activities appropriate to the age of the child and to participate freely in cultural life and the arts." Play is not simply a way to pass the time in between learning academic skills but, rather, a means through which critical thinking and other skills develop (see Figure 6.10).

Cognitive Development

Through play, children learn about the objects in their world, what these objects do, what they are made of, and how they work. To use Piaget's terms, children use symbols to represent their ideas and their world, and also learn behavioral skills that will help them in the future.

Vygotsky believed that play contributes significantly to cognitive development because children learn to use objects and actions appropriately and thus further their ability to think symbolically. Vygotsky (1978) also argued

FIGURE 6.9
Perceived Importance of Play

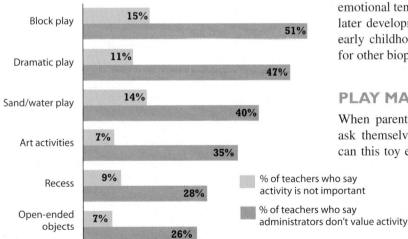

Block play — 15% / 51%
Dramatic play — 11% / 47%
Sand/water play — 14% / 40%
Art activities — 7% / 35%
Recess — 9% / 28%
Open-ended objects — 7% / 26%

% of teachers who say activity is not important

% of teachers who say administrators don't value activity

This graph shows teachers' views versus perceived administration views of the importance of various playful and creative activities.

Source: http://drupal6.allianceforchildhood.org/sites/allianceforchildhood.org/files/file/kindergarten_report.pdf

that children's imaginary situations provide zones of proximal development that function as mental support systems. Children's levels of play change as they are guided by the suggestions, hints, and ideas offered by peers and adults. As Vygotsky noted, children tend to play at a level above their average age and above their daily behavior. The safety afforded by imaginary scenarios allows children to pretend to do things that they would not be able to do in reality, as determined by their developmental abilities.

Social Development

Play helps social development during this period, because the involvement of others demands a give-and-take that teaches early childhood youngsters the basics of forming relationships. Social skills demand the same building processes as cognitive skills, and children begin to share symbolic meanings through their use of pretend play.

At 3 years of age, children prefer playmates of their own sex. Girls show a stronger preference than boys do at this age, but from 4 to 5 years it is boys who show a stronger preference for same-sex playmates, although they still play in mixed-sex groups. Gender differentiation from 3 to 5 years becomes ever more apparent. During free-play sessions in preschool and day-care centers, children of the same sex are the close partners, a trend that underscores the prevalence of sex cleavage.

Why are some 5- and 6-year-olds more popular with their classmates than others are? Watching closely, you can often discover the reasons: decreasing egocentrism, recognition of the rights of others, and a willingness to share. These social skills do not simply appear; they are learned, and much of the learning comes through play.

Emotional Development

Play helps children to master intense, sometimes overpowering, experiences that all children encounter. In their play, they avoid the right-or-wrong, life-and-death feelings that accompany interactions with adults. Children can be creative without worrying about failure and work out their emotional tensions through play. As children transition into later developmental periods of life, the lessons learned in early childhood will accompany them and form the basis for other biopsychosocial interactions.

PLAY MATERIALS

When parents shop for their children's toys, they might ask themselves a basic question: What kind of activities can this toy encourage? Too often, the answer is "nothing good." Today's toys frequently promote violence, involve candy, or depend on electronic technology that turns children into passive observers. As Martha Bronson (1995) noted, the play materials we supply our children are loaded with multiple messages. They not only cause children to do certain things because of the nature of the toy, they also convey messages about what

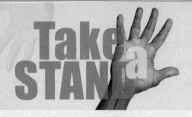

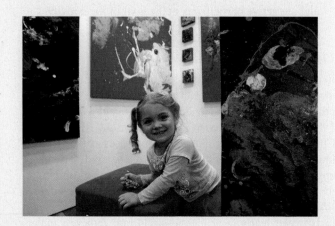

In October 2008, a gallery owner in Melbourne, Australia, was asked to consider showing the abstract paintings of an artist called Aelita Andre. The owner agreed to add them to a group show in his studio, promoting the show and placing ads in art magazines. Only at that point did the owner find out that the artist was not a professional artist but, rather, a 2-year-old—the daughter of artist Michael Andre and photographer Nikka Kalashnikova.

Can a 2-year-old truly create art deemed comparable to the work of professional artists? Is this a practical joke at the expense of the art world or the story of a child prodigy?

parents think is acceptable. For example, some parents would never give a child a toy gun, while others think playing with toy guns is a normal part of growing up.

Play materials are typically grouped into four categories: social and fantasy; exploration and mastery; music, art, and movement; and gross motor play. Social and fantasy play materials include items that encourage the use of imagination and the mental representation of objects and events, as well as a deeper understanding of people and the rules we live by. Play materials in this category are often used in dramatic play, solitary fantasy play, and role play. Exploration and mastery materials such as puzzles, pattern-making games, and sand, water, and string increase children's knowledge about the physical world, encouraging them to devise ways to enrich their comprehension of how things work. Music, art, and movement aid in the development of artistic expression. Gross-motor play materials, including playground and gym equipment, push-and-pull toys, and sports equipment, foster large-muscle development and skills.

Children's Artwork

Children love to draw for the sheer physical act as well as the cognitive stimulation. Their artwork has long attracted the attention of scholars, and culture plays a large role in children's aesthetic development. Young children innately progress from the pincer movements of infancy to random scribbles to skillful creations. Learning to draw is like learning a language: Children acquire increasingly com-

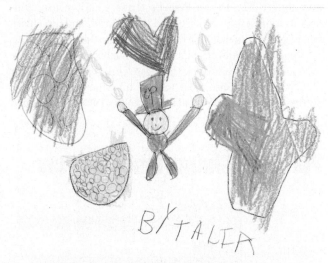

plex and effective drawing rules, which is one of the major achievements of the human mind (Willat, 2005).

The work of Rhoda Kellogg (1970) focused on universals in children's artwork. Kellogg collected more than 1 million children's drawings and paintings, created by thousands of children, and argued that children's drawing passes through the following four stages:

1. *Placement,* which refers to where on the paper the child places the drawing (2 to 3 years)

2. *Shape,* which refers to diagrams with different shapes (about 3 years)

3. *Design,* which refers to a combination of forms (about 3 to 4 years)

Children and Their Drawings

The work of anthropologist Alexander Alland (1983) has focused on cultural differences evident in children's artwork. Studying the drawings of children from Japan, Bali, Taiwan, Ponape, France, and the United States, he argued against theories of specific universal stages of development and proposed that children internalize culturally specific rules that are manifest in their drawings. An example of this influence may be seen in the influence of Manga (a type of comic book) in Japanese culture. These popular books have had an impact on the artwork that children produce. Not only do children re-create the style of Manga in their own work, but they imitate the style of dress and hair as well.

4. *Pictorial,* which refers to representations of humans, animals, buildings, and so on (about 4 to 5 years)

Kellogg concluded that child art contains the aesthetic forms most commonly used in all art.

Children's drawings not only are good clues to their motor coordination but also provide insights into their cognitive and emotional lives. A child who frequently draws violent scenes, featuring bloodshed and dead bodies, might be helped by some conversation about what she is drawing. A child might observe much through television and video games that could inspire drawings with violent content, but might also witness real-life violence in her home and neighborhood, and both situations demand the attention of adults who can help a child process the scenes she's observed and the feelings that result from such images.

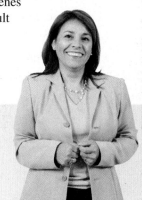

Career Apps

As an art therapist, how might you encourage a child to express herself through art when she might not be able to (or want to) articulate her feelings verbally?

CONCLUSIONS & SUMMARY

Although the rate of physical growth slows in early childhood, it continues at a steady pace. Physical and motor skills become more refined. Cognitive development leads to a world of representation in which children are expected to acquire and manipulate symbols. Language gradually becomes a powerful tool for adapting to the environment.

What are the major physical and motor accomplishments of the early childhood years?

- Growth continues at a steady, less rapid rate during these years.
- Brain lateralization seems to be well established by the age of 5 or 6.
- Height is a good indicator of normal development when heredity and environment are considered in evaluating health.
- Increasing competence and mastery are seen in a child's acquisition of motor skills.

How do Piaget's and Vygotsky's views on cognitive development differ from those of information-processing theorists?

- These years are the time of Piaget's preoperational period and the continued appearance of symbolic abilities.
- During these years children develop a theory of mind.
- Many current early childhood programs have a constructivist orientation.

What types of early childhood education seem most promising?

- Early childhood programs in Reggio Emilia, Italy, emphasize children's competence and curiosity.
- Head Start was originally designed to offer educational and developmental services to disadvantaged children.
- Several positive outcomes seem to be associated with Head Start programs.

How does children's language acquisition proceed during these years?

- Children acquire the basics of their language during these years with little, if any, instruction.

By the end of early childhood, most children enter formal schooling. What role does family play in development during these years?

- The meaning of "family" in our society has changed over time.
- Baumrind's types of parenting clarify the role of parents in children's development.
- Consistent and reasonable discipline is key as children try to gain mastery over themselves and their surroundings.
- Research has demonstrated how divorce affects children.
- Many children attend some form of day care, and the developmental outcomes of these experiences are still in question.

How do children of this age acquire a sense of self and gender?

- The emergence of the self is very much influenced by interactions with family and peers.
- Various theories have been proposed to explain how children achieve their sense of gender.
- Children initially seem to acquire an understanding of gender before they manifest sex-typed behavior.

What is the value of play?

- Play affects all aspects of development: physical, cognitive, social, and emotional.
- The nature of a child's play changes over the years, gradually becoming more symbolic.

KEY TERMS

animism *133*

authoritarian parenting *143*

authoritative parenting *143*

centration *134*

classification *135*

conservation *135*

constructivism *136*

constructivist approach *138*

day care *145*

deferred imitation *134*

egocentrism *134*

expressive language *141*

fine motor skills *132*

gender *146*

gender identity *146*

gender role *146*

gender stereotype *146*

gross motor skills *132*

Head Start *139*

myelination *131*

organization *136*

overextensions *141*

overregularization *141*

permissive parenting *143*

play *148*

preoperational period *133*

receptive language *141*

rehearsal *136*

representation *133*

retrieval *137*

reversibility *135*

scaffolding *136*

sensitive periods *139*

sex *146*

sex cleavage *147*

sibling underworld *144*

social constructivism *136*

symbolic play *134*

theory of mind *137*

uninvolved/neglectful parenting *143*

zone of proximal development (ZPD) *136*

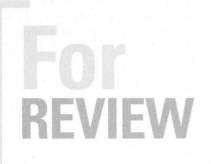

For REVIEW

1. As you can tell from the data presented in this chapter, young children continue their rapid growth, although at a less rapid rate than during infancy. If you were a parent of a child of this age (boy or girl), how much would you encourage him or her to participate in organized, directed physical activities (swimming, dancing, soccer, and so on)? Be sure to give specific reasons for your answer.

2. Given today's expectations for male and female gender roles, do you think children growing up in these times are more or less confused about gender identity? Why?

3. Think back to your own childhood. How would you categorize the parenting style or styles of your parents? Do you think it affected your behavior? Explain your answer by linking your parents' behavior to some of your personal characteristics.

Chapter Review Test

1. By the age of 5 to 6 years, ___ of adult brain weight is present.
   a. 70%
   b. 80%
   c. 90%
   d. 100%

2. When children show a preference for one hand or the other, this illustrates brain
   a. lateralization.
   b. synapses.
   c. dendrites.
   d. initiative.

3. Using the large muscles is referred to as _____ motor skills.
   a. fine
   b. peripheral
   c. gross
   d. anatomical

4. Which of the following behaviors is not associated with the preoperational period?
   a. symbolic play
   b. drawing
   c. language
   d. walking steadily

5. Head Start was initiated in the
   a. 1960s
   b. 1970s
   c. 1980s
   d. 1990s

6. Educators in Reggio Emilia, Italy, consider the _____ to be another teacher in the classroom.
   a. director
   b. environment
   c. parents
   d. siblings

7. About ___ of first marriages end in divorce.
   a. 75%
   b. 80%
   c. 50%
   d. 25%

8. The assumptions that we have about characteristics and behavior associated with "male" and "female" are called
   a. accommodation.
   b. gender practices.
   c. gender stereotypes.
   d. gender equality.

9. True play has no _____ goals.
   a. divergent
   b. coercive
   c. intrinsic
   d. extrinsic

10. Types of play include functional, constructive, make-believe, and games with
    a. balls.
    b. punishment.
    c. rewards.
    d. rules.

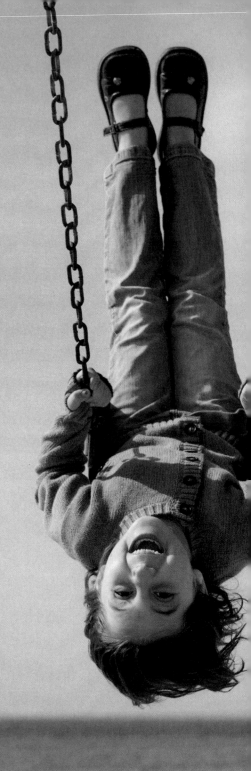

MIDDLE CHILDHOOD

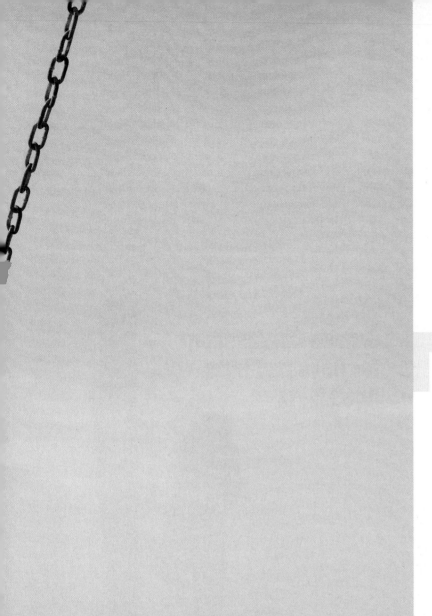

As You READ

After reading this chapter, you should be able to answer the following questions:

- How would you describe physical and motor development during these years?

- What are some of the competing views of cognitive development during the middle childhood years?

- How do children develop thinking and problem-solving strategies?

- How would you trace children's progress in moral development?

- How does children's language change during middle childhood?

- What are the key elements that help children acquire a personally satisfying and competent sense of self?

- How influential are peers during these years?

- What are some effects that different schools and teachers have on children during middle childhood?

- What are some of the major stressors in middle childhood?

In middle childhood, children display many competencies—physical, cognitive, and emotional—and yet they are still children—physically, cognitively, and emotionally. For example, older children are often able to use computers in ways that adults can't, yet they still might expect a bedtime story at night. They may have a pen pal around the world with whom they instant message (IM) each day, yet they don't realize that the ground turkey Mom buys at the grocery store comes from real animals on a working farm. Children's competencies and limitations are greatly influenced by their complex world (see Figure 7.1). As their skills mature, they must also develop a sense of responsibility that equips them to handle increasing independence. Developmental advances that prepare a young person to move from these last years of childhood into adolescence are of great importance for laying foundations that will impact the entire lifespan.

In this chapter, you will learn about many influences on the middle childhood years, affecting many areas of children's lives, including cognitive growth, moral reasoning, and physical and social development. The middle childhood years launch talents that children have been previously nurturing, and budding skills become full-blown if children are given support and opportunity.

Physical Development

Physical development proceeds at a slower pace during middle childhood than in early childhood (see Figure 7.2). Most children gain about 2 inches in height and 5 to 7 pounds in weight during middle childhood. Children in this age group are extremely active physically and gradually display a steady improvement in motor coordination. Fine motor skills assist them with self-help tasks, such as buttoning, zipping, and using eating utensils. Gross motor skills are visible as children exhibit more jumping and climbing, as well as bike riding and gymnastics abilities, for example.

FIGURE 7.2

Growth Curves Chart for Boys and Girls Aged 5–12

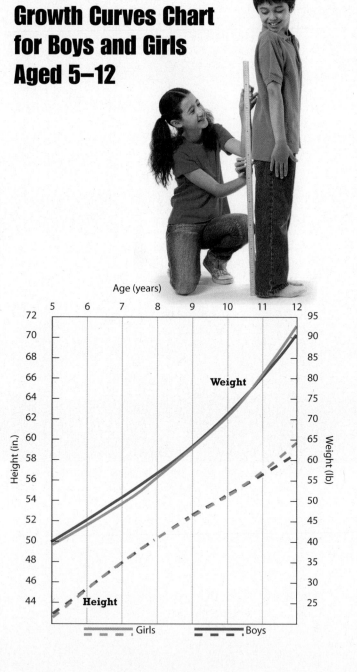

FIGURE 7.1

Uninsured Children in the United States

Other (multi-racial)
149,000
(1.6%)

Asian/Pacific Islander
398,000
(4.4%)

Black
1.5 million
(16.3%)

American Indian
143,000
(1.6%)

Hispanic
3.5 million
(38.3%)

White
3.4 million
(37.8%)

Although older children may seem more mature than in early childhood, they still depend on adults to make decisions that meet their basic needs relating to health, safety, and self-esteem. Health care is one of many controversial topics in our country that directly affect children.

Source: http://www.childrensdefense.org/helping-americas-children/childrens-health/racial-ethnic-disparities.html

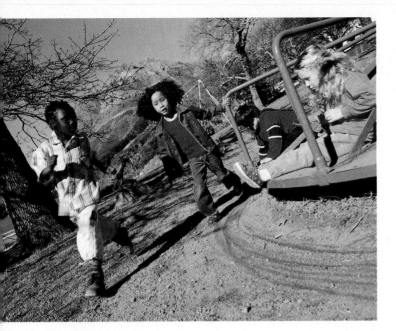

FIGURE 7.3

The Human Brain

The brain at middle childhood and the regions involved in various aspects of development.

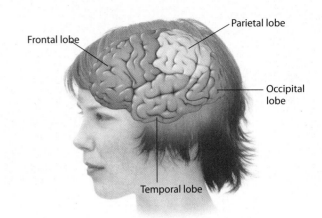

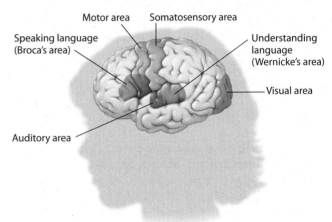

At the end of middle childhood, the body is more proportionate and more like an adult's: The trunk becomes thinner and longer, and the chest becomes broader and flatter. Among the most complex physical changes, however, are those in brain development.

BRAIN DEVELOPMENT

In middle childhood, the brain continues forming stronger connections and neurons become more myelinated. By age 8 or 9, the brain has reached about the size it will be in adulthood. Specifically, the frontal lobes experience significant growth, and children are able to engage in increasingly difficult cognitive tasks (see Figure 7.3).

As their abilities increase, children participate in a broader array of experiences, and the number of synapses increases, forming a vast network of pathways and connections. At this age, the brain also refines existing connections by pruning synapses that are unused. The neurons become more selective in their responses to chemical messages, particularly those deemed unessential, based on the child's experiences with people, materials, and surroundings.

As children learn and experience the world, memory improves, attention sharpens, judgment becomes more mature, and problem solving progresses. The task of adults who are around children during these amazing years is to provide stimulation that will encourage them to participate in this enticing world, thereby adding new connections and strengthening those already present. In this way, biological and environmental forces work together to shape the developing brain.

HEALTH AND NUTRITION

Generally speaking, middle childhood is a period of healthy development. Risks of infancy and early childhood are in the past, and children possess strength and energy that help promote their current development and prepare them for adolescence.

Among the most common reasons for children missing school are asthma and injuries caused by accidents, such as broken bones. **Asthma** is a lung disorder caused by a person's bronchial tubes (tubes connecting the throat to the lungs) reacting to external conditions by filling with mucus and tightening. Children who suffer from asthma experience symptoms including coughing and wheezing, and sometimes problems breathing. Many external conditions can contribute to asthma, such as cold weather, intense physical activity (such as running), allergies, and stress—all of which are commonly experienced in middle childhood. Doctors have also noted connections to pollution and smoking in a child's home in their research to explain the increase in numbers of asthma cases over the past few decades.

Injuries caused by accidents are most often related to riding a bike, because the child either was riding the bike or was struck by someone

asthma Lung disorder resulting in bronchial tubes filling with mucus and tightening.

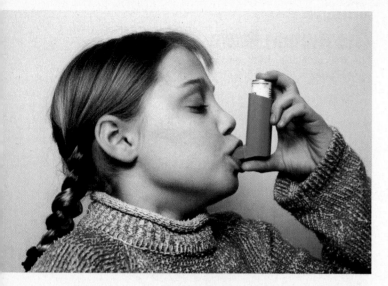

riding a bike. In middle childhood, modeling by teachers and caregivers is the most effective way to send children strong messages about safety rules and safety gear. Injuries are also common when children are playing organized team sports. Many parents push their children to excel at sports at an early age, without considering their physical limitations or lack of developmental readiness. The most direct way for adults to protect children from accidental injury is to be mindful of risk factors and to teach children about practices that will form a foundation for long-term health benefits.

Eating habits are important to a child's long-term health, and school-age children need to eat a well-balanced diet so that they have enough energy to support their learning in school. After-school activities with friends can interfere with plans for healthy, focused mealtimes. However, given children's slower growth rate during middle childhood, less food is needed—it's quality that counts. The 2005 Dietary Guidelines for Americans describe a healthy diet as one consisting of

- fruits, vegetables, whole grains, and fat-free or low-fat milk and milk products;

- lean meats, poultry, fish, beans, eggs, and nuts;

- a limited amount of saturated fats, cholesterol, sodium, and added sugars.

In middle childhood, school schedules influence breakfast and lunch meals, and children often make their own decisions about food. Peer and media influences are important elements in children's decisions about what to eat, but the models that children observe at home have the most influence. Some parents raise children on vegetarian or vegan diets, and some children avoid meat because of their love of animals. The child's body is preparing for the growth spurt that occurs in adolescence, so middle childhood is an ideal time to encourage good eating habits, especially outside the home.

obesity Based on BMI, greater than 85th percentile for sex and age.

body mass index (BMI) Measurement used to compare a person's height and weight to determine a healthy body weight; BMI = weight/height^2.

OVERWEIGHT

Over recent decades, the incidence of obese children has risen in many countries. In the United States, the problem has become increasingly serious, with the rate of **obesity** among children aged 6 to 11 more than doubling from 6.5% in 1980 to 17% in 2006 (CDC, 2009). Estimates are that 25 million children, 17 and under, are overweight. When a child's **body mass index (BMI)** is greater than the 85th percentile for sex and age, the child is considered obese (Miller et al., 2004). (See Figure 7.4.)

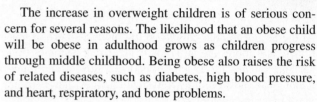

Career Apps

As a nutritionist, how might you recommend healthy eating practices to families on a budget?

The increase in overweight children is of serious concern for several reasons. The likelihood that an obese child will be obese in adulthood grows as children progress through middle childhood. Being obese also raises the risk of related diseases, such as diabetes, high blood pressure, and heart, respiratory, and bone problems.

The causes of childhood obesity involve biopsychosocial forces, such as heredity, mental health, and environment. Obese children often have obese or overweight parents, and therefore grow up with eating practices that make it likely that they will grow up to be overweight. While heredity might account for a predisposition to obesity, the environment plays a major role. Research has shown a connection between low socioeconomic status (SES) and obesity; this is

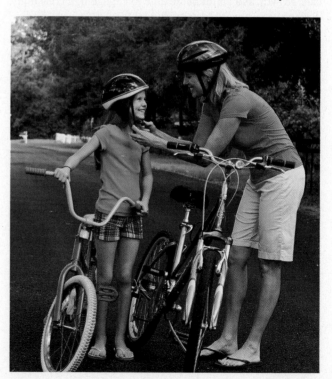

FIGURE 7.4

BMI Calculations Chart

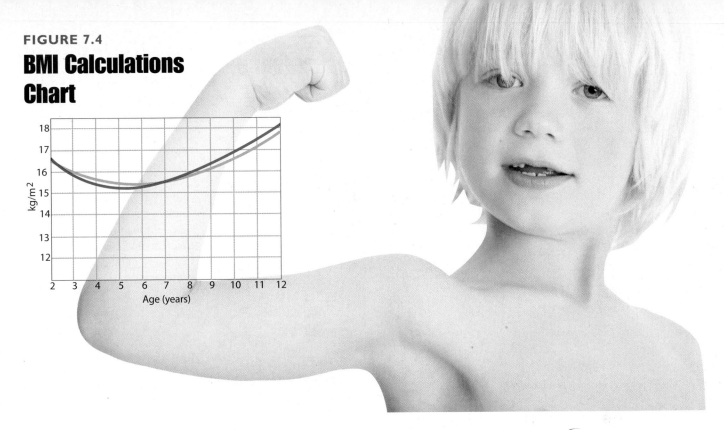

particularly true among ethnic minority groups. Factors such as having less knowledge about healthy nutrition, choosing cheaper, less-healthy foods, and being less physically active are involved. Successful intervention can be accomplished on several fronts, such as encouraging healthy eating habits and exercise, limiting television and computer time, and helping children become aware of their lifestyle choices.

LEARNING DISABILITIES

Children's perceptions of themselves and others include more than visible differences in shape and size. Approximately 10% of school-age children in the United States

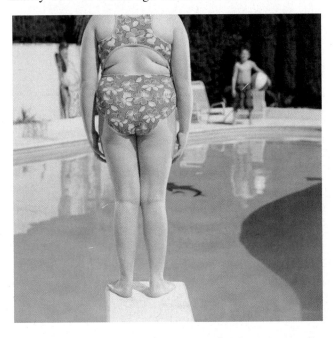

have been identified as having a **learning disability**—a neurological disorder that impacts the brain's functioning. Learning disabilities are defined by three components: (1) a minimum IQ level, (2) significant difficulty in a school-related area, and (3) exclusion of only severe emotional disorders, second-language background, sensory issues, or neurological issues (Siegel, 2003). Approximately 2.6 million children receive special education services in schools in the U.S., which represents 45% of students with disabilities across the nation (www. IDEAdata.org). (See Table 7.1.)

> **learning disability**
> A neurological disorder that impacts the brain's functioning.

Boys are more often diagnosed with a learning disability than girls, perhaps due to teachers' perceptions of boys and behavior issues. Most often, children's learning disabilities are recognized in the academic areas of reading and math.

TABLE 7.1

U.S. Children With a Disability Who Receive Special Education Services

Disability	Number of Children	Percentage of all Children With Disabilites
Learning disabilities	2,846,000	44.4%
Speech/Language impariments	1,084,000	16.9%
Mental retardation	592,000	9.2%
Emotional disturbance	476,000	7.4%

Source: Adapted from the National Center for Education Statistics, 2003.

FIGURE 7.5
ADHD Incidence

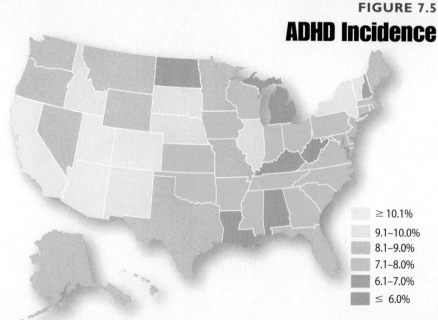

Cognitive Development

Once children begin formal schooling, their growing cognitive abilities help them to meet the increasingly demanding tasks set by the school. Piaget's explanation of cognitive development in the middle childhood years is one lens through which we can learn about children's thinking and how children construct knowledge.

≥ 10.1%
9.1–10.0%
8.1–9.0%
7.1–8.0%
6.1–7.0%
≤ 6.0%

Source: www.cdc.gov/ncbddd/adhd/data.html

decode To pronounce words correctly using knowledge of letters and sounds.

attention deficit hyperactivity disorder (ADHD) A disability related to inattention, hyperactivity, and impulsivity.

attention deficit disorder A disability related to inattention and lack of focus.

concrete operational stage Piaget's third stage of cognitive development, between the ages of 7 and 11 years, in which children's thinking is much more flexible than in early childhood.

Difficulties with attention, specifically being able to focus on relevant information needed to **decode** words or solve a problem, are quite common.

ATTENTION DISORDERS

Attention deficit hyperactivity disorder (ADHD) is one of the more common diagnoses for children who are easily distracted, seem to fidget constantly, and are unable to focus. ADHD is also related to poor impulse control. Children display ADHD differently, and some exhibit lack of attention or focus without hyperactive behaviors, which is called **attention deficit disorder (ADD).** They may seem focused on what someone is saying, or a lesson a teacher is giving, but their minds are a million miles away. The number of children diagnosed with ADD/ADHD has increased tremendously over the past decade, affecting children across the nation (see Figure 7.5).

Although there are no definitive causes of ADHD, heredity, exposure to lead, and biochemical substances (or lack of) have been suggested. Helping children with ADD/ADHD succeed in the classroom context requires consideration of physical, emotional, and environmental factors, lending support to the power of the biopsychosocial approach to human development. Treatment often includes medication (such as Ritalin), behavior plans that help children become less easily distracted, nutrition plans that minimize certain foods (e.g., sugars), and appropriate exercise.

PIAGET'S CONCRETE OPERATIONAL STAGE

The **concrete operational stage,** the third of four stages of cognitive development in Piaget's theory, occurs between the ages of 7 and 11 years. In this stage, children's thinking is much more flexible than in early childhood. For example, children can reverse their mental actions. They understand that rain turns into snow when temperatures drop below a certain level and that, if the weather turns warmer, the snow will melt into the watery state it was before it turned to snow. Children gradually begin to use logical thought processes and are able to reason accordingly with specific, concrete materials—objects, people, and/or events that they can see and touch.

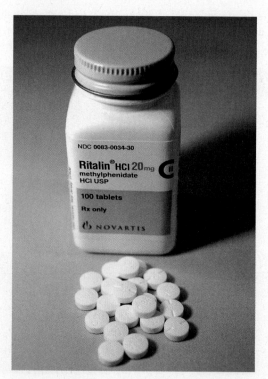

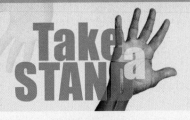

The Ritalin Debate

There is constant debate over whether or not children who have been diagnosed with ADHD or ADD need medication, such as methylphenidate (Ritalin), to be successful in school and in life. Ritalin is a stimulant that works by increasing the activity of the central nervous system. While Ritalin is widely prescribed for ADHD, its value is controversial and its long-term effects on the brain are unknown. The controversy centers on the argument that children who display problematic behaviors are simply overly energetic or otherwise unfocused versus the argument that there is brain-related evidence supporting the success of medication that helps children in ways that behavioral strategies do not. Some parents are hesitant to give their children Ritalin, even when prescribed by medical professionals.

Is prescribing drugs an appropriate response for the child who does not perform well in the modern school environment, or do drugs like Ritalin distract adults from solving important problems in the child's environment?

In middle childhood, children are diagnosed with ADHD more often than other specific learning disabilities.

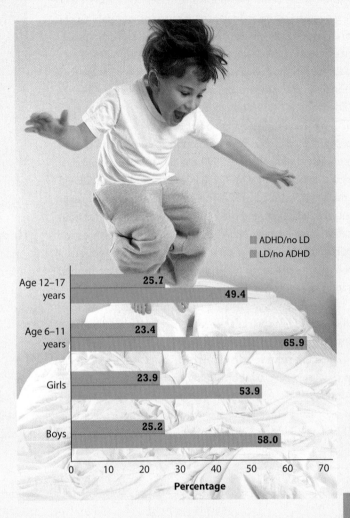

Cognitive Achievements in the Concrete Operational Stage

Recall Piaget's famous task with two identical glasses of water, one of which is poured into a taller, thinner glass (see Figure 6.5 in Chapter 6). Children in the concrete operational stage see that the amount of water in the two glasses is the same, a characteristic called conservation. They can imagine pouring the water back into the first glass. By reversing their thinking in this manner, they conserve the basic idea: The amount of water remains the same.

Conservation involves Piaget's notion of **decentration**—the child's ability to concentrate on more than one aspect of a problem or to connect them. This is seen when a child is able to recognize that in order to win at the card game "Go Fish," she needs not only to make pairs with her cards, but also to have the most pairs at the end of the game. Reversibility, the ability to think through steps involved in a problem and then retrace the mental actions, is evident as children learn math concepts, such as number families (e.g., $3 + 2 = 5$; $5 - 2 = 3$; $2 + 3 = 5$; $5 - 3 = 2$). Other notable features of children's thinking in the concrete operational stage include:

decentration The ability to focus on several features of an object or task.

- Classification – In middle childhood, children demonstrate Piaget's concept of class inclusion—the ability to group objects with some similarities within a larger category (e.g., roses and daisies are all flowers; Red Sox and Yankees are both baseball teams).

perspectives on Diversity

Exceptional Children

Although the term "exceptional" can refer to children who are deemed gifted and talented, it more often refers to children with special needs. At one time, children with special needs were either refused admission to public schools or educated in the public school system but at a different location from mainstream students. In 1975, Public Law 94-142 (Education for All Handicapped Children Act) was passed. This law required public schools accepting federal funds to provide equal access to education for children with physical and mental disabilities. In 1990, the public law developed into the Individuals with Disabilities Education Act (IDEA), and was amended in 1997. Then, in 2004, the law was reauthorized and renamed the Individuals with Disabilities Education Improvement Act. The IDEA governs how states and public agencies provide early intervention, special education, and other services to more than 6.5 million eligible infants, toddlers, children and youth with disabilities.

Some key terms related to the mandates for services that IDEA describes are the least restrictive environment and the individualized education plan:

Least restrictive environment: Students remain in their regular classroom, home, and family as much as possible. Their learning environment should be as similar as possible to that of children who do not have a disability. This is also known as **inclusion.**

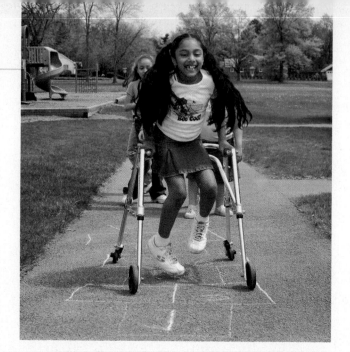

Individualized education plan (IEP): A written document (similar to a contract) that details an educational plan for a child to succeed under the supervision and guidance from the family, teachers and professionals, and administrators.

While best educational practices are designed to benefit all children, there are some children who are at a disadvantage because of several factors, including caregivers' inability to advocate for them, school districts' lack of funding to provide ideal supports, and misperceptions about their abilities due to biases related to culture, language, or poverty.

---

least restrictive environment: A child with a disability must be educated in a setting that is similar to that of children who do not have disability.

inclusion A child with special needs is educated in the regular classroom.

individualized education plan (IEP): A written document (similar to a contract) that details an educational plan for a child to succeed under the supervision and guidance from the family, teachers and professionals, and administrators.

seriation The ability to order items along a quantitative dimension such as length or weight.

transitivity The ability to understand relationships and combine them mentally to draw new conclusions.

• **Seriation** – The ability to order objects along a qualitative dimension, such as increasing or decreasing size or weight, a characteristic of the concrete operational stage. For example, Piaget asked children to place sticks in order of size. An essential aspect of seriation is **transitivity,** which refers to the ability to understand relationships and combine them mentally to draw new conclusions. An example would be in a seriation task, where stick A is longer than stick B, and stick B is longer than stick C. A child who understands the principle of transitivity would infer that stick A is also longer than stick C.

Some of Piaget's strongest conclusions about cognitive development in middle childhood are (1) that children are cognitively active (not passive recipients) as they construct their mental worlds and (2) that children's thinking can be analyzed based on clear evidence with concrete objects, not simply described based on assumptions about their abilities.

Piaget's ideas have inspired others to develop ideas about how children's thinking develops at this stage. For example:

• When the nature of the task is changed, children accomplish specific tasks at earlier ages than Piaget thought. For example, reducing the number of objects children must manipulate in a conservation of number task helps younger children more clearly see the relationship between the number of objects in a row and the length of the row of objects, such as colored plastic bears (often used in children's math games) or seashells.

• When given time and materials to practice, young children can be trained to master concrete operational tasks (see Figure 7.6). The very act of attending school increases children's performance on some tasks (classification, transitivity), while life experience and maturity provide enough experience for children to develop other skills (conservation) (Artman & Cahan, 2006).

- Cognitive development may not proceed through four discrete stages.

Although Piaget has left an enduring legacy, other psychologists have devised new ways of explaining children's cognitive abilities. The broad category of *intelligence* is often used to explore what children know and how we know what they know. **Intelligence** refers to a person's problem-solving skills and use of everyday experiences to inform learning. The work of Howard Gardner and Robert Sternberg has been influential in exploring connections between intelligence and educational practice.

GARDNER AND MULTIPLE INTELLIGENCES

Howard Gardner's **theory of multiple intelligences** challenges the traditional concept of intelligence—either you've got it or you don't—by proposing that everyone has different strengths and areas of growth. Gardner defines intelligence as the ability to solve problems or fashion products that are of consequence in a particular cultural setting or community.

Instead of one general intelligence, Gardner's theory identifies eight equal intelligences:

1. *Linguistic:* The ability to use words and language well to communicate and create. Examples: poet, translator, lawyer, marketing executive.

2. *Musical:* The ability to play an instrument, sing, or otherwise demonstrate sensitivity to rhythm, tone, and melody. Examples: musician, singer, conductor, composer.

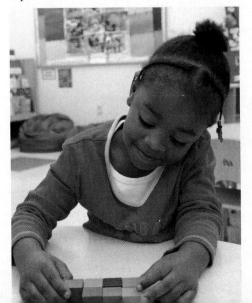

FIGURE 7.6

Conservation Tasks

Conservation of	Example	Approximate age
1. Number	Which has more?	6–7 years
2. Liquids	Which has more?	7–8 years
3. Length	Are they the same length?	7–8 years
4. Substance	Are they the same?	7–8 years
5. Area	Which has more room?	7–8 years
6. Weight	Will they weigh the same?	9–10 years
7. Volume	Will they displace the same amount of water?	11–12 years

Different kinds of conservation appear at different ages.

Source: Originally from John F. Travers, (1982), The Growing Child, Scott Foresman & Co.

3. *Logical-mathematical:* The ability to use and understand objects, numbers, and operations. Examples: accountant, scientist, engineer.

4. *Spatial:* The ability to think about and represent objects in three dimensions. Examples: artist, architect, cartographer.

5. *Bodily-kinesthetic:* The ability to handle objects and use the body skillfully. Examples: surgeon, dancer, acrobat, electrician.

6. *Interpersonal:* The ability to recognize what is distinctive in others; to interact effectively with others. Examples: teacher, politician, therapist, actor.

7. *Intrapersonal:* The ability to understand our own feelings. Examples: psychologist, author, theologian.

8. *Naturalist:* The ability to discriminate among living things; sensitivity to the natural world. Examples: farmer, landscape architect, environmentalist.

Many teachers and parents have embraced Gardner's theory because it suggests children develop and succeed according to their natural abilities and inclinations. Tension

intelligence A person's problem-solving skills and use of everyday experiences to inform learning.

theory of multiple intelligences Gardner's theory that attributes eight types of intelligence to humans.

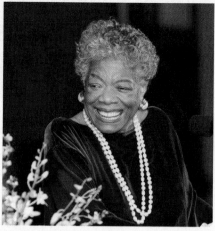

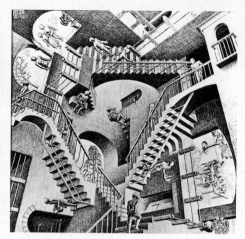

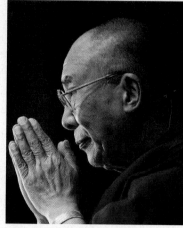

Poet Maya Angelou—linguistic

Art of M. C. Escher—spatial

The Dalai Lama—intrapersonal

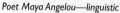

arises when children are assessed using traditional assessments that are typically geared to linguistic and logical-mathematical thinking. Until there is a broadly accepted method of evaluating children's multiple intelligences in a way that translates into the type of data that is used to determine success and funding for school districts, the theory of multiple intelligences may remain something that teachers practice but not be reflected in educational policies.

STERNBERG'S TRIARCHIC THEORY

Robert Sternberg's **triarchic theory of intelligence** focuses on three subtheories of intelligence that are part of information-processing theory (see Figure 7.7):

1. *Componential*. These are the information-processing skills that contribute to intelligent behavior and consist of metacomponents, performance components, and knowledge-acquisition components. **Metacomponents** help plan, monitor, and evaluate problem-solving strategies; **performance components** help execute the instructions of the metacomponents; and **knowledge-acquisition components** help solve problems. For example, consider children planning a field trip to a recycling center. The metacomponents help children decide on the site to visit, plan the day, monitor the surroundings, and evaluate the actual experience. The performance components help with the actual execution of the field trip, such as packing a lunch or snack and bringing recyclables from home to deposit at the center. The knowledge-acquisition components are used to conduct research about recycling and the environment prior to and during the visit.

2. *Experiential*. Life experience improves our ability to deal with novel tasks and to use pertinent information to solve problems. Think of learning to tie your shoes or ride a bike and compare those days to the familiar, expert techniques you now use. As tasks become more familiar, many parts of the task become automatic, requiring little conscious effort.

3. *Contextual*. This refers to the ability to adapt to our environment. We learn how to do those practical things that help us to survive in our surroundings, such as riding a bus and getting along with others. In other words, intelligence must be viewed in the context in which it occurs. The context of intelligence enables us to adapt to our environment, create and/or shape our environment, and select new environments (Sternberg, 2003).

triarchic theory of intelligence Sternberg's theory that intelligence consists of componential, experiential, and contextual parts.

metacomponents Sternberg's term for intelligence components that help us plan, monitor, and evaluate our problem-solving strategies.

performance components Sternberg's term for intelligence components that help us execute the instructions of the metacomponents.

knowledge-acquisition components Sternberg's term for intelligence components that help us learn how to solve problems in the first place.

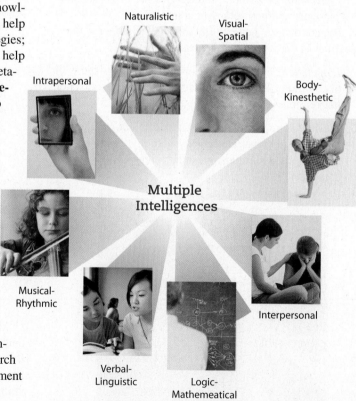

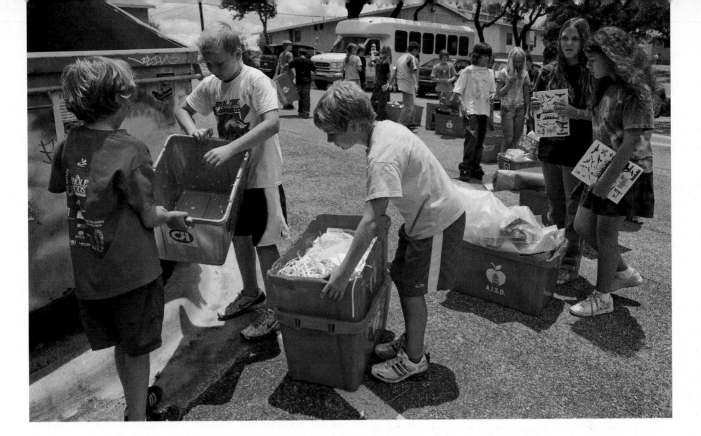

Sternberg argues that successful intelligence demands active involvement by individuals, as opposed to the inert intelligence measured by tests, and consists of analytical, creative, and practical aspects. Successfully intelligent people capitalize on their intellectual strengths and compensate for and correct their weaknesses.

INTELLIGENCE TESTING

Many formal evaluations of intelligence take the form of standardized tests that define and assess children's thinking in ways that are not necessarily developmentally appropriate or culturally sensitive. When intelligence testing incorporates a child's problem-solving skills as well as her or his everyday experiences, then a more valid indication of the child's intelligence may be formed.

When most people hear the phrase "intelligence tests," they think of paper-and-pencil tests designed in the early 20th century by Alfred Binet. Binet developed a measure of assessing children's intelligence to identify children who were unable to perform well in school. His test resulted in a score that reflected a child's **mental age**—an individual's mental development compared to that of others. The concept of an **intelligence quotient**—commonly known as an IQ—was developed by William Stern several years later. An IQ is calculated by dividing a child's mental age by chronological age, and then multiplying by 100. An IQ score of 90–109 is considered average intelligence. Such a method obviously does not work for adults.

The Binet test has been revised many times and is currently known as the Stanford-Binet test. It measures a person's abilities in four areas—verbal reasoning, quanti-

FIGURE 7.7

Sternberg's Triarchic Theory

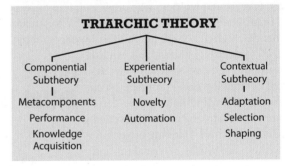

TRIARCHIC THEORY

Componential Subtheory	Experiential Subtheory	Contextual Subtheory
Metacomponents	Novelty	Adaptation
Performance	Automation	Selection
Knowledge Acquisition		Shaping

tative reasoning, abstract/visual reasoning, and short-term memory. Intelligence tests such as the Stanford-Binet are relatively simple to administer and quick to score, but they are widely criticized for not taking into account a child's cultural background, native language, or other individual differences that could render the measure invalid. Furthermore, traditional IQ tests calculate intelligence in an "either you've got it or you don't" general way, rather than viewing intelligence as a multifaceted, complex concept across numerous domains.

Most children score between 70 and 130 on IQ tests. Children who score above 130 are identified as gifted, whereas those who score below 70 are labeled mentally retarded. Gifted children are often

mental age Binet's measure of an individual's mental development compared to that of others.

intelligence quotient (IQ) Stern's concept of a child's intelligence, calculated by dividing mental age by chronological age, and multiplying by 100.

identified as having above-average skills in areas outside of academics, such as art, dance, or sports. Mentally retarded children typically possess limited cognitive abilities, and the disability often has biological roots. For example, as discussed in Chapter 3, Down syndrome is a chromosomal disorder that results in some degree of mental retardation. Brain damage that occurs to a fetus in utero, such as that due to the mother's alcohol or drug consumption, can also result in impaired cognitive functioning. Delays in cognitive development that occur after birth can sometimes be linked to environmental factors, such as malnutrition, neglect, and lack of stimulation in the home.

Critical Thinking and Problem Solving

The skills that children need to adapt to their environments change with the times. Unless adults are able to teach children innovative skills and help them keep up-to-date with technological advances, they will be unprepared to meet the demands of a changing environment. Children need critical thinking skills and problem-solving strategies that enable them to adapt to change.

Once children have accumulated knowledge, they must plan what to do with it. It's not enough just to obtain knowledge; children need to apply what they have learned, to integrate it with other facts, and to evaluate the process and outcomes. Parents and teachers who are attempting to help children improve their thinking skills should try to stretch and challenge children's thinking abilities by encouraging application, analysis, synthesis, and evaluation. These skills are emphasized in the creative work of thinking skills programs, such as Odyssey of the Mind and Project Zero. One example of a thinking protocol is found in Project Zero's Artful Thinking project, in which teachers use works of visual art and music to strengthen student thinking and learning (see Figure 7.8).

Odyssey of the Mind. Begun in 1985 by educators Sam Micklus and Ted Gourley, Odyssey of the Mind aims to help children develop creative thinking skills through brainstorming and collaboration. Children are encouraged to solve long-term problems that fall into five categories: mechanical/vehicle, technical performance, classics, structure, and performance. Problems can range from building a machine to interpreting great literature. Competitions take place on local, state, and global levels. Thousands of teams from throughout the United States and internationally participate in Odyssey of the Mind each year. You can find this year's problems at the Odyssey of the Mind website, http://www.odysseyofthe mind.com.

Project Zero. Begun in 1967 by Nelson Goodman at the Graduate School of Education at Harvard University, Project Zero was later co-directed by David Perkins and Howard Gardner. This program is geared toward creating communities of independent, reflective learners and developing a broad range of thinking skills across several disciplines, including the arts. Designed for individuals as well as institutions, projects include Learning in Out-of-School Settings, Multiple Intelligences, Visible Thinking, and School Change/School Improvement. See http://www.pz.harvard.edu for a description of current research projects.

PROBLEM-SOLVING STRATEGIES

Solving a problem occurs when a child has a particular goal in mind that can't be attained immediately. There are four criteria needed for problem solving to occur: goals, obstacles, strategies, and evaluation (Bjorklund, 2005). Children need to focus their attention on the task at hand in order to recognize what resources are needed to solve the problem and reach a desired goal. An assessment of the obstacles that may lie in the path of task completion helps a child accurately gauge realistic expectations for completing the task successfully. Strategies enable a child to solve a problem through various means, and evaluation provides a means for considering how well the child met her goals. Problem-solving strategies come in many forms, such as the collaborative activity used in Odyssey of the Mind.

FIGURE 7.8

Artful Thinking Palette

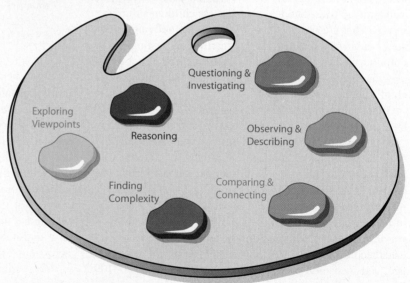

The Artful Thinking program uses an artist's palette as its central metaphor. Much like a palette may hold basic colors that can be combined in multiple ways, these six thinking dispositions can be combined.

Source: http://www.pz.harvard.edu/Research/ArtThink.htm

Memory shows marked improvement in middle childhood. This is largely due to the fact that attention dramatically improves as children learn to shut out distractions and concentrate on the immediate task. Short-term memory span increases as they acquire and use various memory strategies, and older children become more capable of transferring ever-increasing amounts of information to long-term memory by strengthening synaptic connections (Squire & Kandel, 2000).

One memory strategy that children employ is known as **elaboration,** an association between two or more pieces of information that are not necessarily related. This ability helps children engage in a wider range of information processing because they are able to remember more information by organizing it into meaningful units. An example of elaboration could occur when a child is asked to remember the famous opening sentence from Abraham Lincoln's Gettysburg Address, "Four score and seven years ago." The child might remember that he liked to play the game "Four Square" at recess when he was 7 years old. Thus, the opening to The Gettysburg Address can be linked to the child's existing knowledge and memories using the numbers 4 and 7.

OBSTACLES TO SUCCESSFUL PROBLEM SOLVING

Sometimes, despite their best efforts, children have trouble solving problems. Experts often point to cognitive processing as a factor: If children aren't able to process information from the environment accurately, how can they solve a problem successfully? Sometimes, paying attention to critical stimuli is the key to success, and attention deficits pose a challenge.

Other obstacles to successful problem solving include challenges relating to a specific academic area or behavior. Many children develop strategies to compensate for their problems, and they choose the best strategy to fit the situation. For example, a child may realize that she can't concentrate on her homework when there is background noise, so she will always choose a quiet spot to do her homework. Other strategies, such as relying on others in class to help with classroom activities, do not help students retain information, even though the student may experience short-term success on assignments. Strategies that children develop to succeed on their own and that result in success tend to increase in frequency, and motivation increases as well.

Moral Development

Adults are held to a different standard than children when it comes to right and wrong, because we assume adults know better. When investment banker Bernard Madoff was convicted for crimes he committed while running the biggest Ponzi scheme (fraud that uses money from new investors to pay high rates of returns to earlier investors) in history, he addressed some of his victims in the courtroom, saying, "I know this will not help. I'm sorry." Madoff is estimated to have brought financial ruin to about 8,000 people.

In today's regulatory environment, it's virtually **impossible** *to violate* **rules** *... but it's impossible for a violation to go undetected, certainly not for a* **considerable** *period of time.*

BERNARD MADOFF, INVESTMENT BANKER, OCTOBER 20, 2007 (CONVICTED OF FRAUD, MONEY LAUNDERING, PERJURY, AND OTHER CHARGES JUNE 30, 2009)

Morality will always be of primary concern to humans, yet the concept is hard to define because its developmental pathways are numerous, complex, and interactive. We want children to be kind, truthful, wise, courageous, and virtuous. We also want them to behave according to an internalized code of conduct that reflects such desirable characteristics. **Moral development,** therefore, entails thinking, feeling, and behaving based on rules and customs about how people interact with others.

Children internalize moral standards, and they also develop an evolving moral capacity that influences how they think about moral issues, how they feel about moral matters, and how they behave in complex situations. This mixture of *cognition* (thinking about what to do), *emotion* (feelings about what to do or what was done), and *behavior* (what is actually done) is reflected in theories of moral development.

PIAGET'S EXPLANATION

Piaget explained children's moral development from his cognitive perspective. He based his ideas on close observations of children playing a game of marbles. Watching the children, talking to them, and applying his cognitive theory to their actions, he interpreted how children conform to rules. Young children (under 5) played with no specific rules, children aged 5 to 10 played with rules they viewed as nonnegotiable, and by age 10 children felt comfortable modifying rules and creating their own.

While observing the marbles game, Piaget also asked children about fairness and justice, breaking the rules, and punishment. From this information, he devised a theory of moral development:

elaboration An association between two or more pieces of information that are not necessarily related.

moral development Thinking, feeling, and behaving based on rules and customs about how people interact with others.

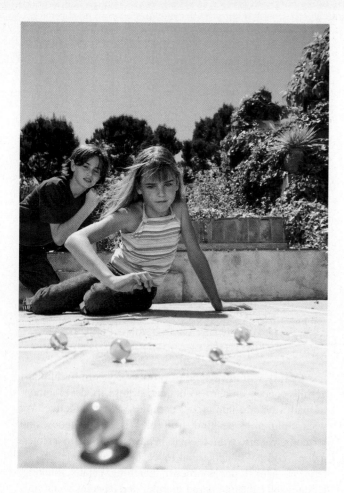

A man does what he must—in spite of personal **consequences**, in spite of obstacles and **dangers**—and this is the basis of all human **morality**.

JOHN F. KENNEDY

KOHLBERG'S THEORY

Piaget's ideas influenced a more elaborate theory devised by Lawrence Kohlberg (see Table 7.2). Kohlberg's theory traces moral development through six stages, each reflecting development of cognitive structures. In middle childhood, children are typically at Kohlberg's preconventional level of morality, where authority dictates whether something is right and wrong, reward and punishment are key, and a child's self-interest heavily influences decisions. As children reach adolescence, they begin to edge into the conventional level of morality, where they consider society's views and expectations before rendering judgment. In the postconventional level of morality, typically reached after adolescence, people consider options and weigh them against their own personal code and the notion of a social contract that exists among humankind.

- Up to about 4 years, children are not concerned with morality. Rules are meaningless, so they are unaware of any rule violations.

- Around 4 years, children believe that rules are fixed and unchangeable. Rules come from authority figures and are to be obeyed without question (**heteronomous morality**). Children make judgments about right or wrong based on the consequences of behavior; for example, it is more serious to break five dishes than one. They also believe that anyone who breaks a rule will be punished immediately (**immanent justice**).

- From around 7 to 11 years of age, children begin to realize that because rules are made by people, they can be changed. At this age, children think punishment for any violation of rules should be linked to the intent of the violator. Older children realize that opinions and feelings of others matter and that what they do might affect someone else. By the end of middle childhood, children clearly include intention in their thinking. For 6-year-olds, stealing is wrong because they might get punished; for the 11-year-old, stealing is wrong because it takes away from someone else (**autonomous morality**).

heteronomous morality Piaget's term for moral development in children aged 4 to 7; they conceive of rules as unchangeable.

immanent justice Piaget's term for a child's belief that broken rules will be punished immediately.

autonomous morality Piaget's term for moral development in children after age 11; actions must be thought of in terms of intentions and consequences.

TABLE 7.2
Kohlberg's Stages of Moral Development

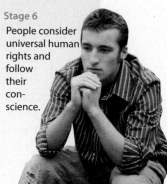

Level 1 Preconventional	Level 2 Conventional	Level 3 Postconventional
Stage 1 Children follow rules because adults tell them to do so. Fear of punishment motivates actions.	**Stage 3** People value trust, loyalty, and kindness. This impacts their judgments.	**Stage 5** People realize that there are greater rights and principles that support or are above the law.
Stage 2 Children develop and pursue their own interests. The notions of reciprocity and mutual satisfaction emerge.	**Stage 4** Moral judgments include attention to justice and authority.	**Stage 6** People consider universal human rights and follow their conscience.

According to Kohlberg, children must overcome their egocentrism before they can make true moral judgments. Cognitive development is just one of many factors that influence moral thinking. Cultural beliefs, family values, gender, and society also shape children's morality. It's important to note that moral development is not the same as moral behavior. In a given situation, children may know what is right, yet do things they know are wrong, similar to Bernie Madoff's behavior described earlier. Research suggests that when children are in a stage of developmental transition, they are less sure how to interpret and act on actual events.

GILLIGAN'S ETHICS OF CARE

A well-known critic of Kohlberg's stages is Carol Gilligan. Noting that most of Kohlberg's research was with males rather than females, Gilligan argued that Kohlberg's theory reflects a gender bias and a focus on justice rather than interpersonal relationships. She stressed the idea that people do not make moral decisions in a vacuum but, instead, make them in light of relationships and concern for others.

Gilligan argued for a different sequence of moral development of girls and women that focuses on the **ethics of care,** a view of people in terms of relationships and responsibilities to others:

- Initially, a girl's moral decisions center on the self and related concerns: "Will it work for me?"

- Gradually, as her attachment to her parents strengthens and loyalty develops, self-interest is redefined in light of "what one should do." A sense of responsibility for others appears (the traditional view of women as caretakers), and goodness is equated with self-sacrifice and concern for others. Gilligan believes that women consider whether it is possible to be responsible to one's self as well as to others. Women come to realize that recognizing one's needs is not selfish, but honest and fair.

- Finally, women resolve the conflict between concern for self and concern for others because of their maturing ability to view relationships from a broader perspective, including a guiding principle of nonviolence.

Neither Gilligan nor Kohlberg argued for the superiority of a male or a female sequence of moral development. Yet the difference in emphasis on justice versus care as the basis of moral development raises interesting questions about how society views men and women and about expectations for behavior. Children incorporate these ideas into their growing body of knowledge and desire to gain mastery over their environment.

Language Development

Children's skills across domains are not simultaneous accomplishments. This is true of vocabulary and language

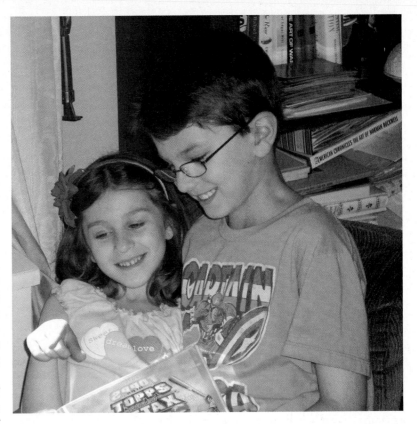

skills—reading is built on solid skills and helped by growing cognitive abilities (Bjorklund, 2005; Siegler & Alibali, 2005).

CHANGES IN VOCABULARY

During middle childhood, children communicate constantly with their peers, using language rich with humor and expressions they learn from the media. They are quite sophisticated in their knowledge of language because they use language to express thoughts and emotions and use inflection and intonation. By the end of middle childhood, they understand about 50,000 words and are similar to adults in their language usage.

One of the most obvious examples of children's developmental change is reflected in their use of language in ways that are culturally appropriate. They have internalized *pragmatics,* the use of language in different social contexts and environments. For example, a child may refer to a friend's mother as "Mrs. Kane" when in the presence of her own mother, but when playing at the friend's house, the child may address her friend's mother by using the parent's first name.

THEORIES OF READING ACQUISITION

Theorists are divided over two models of how reading skills are acquired: via a stage model of reading acquisition or via a nonstage model. **Stage theorists** believe children's abilities and tasks change

ethics of care Gilligan's perspective on moral thinking in which people view moral decisions in terms of relationships and responsibilities to others.

stage theorists Reading theorists who argue that reading occurs in distinct developmental stages.

Can Popular Literature Increase Literacy?

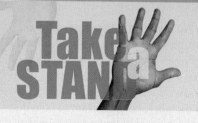

There is no doubt that the Harry Potter phenomenon, which began in 1998, ignited a passion for reading among readers of all ages—one that continues today as J. K. Rowling's stories and characters continue to resonate with fans on paper and on-screen in feature films. What is less clear is whether the excitement over popular literature is strong enough to transfer to other books and develop into a lifelong love of reading.

With the popularity of texting and email, there has been a downward trend in the number of students reading "for fun." The Harry Potter series is a clear exception. Research has showed that almost 60% of children in the United Kingdom believe that the Harry Potter books are responsible for their improved reading skills, and nearly half say that the books have fueled their desire to read more often (Hallett, 2005). The books have also proved to be motivating to struggling readers.

What is the appeal of the Harry Potter books and similar series that are helping create a generation of readers? What factors might compel readers of various ages to confront their reading challenges, and what are the rewards of meeting those challenges?

non-stage theorists Reading theorists who argue that reading develops naturally, as does language.

No Child Left Behind Act Federal legislation based on the notion that high standards and measurable goals improve individual educational outcomes; requires assessments in basic skills to be given to all students in certain grades.

emergent readers Children who possess skills, knowledge, and attitudes that are developmental precursors to formal reading.

according to specific stages of development, each stage qualitatively different from the preceding stage. **Nonstage theorists** argue that reading should unfold naturally, much as a child's language develops, according to the individual child's own readiness and abilities.

An example of stage theory is seen in the work of a leading reading specialist, Jeanne Chall, who has proposed a stage model leading to reading proficiency (Chall, 1983; Chall, Jacobs, & Baldwin, 1990). The features of middle childhood stages are as follows:

- *Ages 6 to 7 years.* Children learn the relationship between letters and sounds and begin to read simple text. They usually experience direct instruction in letter-sound relations (phonics) and use high-frequency words in their reading. For example, many kindergarten and first-grade classrooms feature a "word wall," where commonly used words are displayed so that children have ample opportunities for recognition.

- *Ages 7 to 8 years.* Children demonstrate greater fluency in reading simple stories. They combine improved decoding skills with fast mapping, using context to figure the meaning of words, in their reading.

- *Ages 9 to 13 years.* Reading is now used as a tool to obtain knowledge.

The two major goals of reading acquisition are efficient word identification and the comprehension of increasingly difficult material. Nonstage theorists describe reading acquisition as continuous development within different reading categories. Reading is viewed as the assembly, coordination, and automatic use of several processes (Paris & Paris, 2006). With regard to reading instruction, children in today's public schools experience the impact of the "top five" components identified in the federal **No Child Left Behind Act** of 2001: the alphabetic principle, phonemic awareness, oral reading fluency, vocabulary, and comprehension.

In another, but similar nonstage model, Whitehurst and Lonigan (1998) have proposed nine components of successful reading: familiarity with the child's language, knowledge of the conventions of print (left to right, top to bottom), knowledge of letters, linguistic awareness (awareness of phonemes, syllables, and so on), the relationship of sounds to letters, emergent reading (pretending to read), emergent writing (pretend writing), print motivation (interest in and attention to "breaking the code"), and a mixture of other cognitive skills. Interestingly, the continuous nonstage theory often translates into practices that break reading experiences into distinct, seemingly unrelated units.

THE ISSUE OF LITERACY

School-age readers are typically classified as emergent, developing, or independent readers. These categories are helpful descriptive tools for teachers and families.

- **Emergent readers** are at the beginning of the reading adventure. They know that books tell interesting stories and that words and pictures aid understanding. The skills, knowledge, and attitudes that are the developmental precursors to formal reading are formed at this stage (Whitehurst & Lonigan, 1998).

- **Developing readers** are becoming true readers. They have established the habit of reading for meaning and use their own experiences to enrich the meaning of stories. They have learned to use letter sounds, words, illustrations, and their own knowledge to predict meaning.

- **Independent readers** are those who read on their own and when they are alone. These children are competent, confident readers who use all their skills to derive as much meaning and enjoyment from their reading as possible.

Literacy can be a stressful topic for parents, educators, and children. Parents may become worried if their child is not reading fluently by the time they expect her to. Likewise, if a child is not reading as well as friends in his age group, he may feel embarrassed. With the strong emphasis on literacy and math skills in schools, teachers and administrators may feel responsible to families as well as state and national authorities for their students' success.

Other types of literacy are equally important but receive much less formal attention:

- Technological literacy—ability to understand and work with computers, software, and the Internet

- Visual literacy—ability to decipher, interpret, and express ideas using images, charts, graphs, and video

- Cultural literacy—knowledge and appreciation of the diversity of people and cultures

- Global awareness—understanding and recognition of the interrelations of nations, corporations, and world politics

If children are to be citizens of the world in the 21st century, multiple literacies must be considered and supported in schools.

> **developing readers** Readers who use letter sounds, words, illustrations, and their own knowledge to predict meaning.
>
> **independent readers** Competent, confident readers who use skills to derive meaning and enjoyment from reading.

BILINGUALISM

The United States has become more ethnically and linguistically diverse than ever before. Many children in the U.S. do not speak or write English as their primary language. Estimates of the number of English language learners (ELLs) in school range from 2 million to 6 million (Marshall, 2002). But this figure is deceptive owing to differences within the ELL population that represent a wide range of economic and ethnic diversity (see Figure 7.9). For many children, economic conditions dictate their access to resources that contribute to the acquisition of necessary English language skills. Although the largest number of ELL students are of Hispanic/Latino origin (approximately

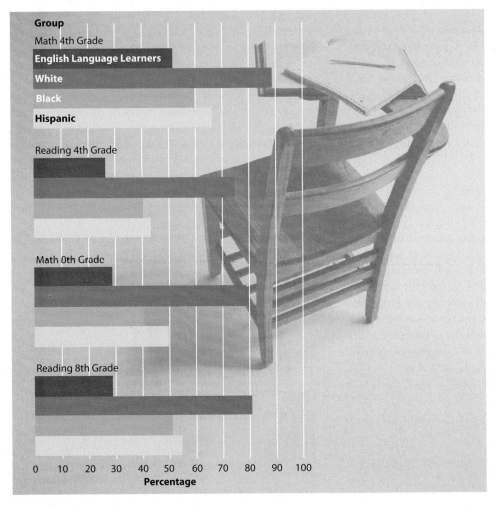

FIGURE 7.9

ELL Test Scores

This graph shows the percentage of basic and above academic skills by student demographic group in 2005.

Source: 2005 National Assessment of Educational Progress.

Culturally Sensitive Practice

Many schools in the country work with immigrant families. Through a special certification called TESOL (Teaching English to Speakers of Other Languages) (Wong, 2006), teachers are encouraged to use their students' families and communities as resources (Kachru, 2005). Three questions guide teachers' work:

1. What do we know about the nature of the language?
2. What do we know about the nature of the learner?
3. What are the aims of your instruction?

Adults who work with immigrant children can better appreciate the needs, attitudes, and values underlying children's behaviors when they obtain as much information as possible about children's cultures. Parents, grandparents, and other interested adults should be encouraged to share books with children even though they may not read or write English.

Many books by well-known authors and illustrators are available in other languages and bilingual editions. Rebecca Emberley's *My Numbers/Mis Números* uses everyday objects and paints the objects in bright, vivid colors to encourage children to match English words with Spanish words. At each stage in the reading acquisition process, teachers, librarians, and interested adults are constantly exploring many innovative ways to encourage and motivate *all* children to be readers.

CDs, audiotapes, and videotapes of books are available at public libraries. The American Library Association annually selects videos, recordings, and software for all ages based on the recommendations of committees of librarians and educators from across the country who consider their originality, creativity, and suitability.

74%), the number of languages spoken within the ELL population is boundless.

The major question facing educators is: "What is the most effective way to teach English to non-English speakers while maintaining the richness and cultural values of their own languages?" Two approaches are at the heart of the discussion: immersion, which places non-English-speaking students in classrooms where the dominant language is spoken exclusively, and bilingual instruction, which emphasizes learning in a child's native language and English.

Bilingual Education Programs

In a landmark decision in 1974 (*Lau v. Nichols*), the U.S. Supreme Court ruled that limited English proficiency (LEP) students in the San Francisco school district were being discriminated against because they were not receiving the same education as their English-speaking classmates. The school district was ordered to provide means for LEP students to participate in all instructional programs. The manner of implementing the decision was left to the school district under the guidance of the lower courts. This decision provided the impetus for the implementation of bilingual education programs in the United States.

With the bilingual technique, three major goals are identified:

1. Continued development of the student's primary language

2. Acquisition of a second language, usually English

3. Instruction in content using both languages

Because students in bilingual education programs are taught partly in English and partly in their native language, they acquire subject matter knowledge simultaneously with English. Bilingual programs also allow students to retain their cultural identities while simultaneously progressing in their school subjects. In today's schools, bilingual education has become the program of choice, and there are several ways to implement bilingual practice. Political policies sometimes impede bilingual instruction, however. Many states have recently passed laws that, on the surface, attempt to get English language learners into solely English-speaking classrooms quickly. However, the actual practice often leaves English language learners at a huge disadvantage in terms of academics, social and emotional development, and family engagement.

As children experience physical and cognitive challenges, their developing sense of self is affected.

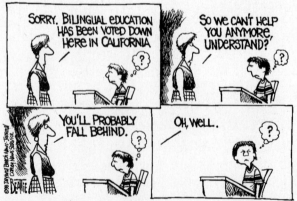

By permission of Bruce Beattie and Creator's Syndicate, Inc.

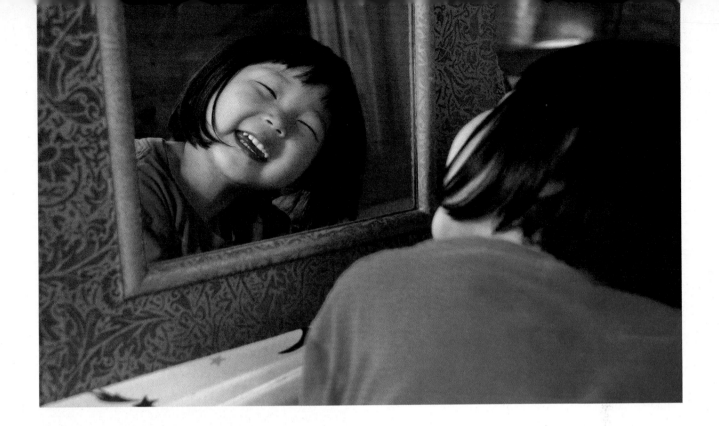

The Changing Sense of Self

The developmental pathway of the self reflects a child's growing complexity, the gradual transformation of physical features of self (I have blonde hair, brown eyes) into more subtle characterizations (I'm a true friend, I get along well with others). These different shadings of the self continue to develop as cognitive and social awareness sharpen. Both self-concept and self-esteem contribute to a child's understanding of who and what "I" am.

THE DEVELOPING SELF-CONCEPT

Self-concept a person's evaluation of him- or herself—is not something that a person is born with, and it is not unchanging over the course of the lifespan (Harter, 2006). Rather, the self develops through the years as the result of life experience.

The self can be described as both a *cognitive* and a *social* construction (Harter, 2006). Erikson (1963, 1968) described middle childhood in the life stage he called industry versus inferiority. It is a time when children use their tools and skills and acquire a feeling of satisfaction at the completion of satisfactory work. If children are encouraged to engage in work they find fulfilling, such as building, creating art, cooking, or solving math problems, their feeling of industry increases. Their developing sense of competency leads them to understand the perspective of others, which then influences further development of self.

SELF-ESTEEM AND COMPETENCE

Self-esteem can be described as the sense of worth and value that children place on themselves. During middle childhood, children's developing sense of self helps to shape their personal goals. Any discrepancy between the perceived ideal self and the real self can be a strong motivating force. For example, children begin to compare their achievements with those of others. They come to realize that although they may excel in one area (math), someone else is much stronger in a different area (art). This discrepancy can serve as a motivating force for some children to work harder, whereas others register the information and accept it without desire for change.

As older children begin to assess their personal strengths and weaknesses, they recognize that they have both desirable and undesirable qualities. Their perceptions of self and self-esteem are tightly woven with their satisfaction with their physical appearance, their need for support from those they love and trust, and a belief in their own competence.

Developmental psychologist Susan Harter has been a longtime student of the concept of self-esteem. Studying 8- to 13-year-old children, Harter and her colleagues developed a Self-Perception Profile for Children (SPPC) that tested five types of **competence,** the ability to do something well, as a measure of self-esteem: scholastic competence, athletic competence, social competence, physical appearance, and behavioral conduct (Harter, 1999).

self-concept A person's evaluation of himself or herself.

self-esteem One's personal sense of worth and value.

competence The ability to do something well.

The results indicated that children don't feel they do equally as well in all the five types of competence that Harter identified. Most children feel good about themselves in some types of competence but not so good in others.

In the second phase of her study, Harter explored how what others think about children affects children's self-esteem. Children who received much support from the important people in their lives had a high regard for themselves. Those who obtained little, if any, support from significant others showed the lowest self-esteem. These findings provide important insights into how children acquire their sense of self-esteem.

Harter noted a strong link between what children thought of their physical appearance and their level of self-esteem. Researchers Diane Levin and Jean Kilbourne (2008) argue that children are bombarded by sexualized content in popular culture and technology, and companies aggressively produce and market products to children that sustain images of sex and desirability based on appearance and sexuality. They stress how critical it is for adults to communicate with children about these issues and to build children's confidence and self-concept based on developmentally appropriate, respectful experiences.

Praise and recognition for effort and honest achievements go a long way in building children's self-esteem. Honest critique and thoughtful suggestions for improvement also teach children that they don't need to be perfect. For example, "You didn't do that well this time, but I know if you practice, you'll do better next time." The discipline and desire required to improve one's self are related to another quality—self-regulation.

SELF-REGULATION

As you may imagine, self-regulation refers to many situations: mastering fear, controlling eating and drinking, monitoring one's responses, and refusing dangerous substances. **Self-regulation** is based in our psychology and reflects higher-level-thinking—an individual's capacity to initiate, terminate, delay, modify, or redirect thought, emotion, behavior, or action (Compas et al., 2002). Developing these vital coping skills is a key part of psychosocial development (Dacey & Fiore, 2000).

For children to be successful in work and relationships, they must exercise restraint in deciding what to do, how to

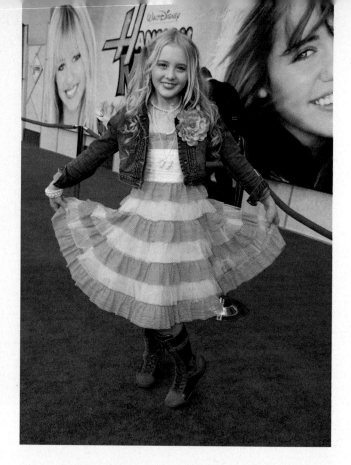

do it, what to say, and how to say it. Children's temperament and perceptions of others impacts how they respond to others and how others respond to them. Research in this area has shown that children who display impulsivity at a young age tend to be troubled adolescents, with few friends and great psychological difficulties. Young children who delay gratification can later handle frustration well, are focused and calm in the face of challenges, and are self-reliant and popular adolescents (Peake, Hebl, & Mischel, 2002).

Social Development

Children in middle childhood bring characteristics they formed within their family surroundings to their interactions with those outside the family. Although parents typically spend less time with children in middle childhood than in early childhood, due to children's increasing competencies and budding desire for independence, they remain a strong influence in their lives. With this in mind,

The capacity for **conscious** *and voluntary* **self-regulation** *is central to our understanding of what it is to be human. It underlies our assumptions about* **choice,** *decision making, and planning. Our conceptions of* **freedom** *and* **responsibility** *depend on it.*

MARTHA BRONSON, EARLY CHILDHOOD EDUCATOR AND ADVOCATE

let's examine the impact of families and peers on development in middle childhood.

THE ROLE OF FAMILY AND FRIENDS

Children focus energies in new directions during middle childhood, such as school activities and peer relationships. Their cognitive abilities allow them to reason with their parents about rules, chores, discipline, and countless other topics. They tend to practice their self-regulation skills on a daily basis, such as choosing to complete their homework before watching a favorite television program, and gradually internalize their parents' values and expectations.

Children whose parents divorce or who live in a stepfamily face some additional challenges in their development. They must also cope with realities of fewer or shared resources and different levels of attention from their biological parents. In a divorced family, a child may be forced to adjust to less time with a mother who used to spend much time at home, but who has taken a job or is working extra hours to pay the bills. Similarly, a father who is trying to forge a relationship with new stepchildren may spend less time with his biological child during the adjustment period.

Another focus of research on the role of family in children's social development is lesbian, gay, bisexual, and transgender (LGBT) parenting. Findings indicate that parents' sexual orientation is in no way connected to parenting skills. Many professional organizations have issued statements underscoring that a parent's sexual orientation is unrelated to parenting roles and functions (see http://www .hrc.org/issues/professional-opinion.asp for a list of professional organizations and their position statements).

One common function that parents serve is acting as chaperone (and/or chauffeur) for children and their peers. During middle childhood, peer interactions increase dramatically to about 30% of all social interactions. The decreasing amount of adult participation in a variety of settings, including schools, interests, and phone and online exchanges, parallels the increase in peer interactions. Getting along with peers is a major step in social development, and research findings are consistent with the conclusion that peer rejection directly impairs children's adjustment. Peers more often direct negative behaviors and verbal harassment toward rejected children (Buhs & Ladd, 2001), which also makes it more likely that rejected children will be excluded from social activities (Dodge et al., 2003).

Aggression becomes more verbal and personally hostile in middle childhood, with friendship assuming a greater role in acceptance or rejection (Rubin, Bukowski, & Parker, 2006). Children who have friends are less likely to be picked on or rejected by others. **Bullying,** the act of using verbal or physical means to intimidate or embarrass someone else, is a common challenge in schools and neighborhoods. The challenge is further complicated by technology, specifically incidents of "cyberbullying"—bullying conducted online or via text messages. Of immediate concern

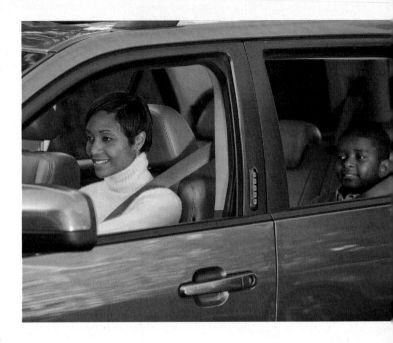

is the danger that a child's zones of safety become violent, scary places. Many schools and communities are making greater efforts to adhere to zero tolerance policies with bullying, and this requires a coordinated effort among adults and children.

> **bullying** The act of using verbal or physical means to intimidate or embarrass someone else.

Lisa: Why does she only go after the smart ones?
Nelson: That's like asking the square root of a million. No one will ever know.
Lisa: Someone will—I'm going to crack the bully code.

—THE SIMPSONS, EPISODE 264

THE ROLE OF SCHOOLS

There are many issues facing schools today, including funding, high-stakes testing, and family involvement in and support of children's education. Common sense dictates that any environment in which children sharpen their intellectual skills, learn how to get along with others, work with a diverse cultural group of peers, and assess their self-concepts in competition with others must have a powerful effect on development. Researchers have looked beyond the academic aspects of school to examine how school influences a child's identity, self-esteem, beliefs, and behavior.

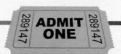
To examine schools' effects on development, Michael Rutter (1983) conducted a study of school effectiveness and found startling differences between schools in terms of their impact on children. His data led to several conclusions:

- Schools that encourage moderate risk-taking and ample opportunities for social and academic success lead to increased motivation for students.

- Differences between schools are due to a school's emphasis on academic success, teacher expectations of student success, time-on-task, skillful use of rewards and punishment, teachers who provide a comfortable and warm classroom environment, and teachers who insist on student responsibility for their behavior.

- Differences between schools are not due to the size or age of the buildings.

Clearly, there are different ways to teach children and to hold teachers and schools accountable for the success that students experience. In middle childhood, teachers play a particularly important role as children grapple with both the

desire to succeed and feelings of incompetence. Teachers, like parents, help children cope with academic and social demands, and transmit a set of values and expectations in the classroom (see Figure 7.10). The classroom context is one of many systems that influence a child's development (see Chapter 2).

As children pass through the elementary grades, they experience steady developmental changes, as well as constantly changing subject matter. Recognizing the developmental pathways that children follow, schools must focus on some critical, timeless themes that help children learn:

1. To develop good relationships

2. To acquire effective thinking skills

3. To be part of the solution, not the problem

4. To look at things differently

5. To be goal-oriented

6. To achieve academic success

7. To recognize the difference between right and wrong

8. To know and accept differences in others

9. To see the true self

10. To bounce back and keep trying

Summarizing 40 years of research on schooling, Eccles and Roeser (1999) reach several conclusions about school's impact on children:

FIGURE 7.10

Ecological Model of Schooling and Development of Self

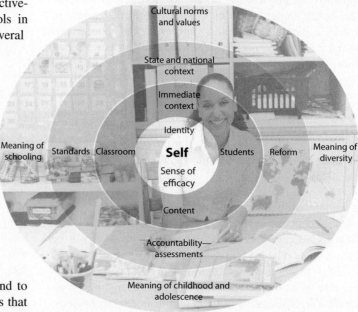

Source: Bronfenbrenner, U. (1986). Ecology of the family as a context for human development: Research perspectives. Developmental Psychology, 22, 723–742.

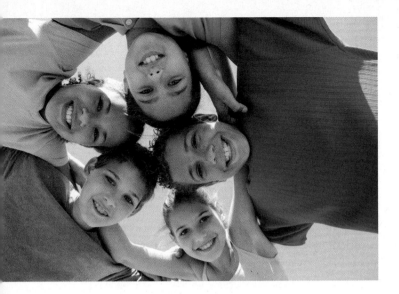

- Although school resources are important, the organizational, social, and instructional processes have the greatest impact on children's development.
- Schools produce their effects at different levels: the school as a whole, the classroom, and interpersonal interactions.
- Children's perceptions of the school are powerful predictors of their adjustment, adaptation, and achievement.
- A school's effects on behavior are determined by individual, psychological processes.

Expectations and Achievement

Research has demonstrated a powerful relationship between poverty and a child's health, behavior, and achievement. For example, poor children repeat grades and drop out of high school at a rate that is more than double that of wealthier peers (Duncan & Brooks-Gunn, 2000). In *Savage Inequalities*, Jonathan Kozol (1991) drew some vivid comparisons between urban schools and those in affluent suburbs. An inner city school he describes is situated among piles of garbage, raw sewage, and fumes from local chemical plants. Teacher and staff layoffs are common. School buildings are in disrepair and have only a few windows; the few windows are barred, many doors are chained. Thirty students are crammed into a classroom designed to seat 15.

A more affluent district in the same state presents a different picture. A greenhouse is available for students interested in horticulture; there are more than 30 science electives. The school's orchestra has traveled to the former Soviet Union. Beautifully carpeted hallways encourage students to sit and study; every student has access to a computer. The ratio of counselors to students is 1 to 150. Given these different conditions, is it any wonder that different educational outcomes are inevitable?

These conditions can be either improved or made worse by the family's belief in education. As Garbarino and Benn noted (1992), parents may not be present in the classroom, but they have a profound influence on the way their

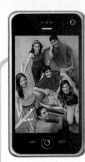

TECH TRENDS

Online Peers and Safety Precautions

The term *social media* is a relatively new term referring to software applications that allow people to communicate and share data. Older children are often more familiar with these forms of communicating than adults, and schools and teachers must keep up with the technology to equip children to use the tools safely and effectively.

Instant messaging (IM): A form of real-time text-based communication between two or more people using personal computers or other devices.

Internet forum (also called a message board): A separate, virtual room where children can talk about topics of interest. Someone starts by thinking of a question or conversation topic and posts it in the forum, and others respond accordingly.

Blogs: Online journals for individuals. Some blogs permit others to leave comments, which keeps a record of the flow of the conversation.

Wikis: A wiki is a webpage whose content can be edited by visitors. Visitors edit and share thoughts with others online.

Facebook: A social networking website in which users can add friends, send them messages, and post updates to their status and profiles to let friends know what's going on in their lives.

Of most concern to parents is the threat of sexual predators online who may take advantage of a child's desire for independence, friendship, and social acceptance, and potentially harm a child. Online bullying (cyberbullying) is another concern. Close supervision and monitoring of children's online activities is vital for adults to ensure that a child's desire to wed social activity and technology results in positive socialization opportunities.

Career Apps

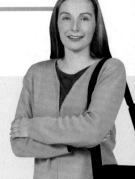

As a town ombudsperson, how might you advocate for children's rights in the educational system and inform families of available services?

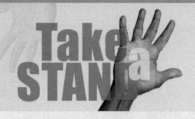

Most children watch television with few, if any, parental restrictions. Educator James Garbarino (1999) summarizes the potential danger of television viewing:

> Psychological, physical, and sexual violence exists in homes and neighborhoods throughout the country, regardless of geography. Such violence occurs in small towns and suburbs, in cities and rural areas. And images of it are accessible to almost every child in America simply by turning on the television. (p. 107)

The effects of viewing televised violence are more intense for children than for adults, especially if the children believe that the televised violence is real. Another major concern, of course, is the possibility of children becoming desensitized to real-life violence because of their exposure to a steady diet of televised violence.

However, television can also have positive effects on children's development. Educational programs can foster an appreciation for global issues and cultural differences. Certain programs also teach children prosocial behaviors in the exact same manner that people fear children will learn violence and aggression. By simply watching television, children can learn alternative ways to solve conflicts, identify and contradict stereotypes, and reduce anxiety by watching others conquer fearful situations.

Do the positive effects of television viewing outweigh the risks? What guidelines should determine the amount of television children watch?

---

stress Anything that upsets a person's equilibrium—psychologically and physiologically.

children view school and learning. The extent to which the family supports the school's objectives directly affects their child's academic performance. Too often, low parental expectations for their children reflect the parents' own educational experiences.

THE ROLE OF TECHNOLOGY

Although today's children are immersed in a media world (movies, television, video games, CDs, audiotapes, videotapes), television is the most widely used medium and undoubtedly has a greater effect on development than do other media (see Figure 7.11). In 2005, children 2 to 11 years of age watched on the average 23.4 hours per week, according to Nielsen Media Research (2006).

Research findings indicate the following:

- Television viewing seems to have little effect on vocabulary during middle childhood and has little impact on creativity.

- Amount of time spent looking at the screen is directly related to age. During middle childhood, viewing time remains steady and begins to decline after age 12.

- Television viewing and school achievement are positively and negatively related. Educational programs can boost literacy skills. More than 30 hours of TV viewing per week seems to interfere with academic achievement.

Stress in Middle Childhood

Children today are growing and developing in a climate of **stress**—anything that upsets a person's equilibrium, psychologically and physiologically—that impinges on every part of their lives.

When children are stressed, they encounter four problems:

1. They find it harder than other children do to calm themselves in stressful situations.

2. They can't use their abilities to the maximum extent.

3. They become discouraged easily and tend to generate feelings of helplessness.

4. Even when successful—academically, emotionally, athletically—children who are stressed don't recognize and accept their progress (Dacey & Fiore, 2000).

Adults can help to provide children with critical emotional security in stressful times and help them develop the coping skills that will serve them well in times of need.

CHILD ABUSE

Although **child abuse** is an age-old problem, but not until the last two decades did it become widely publicized.

FIGURE 7.11
Children Who Watch Television

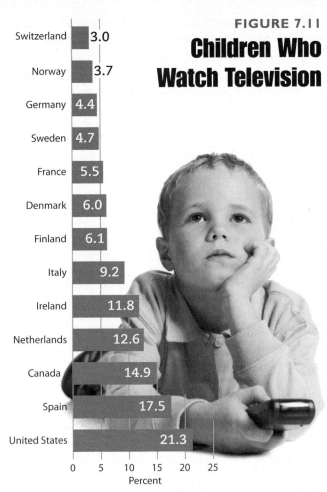

Country	Percent
Switzerland	3.0
Norway	3.7
Germany	4.4
Sweden	4.7
France	5.5
Denmark	6.0
Finland	6.1
Italy	9.2
Ireland	11.8
Netherlands	12.6
Canada	14.9
Spain	17.5
United States	21.3

Percent: 0 5 10 15 20 25

This graph shows the percentage of 9-year-old children who reported watching more than 5 hours of television per weekday in 2005 in 13 countries.

Four major types of child abuse are commonly identified: physical abuse, sexual abuse, emotional abuse, and child neglect. Among these types, a review of research conducted between 2000 and 2009 concluded that 4–16% of children are physically abused in high income nations, such as the United States, the United Kingdom, Australia, and Canada. An additional 10% of girls and 5% of boys are victims of sexual abuse (Sharples, 2008).

Unfortunately, there are no universal legal or scientific definitions of child abuse (Emery & Laumann-Billings, 2002). As Figure 7.12 shows, child abuse affects children of all ages. Physical and sexual abuses, if reported, leave evidence to detect and describe. In 1961, C. Henry Kempe and his associates startled the annual meeting of the American Academy of Pediatrics by their dramatic description of the **battered child syndrome,** a combination of physical and other signs indicating that a child's injuries stem from physical abuse. Other forms of abuse that emotionally wound youngsters may never be detected. In a diverse population, some parents may not consider certain practices as abusive. For example, Cambodian families may treat fever with cao gao, a practice of rubbing hot coins over a child's back or chest that leaves a symmetrical pattern of bruises (Wyckoff, 1999).

RESILIENT CHILDREN

Many children can adapt to stress and develop competent social, emotional, and cognitive functioning despite the challenge of powerful stressors (Friedman & Chase-Lansdale, 2002). Resilience is characterized by the ability to recover relatively quickly from setbacks.

Resilient children have endured terrible circumstances and come through, not unscathed but skilled at fending off feelings of inferiority, helplessness, and isolation (Heller et al., 1999). What we know about these children points to their ability to recover from either physiological or psychological trauma and return to a normal developmental path (Cicchetti & Toth, 1998).

What personal characteristics distinguish resilient children? The following features are the results of many years of research (Garmezy & Rutter, 1983, 1985; Werner & Smith, 1992, 2001):

- *They have temperaments that elicit positive responses from those around them.* They are "easy" children: Their eating and sleeping habits are quite regular, they show positive responses when people approach them, they adapt to changes in their environment, and they

child abuse Infliction of injury to a child; commonly includes physical, sexual, and emotional abuse, or neglect.

battered child syndrome A combination of physical and other signs that indicate a child's injuries result from physical abuse.

resilient children Children who sustained some type of physiological or psychological trauma yet return to a normal developmental path.

FIGURE 7.12
Child Abuse and Neglect

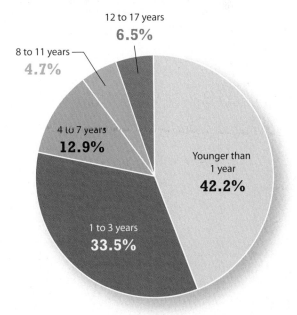

- 12 to 17 years: 6.5%
- 8 to 11 years: 4.7%
- 4 to 7 years: 12.9%
- 1 to 3 years: 33.5%
- Younger than 1 year: 42.2%

This graph shows child abuse and neglect fatality victims by age, 2007.

Source: http://www.childwelfare.gov/pubs/factsheets/fatality1.gif

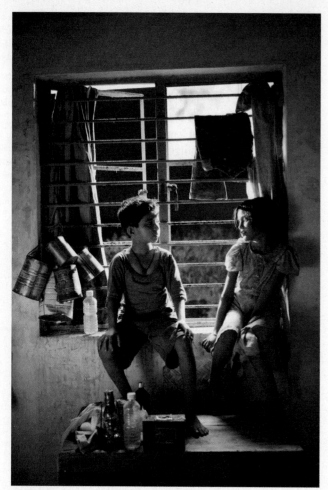

The main characters in the film Slumdog Millionaire *exhibit resilience despite tremendous challenges.*

exhibit a considerable degree of self-regulation. Despite the trauma they have suffered, they are friendly, likable children who possess an inner quality that protects them from their hostile surroundings and enables them to reach out to an adult who could offer critical support.

- *They have special interests or talents.* Some might be excellent swimmers, dancers, and artists, and others might have a special knack for working with animals or a talent with numbers. Whatever their interest, it serves to absorb them and help shelter them from their environment. These activities seem to provide the encouragement and stability often lacking in their home lives.

- *They are sufficiently intelligent to acquire good problem-solving skills,* which they then use to make the best of things around them. They attract the attention of helpful adults, do well in school, and are often popular.

Their competence elicits support from others, which produces a good sense of self.

When adults who come from troubled families look back on the struggles they had during childhood, they usually mention some person—grandparent, aunt, neighbor, teacher, religious figure, coach—who helped them. The support, warmth, advice, and comfort offered by this person was crucial (Dacey & Fiore, 2000).

Such characteristics—a genuinely warm, easygoing personality, an absorbing interest, and the ability to seek out a sympathetic adult—help to buffer children from an abusive parent or other hardships. Efforts to learn more about resilient children also help identify paths of intervention and prevention of undesired outcomes of adverse conditions (Von Eye & Schuster, 2000). There is no single set of qualities or circumstances that characterizes all such resilient children. But psychologists are finding that they stand apart from their more vulnerable siblings almost from birth. They seem to be endowed with innate characteristics that insulate them from the turmoil and pain of their families and allow them to reach out to some adult—a grandparent, teacher, or family friend—who can lend crucial emotional support (Werner & Smith, 1992).

CONCLUSIONS & SUMMARY

In middle childhood, children can assimilate and accommodate material they encounter at their developmental level. They are capable of representational thought, but only with concrete objects. They find it difficult to fully comprehend abstract subtleties in reading, social studies, or any subject.

With all of the developmental accomplishments of the previous 6 or 7 years, youngsters want to use their abilities, which means that they sometimes experience failure as well as success, especially in their schoolwork. Now that they are physically active, cognitively capable, and socially receptive, much is expected of these children, especially in school. During these years, children move away from a sheltered home environment into a world of new friends, new challenges, and new problems. Whether the task is adjusting to a new sibling, relating to peers and teachers, or coping with difficulties, children of this age enter a different world. Children deal uniquely with stress, using temperamental qualities and coping skills as best they can.

How would you describe physical and motor development during these years?

- Children consolidate their height and weight gains.
- Children develop considerable coordination in their motor skills.

What are some of the competing views of cognitive development during middle childhood?

- Among the major cognitive achievements of this period are conservation, seriation, classification, numeration, and reversibility.
- Children of this age show clear signs of increasing symbolic ability.
- Gardner and Sternberg have proposed new ways of explaining intelligence.

How do children develop thinking and problem-solving strategies?

- Children today need critical thinking skills to adapt to sophisticated, technological societies.

How would you trace children's progress in moral development?

- Piaget formulated a theory of moral development that is tightly linked to his explanation of cognitive development.
- Kohlberg proposed six levels of moral development that follow a child's progress from about 4 years of age to adulthood.
- Gilligan has challenged the male-oriented basis of Kohlberg's work.

How does children's language change during these years?

- Children's language development during these years shows increasing representation and facility in conversing with others.
- Children develop several strategies to help them with their reading.

What are the key elements in children acquiring a personally satisfying and competent sense of self?

- The link between self-esteem and competence grows stronger.
- The development of self-regulation becomes a key element in a child's success.

How influential are peers during these years?

- Children begin to form close friendships.
- Children form and test social relationships.

What are some effects of schools and teachers?

- Children encounter considerable change in both curriculum and instructional methods.

How does technology affect children's development?

- Television rivals school for children's time and attention.
- Controversy surrounds the issue of the effects of television violence.
- Television also has potential for encouraging prosocial behavior.

What are some of the major stressors of the middle childhood years?

- Children react differently to stress according to age, gender, and temperament.
- Some children, determined to be resilient, overcome adverse effects of early stressors.

KEY TERMS

asthma *157*

attention deficit disorder *160*

attention deficit hyperactivity disorder (ADHD) *160*

autonomous morality *168*

battered child syndrome *179*

body mass index (BMI) *158*

bullying *175*

child abuse *178*

competence *173*

concrete operational stage *160*

decentration *161*

decode *160*

developing readers *171*

elaboration *167*

emergent readers *170*

ethics of care *169*

heteronomous morality *168*

immanent justice *168*

inclusion *162*

independent readers *171*

individualized education plan (IEP) *162*

intelligence *163*

intelligence quotient (IQ) *165*

knowledge-acquisition components *164*

learning disability *159*

least restrictive environment *162*

mental age *165*

metacomponents *164*

moral development *167*

No Child Left Behind Act *170*

non-stage theorists *170*

obesity *158*

performance components *164*

resilient children *179*

self-concept *173*

self-esteem *173*

self-regulation *174*

seriation *162*

stage theorists *169*

stress *178*

theory of multiple intelligences *163*

transitivity *162*

triarchic theory of intelligence *164*

For REVIEW

1. Imagine a 9-year-old boy (Tim) who lives in the suburbs of a large city. He shows signs of becoming a great baseball player, and his father believes that his son could eventually win a college scholarship and go on to become a professional someday. He decides that Tim should not play pickup games with his friends, because he might hurt himself. He also decides that the family should move to the South so that Tim can play ball all year. How can you relate this scenario to the notion of competence? To family and peer relationships?

2. You are a first-grade teacher and you turn to six-year-old Talia and say, "Talia, Matthew is taller than Sam, who is taller than Ella. Who's the tallest of all?" Talia looks at you quizzically. How would you explain Talia's behavior in light of Piaget's theory?

3. Great concern exists today about the increasing rate of violence among children. Do you think the problem is as serious as researchers indicate? From your knowledge of this topic, do you think the predictors of early criminal behavior are useful?

Chapter Review Test

1. Psychological characteristics of middle childhood include all except
   a. seriation.
   b. conservation.
   c. moral reasoning.
   d. random scribbling.

2. Sternberg's triarchic theory includes metacomponents, knowledge-acquisition components, and _____ components.
   a. gender
   b. performance
   c. age
   d. chromosome

3. Two creative thinking skills programs are Odyssey of the Mind and
   a. Triarchic Theory.
   b. Multiple Intelligence.
   c. Piaget's Program.
   d. Project Zero.

4. Howard Gardner's theory of multiple intelligences includes _____ equal intelligences.
   a. four
   b. five
   c. eight
   d. ten

5. Recognizing what is distinctive in others is an example of which of Gardner's intelligences?
   a. linguistic
   b. interpersonal
   c. logical-mathematical
   d. bodily-kinesthetic

6. One problem with intelligence tests is that the _____ of test takers and test makers may differ.
   a. relationships
   b. circumstances
   c. conditions
   d. values

7. Gilligan's developmental sequence is based on
   a. social justice.
   b. female superiority.
   c. ethics of care.
   d. moral reasoning.

8. Children who have similar levels of competence may have quite different levels of
   a. self-esteem.
   b. friendship.
   c. television viewing.
   d. cognitive development.

9. Friends provide certain resources for children. Which of these is not a resource provided by friends?
   a. membership in the sibling underworld
   b. opportunity for learning skills
   c. chance to compare self with others
   d. chance to belong to a group

10. Among the protective factors for resilient children is
   a. temperament.
   b. interactive error.
   c. geographic mobility.
   d. assimilation.

Answers: 1d, 2b, 3d, 4c, 5b, 6d, 7c, 8a, 9a, 10a

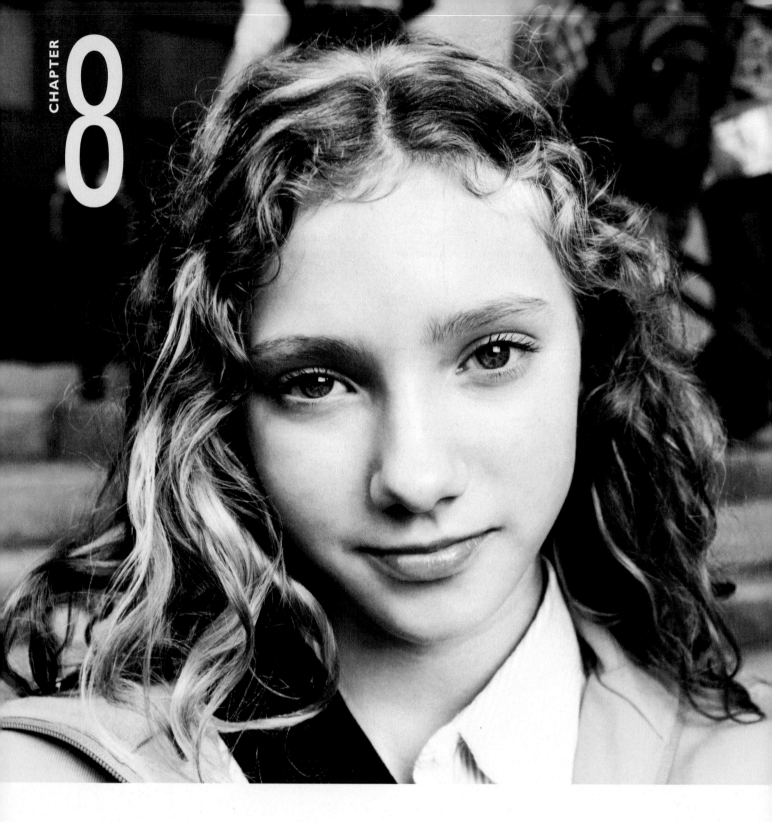

ADOLESCENCE

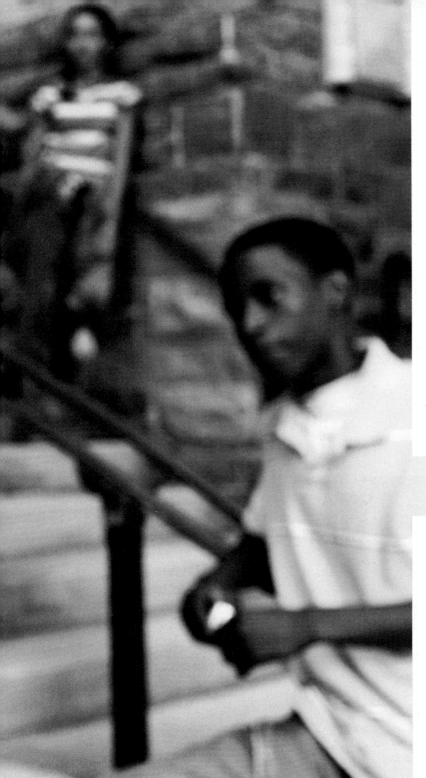

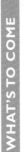
As You READ

After reading this chapter, you should be able to answer the following questions:

- How is adolescence defined?

- What are the leading theories that attempt to explain adolescence?

- What are the key factors of physical development in adolescence?

- How does cognition develop during the adolescent years?

- What changes have occurred to American families and their roles in adolescent life in recent years?

- What is the nature of peer relations during the teen years?

- How do teens deal with sexual relations?

- What recent information do we have on adolescent illegal behavior?

"Who are you?" said the caterpillar. Alice replied, rather shyly, "I—I hardly know, Sir, just at present—at least I know who I was when I got up this morning, but I must have changed several times since then."

LEWIS CARROLL, *ALICE IN WONDERLAND* (1865)

The musical *Spring Awakening* has become a powerful experience for audiences of all ages. The creators have opened doors for conversations among parents and children about topics they may be nervous to discuss, attempt to ignore, yet yearn to talk about. Research argues that youths are under greater stress than in previous decades (for example, Reisberg, 2000), but *Spring Awakening* testifies to the fact that adolescence has long been a unique and challenging period for young people and their families.

What Is Adolescence and When Does It Start?

Frank Wedekind (1864–1918) and Lewis Carroll (1832–1898) both captured elements of adolescence that still ring true today. Adolescence is a time of life marked by transitions. As exemplified in *Spring Awakening* and supported by research, key biological, psychological, and social transitions signal the entry into adolescence.

When did your adolescence begin?

- When you began to menstruate, or when you had your first ejaculation.

- When the level of adult hormones rose sharply in your bloodstream.

- When you first thought about dating.

- When your pubic hair began to grow.

- When you turned 11 years old (girl) or 12 years old (boy).

- When you developed an interest in sex.

- When you passed societal initiation rites (e.g., Jewish bar or bat mitzvah; Catholic confirmation)

- When you became really moody.

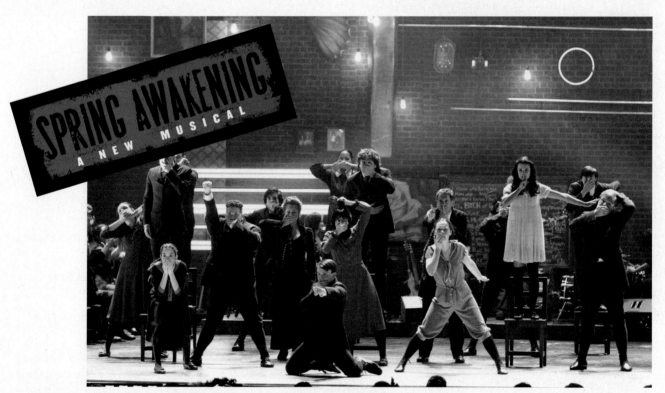

Spring Awakening, the Broadway musical, is inspired by a piece of work that was considered so dangerous when it was written by German playwright Frank Wedekind over 100 years ago that it was banned from public viewing on the stage. The play, written in 1891, concerns adolescents who are coming to terms with their sexuality and deals with such topics as masturbation, sexual abuse, homosexuality, abortion, rape, and suicide.

The controversy begins simply enough when the female protagonist, Wendla, becomes curious about her changing body and asks her mother how babies are born. Her mother responds with a curt, diversionary fib that foreshadows unintended consequences.

Only the smart and radical male protagonist, Melchior, is able to embrace the changes that puberty brings, and he attempts to help his good friend Moritz, who is paralyzed with fear over the implications of his new urges and his failing grades. If Moritz can't keep up academically, he worries about how he will measure up . . . in other ways.

- When you thought about being away from your parents.
- When you worried about the way your body looked.
- When you could judge actions independent of your own opinions.
- When your friends influenced you more than your parents.
- When you began to wonder who you really are.

It's possible that there are many adolescence-defining moments, and they don't provide a clear starting point for a clear entry into the rest of life. What is quite clear, however, is the biopsychosocial nature of adolescent experiences. For example, a girl's first menstruation, called **menarche,** can occur at any time from 8 to 16 years of age. A menstruating 8-year-old would not likely be considered an adolescent, but a nonmenstruating 16-year-old would likely be considered one. Cognitive factors relating to social values and expectations join with physical realities when considering a girl a child or an adolescent.

In his two-volume set called *Adolescence* (1904), American psychologist G. Stanley Hall was the first to offer a specific theory to explain development in the teen years. Based almost entirely on biology, a major aspect of his theory was his speculation that this stage of life is characterized by "storm and stress" because of the amount of change a person experiences in physical, cognitive, and social domains. This stereotype has been perpetuated in the media, but refuted in research and personal accounts. Figure 8.1 illustrates adolescent behaviors that translate into perceptions and stereotypes about teenagers.

Physical Development

To better understand physical development in adolescence, let's start with the following questions: What parts of the body are involved? When does puberty start? What are the effects of timing?

Adolescents have many questions about puberty, such as how the organs of our reproductive system function. The musical *Spring Awakening* is a perfect illustration of the degree to which adolescents' healthy biopsychosocial development depends on accurate communication with adults about this topic. Misunderstandings about physical development can impact cognitive and social functions. Figures 8.2 and 8.3 depict the female and male sexual systems.

menarche A girl's first menstruation.

puberty The process of physical changes by which a child's body becomes an adult body capable of reproduction.

hormonal balance Change in hormone levels, one of the triggers of puberty.

WHEN DOES PUBERTY START?

The sequence of bodily changes in **puberty** is surprisingly constant. This holds true whether puberty starts early or late, and regardless of the culture in which the child is reared.

Change in hormone levels, called **hormonal balance,** is one of the triggers of puberty, but its beginning is difficult to pinpoint. Measuring skeletal growth, genital growth,

> Gretchen, *my friend, got* her **period.** *I'm so jealous,* *God. I hate myself for being* so **jealous,** *but I am. I wish* *you'd help me just a little.*

JUDY BLUME, *ARE YOU THERE, GOD? IT'S ME, MARGARET* (1981)

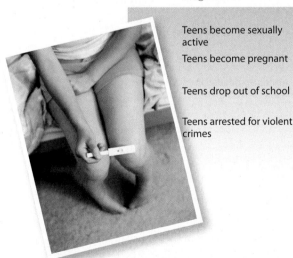

Adolescents have been viewed through lenses that reflect altruistic and negative behaviors.

FIGURE 8.1

An Average Day in the Life of Some North American Teens

Negative behaviors	Altruistic behaviors
Teens become sexually active	Teens join service club
Teens become pregnant	Teens join Students Against Drunk Driving
Teens drop out of school	Teens volunteer at a homeless shelter
Teens arrested for violent crimes	Teens work a part-time job

FIGURE 8.2

Female Sexual System

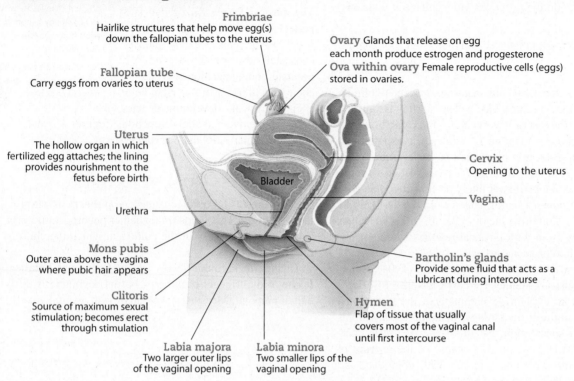

Frimbriae
Hairlike structures that help move egg(s) down the fallopian tubes to the uterus

Ovary Glands that release on egg each month produce estrogen and progesterone
Ova within ovary Female reproductive cells (eggs) stored in ovaries.

Fallopian tube
Carry eggs from ovaries to uterus

Uterus
The hollow organ in which fertilized egg attaches; the lining provides nourishment to the fetus before birth

Cervix
Opening to the uterus

Bladder

Vagina

Urethra

Mons pubis
Outer area above the vagina where pubic hair appears

Bartholin's glands
Provide some fluid that acts as a lubricant during intercourse

Clitoris
Source of maximum sexual stimulation; becomes erect through stimulation

Hymen
Flap of tissue that usually covers most of the vaginal canal until first intercourse

Labia majora
Two larger outer lips of the vaginal opening

Labia minora
Two smaller lips of the vaginal opening

FIGURE 8.3

Male Sexual System

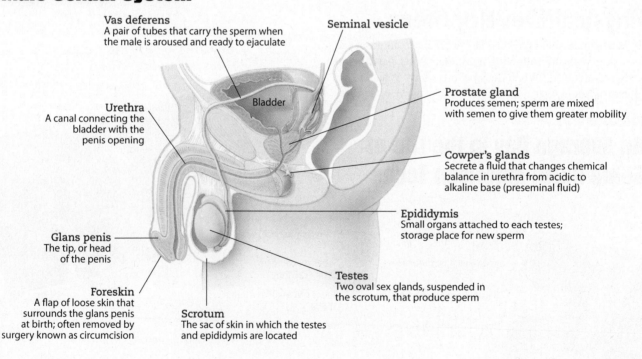

Vas deferens
A pair of tubes that carry the sperm when the male is aroused and ready to ejaculate

Seminal vesicle

Urethra
A canal connecting the bladder with the penis opening

Bladder

Prostate gland
Produces semen; sperm are mixed with semen to give them greater mobility

Cowper's glands
Secrete a fluid that changes chemical balance in urethra from acidic to alkaline base (preseminal fluid)

Epididymis
Small organs attached to each testes; storage place for new sperm

Glans penis
The tip, or head of the penis

Testes
Two oval sex glands, suspended in the scrotum, that produce sperm

Foreskin
A flap of loose skin that surrounds the glans penis at birth; often removed by surgery known as circumcision

Scrotum
The sac of skin in which the testes and epididymis are located

FIGURE 8.4

Typical Age Ranges for Signs of Puberty

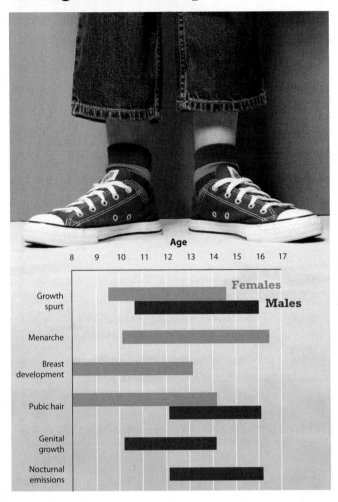

FIGURE 8.5

Adolescent Growth Chart

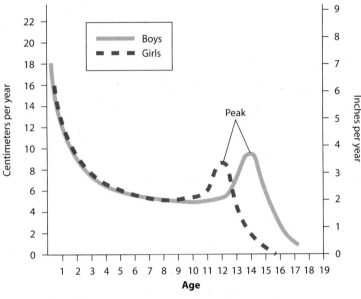

Rate of height increase

pubic hair, breast development, voice change, or a growth spurt requires recording over a period of time. Menarche has been suggested as the major turning point for girls, and first ejaculation as the beginning of adolescent puberty for males, but these are not often remembered as events that felt like entry into adulthood. Figure 8.4 illustrates the typical age ranges for events in puberty

The relatively slow and steady growth patterns of childhood are replaced with a growth spurt in adolescence, as shown in Figure 8.5, and girls tend to grow taller sooner than boys. Adolescent changes in height, soon followed by changes in weight, last for approximately 2 years, and adolescents' eating habits reflect their bodies' energy requirements and demand more fuel. By the time teenagers start high school, girls' and boys' bodies have begun to resemble adults' bodies. Most noticeably, girls develop broader hips and boys develop broader shoulders. The psychological impact of these events, however, can be quite significant. This is especially true with menstruation. When menarche comes early (before 11 years of age), it is more likely to be associated with depression and substance abuse than when it comes later (Beausang & Razor, 2000; Stice, Presenell, & Bearman, 2001).

secular trend The decreasing age of the onset of puberty.

THE SECULAR TREND

In Western countries, the average age of menarche has declined about 3 months per decade over the past 100 years. This phenomenon is called the **secular trend,** which refers to the decreasing age of the onset of puberty. Girls especially are reaching menarche at younger ages. In the United States, in the late 18th and early 19th centuries, the average age of menarche was 17. Today, the average age of

anorexia nervosa An eating disorder characterized by low body weight and distorted body image.

menarche is 12.5 (Posner, 2006). Some researchers have linked childhood obesity with early onset of menarche (Anderson, Dallal, & Must, 2003; Lee et al., 2007).

Ellis and associates (1999) found that factors of family relationships are associated with starting puberty later. These include fathers' presence in the home, fathers providing more child care, greater supportiveness from both parents, and more affection from both parents for the daughter. It is clear that the processes of development and the role of puberty are complicated and occur concurrently (Dorn et al., 2003).

Although there is a trend for later onset of puberty, some boys and girls mature earlier than usual. For boys, this is often associated with self-confidence and popularity, as their increased physical capacity sometimes prepares them to be more skilled at sports and other activities. On the other hand, greater physical ability is sometimes linked with aggression and misbehavior. Early puberty tends to be more difficult for girls than it is for boys in that the sexual attention adolescent girls receive is often unwelcome and unwanted.

In summary, most humans proceed toward maturity in the same way, but in the last few centuries the timing of the process in females has changed radically. Although timing is affected mainly by biology, psychological and social forces clearly influence it, too.

BODY IMAGE AND EATING DISORDERS

At a time when adolescents are preoccupied with their bodies and judging themselves against others, the physical changes of puberty can lead to dissatisfaction with physical appearance. Eating disorders are the third most common chronic condition among adolescents. The two main types, anorexia nervosa and bulimia, have in common a deep concern about weight (Jimerson, Pavelski, & Orliss, 2002). While some symptoms are unique to one disorder, there are many parallels between anorexia nervosa and bulimia.

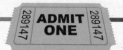

FEATURED MEDIA

Love and Adolescence

***High School Musical* (2006)** – The status quo is challenged when basketball star Troy and science whiz Gabriella break clique barriers and audition for their school play. Musical numbers capture the internal struggles the characters are grappling with as they try on different aspects of their identities and explore friendship, love, and cafeteria politics.

***Nick and Norah's Infinite Playlist* (2008)** – How does a plan to spite less-than-faithful partners turn into the ultimate recipe for romance (not to mention great music)?

***Romeo and Juliet* (1996)** – A modern take on Shakespeare's classic play, set in a modern suburb. The film retains the original dialogue, and presents timeless tensions between teens and their parents.

***Twilight* (2008) *New Moon* (2009) and *Eclipse* (2010)** – These films are based on the series of popular romance novels by Stephanie Meyer, which tell the story of teenage Bella and her (much older!) vampire boyfriend Edward. Bella takes many risks to love, and be loved by, Edward.

Anorexia nervosa is a syndrome of self-starvation that mainly affects adolescent and young adult females, who account for 95% of the known cases. Professionals suspect that many males may also be victims (for example, those who must maintain a low weight for sports), but their anorexia is not as obvious and/or publicly discussed

perspectives on Diversity

Racial and Ethnic Differences in Onset of Puberty

Researchers have cited racial and ethnic differences in the onset of puberty (Chumlea et al., 2003; Obeidallah et al., 2000). The secular trend for earlier onset of puberty in the last century is most noticeable among African American girls, followed by Mexican American girls and then Caucasian girls. African American girls tend to experience puberty 1½ years earlier than Caucasian girls—approximately age 9 compared to age 10½ for breast development and age 12 (African Americans) compared to almost 13 (Caucasians) for menarche.

The reasons for racial differences are not clear, but lifestyle factors such as diet, use of hormone-enhanced products, and exposure to environmental agents could contribute to the differences.

(O'Dea & Abraham, 1999). Some key features of anorexia nervosa are inability to sustain a healthy weight, fear of any weight gain, and a greatly inaccurate perception of body image (American Psychiatric Association, 2000).

Health professionals have seen an alarming rise in the incidence of this disorder among young women in the past 15 to 20 years. Whether anorexia nervosa has actually increased or whether it is now being more readily recognized has yet to be determined.

Bulimia nervosa is a disorder related to anorexia nervosa and sometimes occurs with it. It is characterized by binge eating followed by purging to prevent weight gain. In addition, the self-evaluation of individuals with bulimia nervosa is excessively influenced by body shape and weight. Bulimia has been observed in women above or below weight, as well as in those who are of average weight, and detailed criteria may be found in the *Diagnostic and Statistical Manual of Mental Disorders,* 4th edition, or (DSM-IV) (American Psychiatric Association, 2000).

Despite their clinical differences, anorexics and bulimics share some emotional and behavioral traits. The preoccupation with food and the desire to be thin sometimes mask deep psychological issues that lie beneath the surface (Jimerson et al., 2002). A history of abuse—ranging from emotional to sexual—can prompt eating disorders, as can a home environment where children are raised with expectations of perfection.

Cognitive Development

Adolescence is a complex process of growth and change. Because biological and social changes are often the focus of attention, changes in the young adolescent's ability to think may go unnoticed, yet growth spurts in the parietal and frontal lobes of the brain, as well as subcortical regions, make possible tremendous changes in the quality of a teenager's thinking. During early and middle adolescence, thinking ability reaches Piaget's fourth and last level—the level of abstract thought.

VARIABLES IN COGNITIVE DEVELOPMENT: PIAGET

Recall from Chapter 2 that Jean Piaget proposed that the ability to think develops in four stages: the sensorimotor stage (birth to 2 years old); the preoperational stage (2 to 7 years old); the concrete operational stage (7 to 11 years old); and the formal operational stage (11 years old and up). In the **formal operational stage,** individuals can think abstractly, reason logically, exhibit hypothetical thinking, and combine groups of concrete operations. For example, the adolescent comes to understand democracy by combining concepts such as putting a ballot in a box and hearing that the Senate voted to provide funding to help the homeless.

It was Piaget who first noted early adolescents' bent toward democratic values because of this new thinking

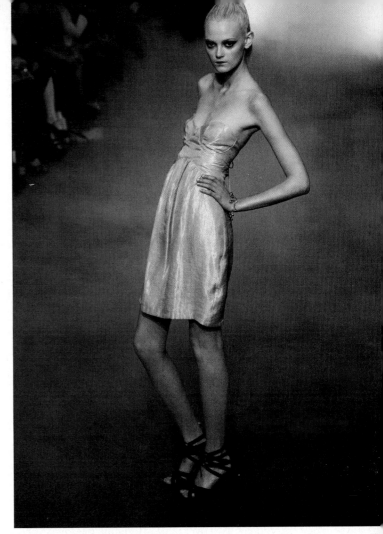

The image of femininity has changed over the years. How might this affect teens' perceptions of their bodies?

capacity. This is the age when youths first become committed to the idea that members of a group may change the rules of a game, but once agreed on, all members must follow the new rules. This tendency, Piaget believed, is universal; all teenagers throughout the world commit to this idea.

However, culture and gender also influence cognitive development. Many theorists focus on an ideal developmental progression that reflects their own values and beliefs about maturity. Piaget (1973) acknowledged that his descrip-

bulimia nervosa An eating disorder featuring binge eating and purging.

formal operational stage Piaget's fourth stage of cognitive development, featuring abstract thought and scientific thinking.

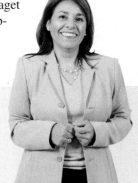

Career Apps

As a school nurse, what resources could you share with young men and women to give them an accurate reference relating to body proportions and optimal health?

tion of the final stage might not apply to all cultures, as evidence showed cultural variation. The influence of context (sociocultural and individual) on development (Rogoff, 1991; Vygotsky, 1978) supports multiple directions for development rather than only one ideal end point. For example, it may be that for some agricultural societies, sophisticated development of the concrete operational stage would be far more useful than development of formal operational thinking. That is, an understanding of the complicated workings of a machine may be concrete, but that does not make that type of thinking inferior to another person's ability to write haiku.

Chavous and associates (2003) studied the effects of culture on cognition, specifically on the academic achievement of African Americans. They compared Black adolescents on educational beliefs, performance, and level of later attainment (completing high school and college attendance). They found that African American youths have different interpretations of their racial identities, and these beliefs may lead them down different paths of educational achievement. For instance, some adolescents who were proud of their race but felt as though society viewed their race negatively had the highest rates of post–high school achievement. Perhaps, in this case, they were motivated by their determination to overcome discrimination.

Gender also plays a role in defining formal operations. According to Gilligan (1982), most theories of development define the end point of development as being male only and they overlook alternatives that more closely fit the mature female. She believed that if the definition of maturity changes, so does the entire account of development. Using men as the model of development, researchers see independence and separation as the goals of development. If women are used as the models, the goals of development are relationship with others and interdependence. Gilligan argues that this gender difference also leads to distinctions in development of thinking about morality.

EMOTIONS AND BRAIN DEVELOPMENT

Researchers continue to study how the brain initiates complex emotions such as self-awareness, morality, feelings of free will, and social emotions. Some believe that neurons known as **spindle cells** play a large part in how the brain creates emotion (Blakeslee, 2003). These cells are responsible for sending socially relevant signals across the brain. This function, whereby the subcortex filters out all but new and/or really important information, is known as the **reticular activation system (RAS).** The RAS protects the brain from being overwhelmed by irrelevant data. Despite great

similarities among various mammals' brains, only humans and great apes have spindle cells. These cells are not even present at the time of birth. Instead, they gradually appear as children develop a concept of moral and social judgments, and then develop more rapidly during adolescence.

Connections between neurons are responsible for communication between the body and the brain. As these connections become more established and complex in adolescence, information is transformed into more sophisticated understandings. Concrete information becomes associated with more intangible emotions along the path. It is through this pathway that the most basic aspects of human nature such as love, sadness, fear, excitement, and anger are processed (Blakeslee, 2003).

In a study conducted by Yurgelun-Todd (1998), adults and adolescents were shown photos depicting fear. The adults accurately identified the emotion, but most adolescents incorrectly identified the pictured emotion as anger and worry. After studying brain scans of the teens and adults, Yurgelun-Todd found that the amygdala (the part of the brain that is responsible for emotional responses) played a large role in the teens' reactions (see Figure 8.6). In contrast, the prefrontal cortex (the part of the brain that is responsible for reason and thought) played a large role in the adults' responses. Such differences between adolescent and adult brain function may impact why teens' experiences are often described as turbulent (Killgore & Oki, 2001).

ADOLESCENT EGOCENTRISM

Parents often feel frustrated by the attitudes and behaviors of their adolescent children. One explanation is the reemergence of a pattern of thought that marked early childhood—egocentrism. **Adolescent egocentrism,** a term coined by Elkind (1978), refers to adolescents' tendency to exaggerate the importance, uniqueness, and severity of their social and emotional experiences. Their love is greater than anything others have experienced. Their suffering is more painful and unjust than anyone else's. Developmentally speaking, adolescent egocentrism seems to peak around the age of 13, followed by a gradual and sometimes painful decline (Elkind & Bowen, 1979).

Elkind sees two parts to this egocentrism. First, teenagers tend to create an **imaginary audience** (Vartanian & Powlishta, 2001). They feel they are on center stage and that other people are constantly scrutinizing their behavior and physical appearance. This accounts for some of the mood swings in adolescents. One minute a glance in the mirror launches an elated, confident teenager ready to take on the world, and the next minute a pimple can be cause for staying inside the house all day. In fact, school phobia can become acute during early adolescence because of concerns over physical appearance.

The second component of egocentrism is the **personal fable.** This refers to adolescents' tendency to think of themselves in heroic or mythical terms (Frankenberger, 2000; Vartanian & Powlishta, 2001). The result is that they

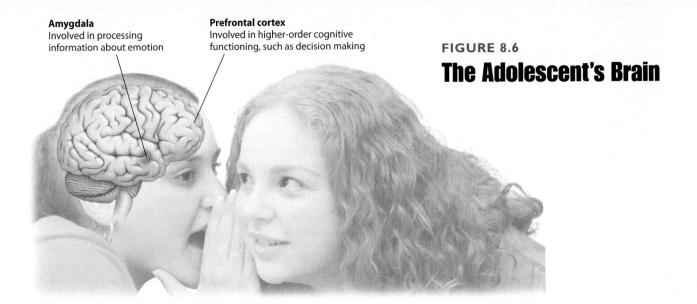

Amygdala
Involved in processing information about emotion

Prefrontal cortex
Involved in higher-order cognitive functioning, such as decision making

FIGURE 8.6
The Adolescent's Brain

exaggerate their own abilities and their invincibility. The personal fable sometimes leads to increased risk-taking, such as drug use, dangerous driving, and disregard for the possible consequences of sexual behavior. Many teenagers simply can't imagine an unhappy ending to their own special story.

INFORMATION PROCESSING

As children transition into adolescence, one of the cognitive changes that is markedly different from that of earlier years is their improved **executive functioning.** Executive functioning includes efforts aimed at allocating attention, cognitive resources that can impact physical and emotional resources, and critical thinking strategies. As teens acquire more strategies for evaluating and solving problems, they can apply these skills to everyday decision making in various situations (Byrnes, 2005). For example, teens must make decisions about whether or not to experiment with drugs and alcohol, which friends to bring into their close trust, and how to best prepare for college or career.

As with any skills that initially require practice before they become effortless, decision-making skills require practice in real-life situations in order for adolescents, and the adults who care for them, to become confident in their abilities. This holds true for trial-and-error experiences

we experience at any age, but in adolescence, when teens are poised on the verge of adult recognition and responsibility, decision-making skills come under closer scrutiny and can have larger consequences. A decision to ride in a car with a close friend who has been drinking and now wishes to drive home may result in a life-threatening accident.

executive functioning Cognitive efforts involving attention and critical thinking.

convergent thinking Thinking used when a problem to be solved has one correct answer.

divergent thinking Thinking used when a problem to be solved has many possible answers.

CRITICAL THINKING

The role of critical thinking is highlighted in adolescence as teens are able to think about a problem or situation from multiple perspectives. Critical thinking involves two abilities: convergent thinking and divergent thinking.

Convergent thinking is used when we solve a problem by following a series of steps that close in on the correct answer. Only one answer is correct. **Divergent thinking** is just the opposite: This type of thinking is used when a problem to be solved has many possible answers. Divergent thinking can be right or wrong, too, but much more leeway exists for personal opinion than with convergent thinking. Not all divergent thinking is creative, but it is more likely to produce a creative concept.

Young teenagers today are being forced *to make decisions that earlier* generations *didn't have to make until they were older and more* mature, *and today's teenagers are not getting much support and* guidance.

DAVID ELKIND

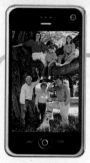
Identity in Adolescence

The theories of three psychologists, Erik Erikson, James Marcia, and John Hill, represent different views on adolescence and capture the complexities of this developmental period. Considered together, their theories provide a perspective on adolescence as a multidimensional period in the lifespan.

ERIKSON'S PSYCHOSOCIAL THEORY

For Erik Erikson (1902–1994), adolescence is the fifth stage in his psychosocial theory of development, that of identity versus identity confusion. The main task is to achieve a state of identity, something to which one strives, rather than a final, definitive identity. Erikson saw adolescence as a time of intensive exploration and analysis of ways of looking at oneself. He used the term **identity crisis** to capture the essence of confusion a person feels when she experiences discomfort about herself. For example, a teen who is very smart and competent, but not part of the "popular" crowd at school, may aspire to popularity even though she knows that the group often behaves in ways that go against her personal values. She must grapple with the importance of being true to what she deems correct and what she perceives as being prized and rewarded by others.

Erikson suggested that identity confusion is likely in a democratic society because so many life choices are available. In a totalitarian society, youths are typically given an identity that they are forced to accept. For example, the paramilitary Hitler Youth of Germany in the 1930s is an example of a mandatory national effort backed by intense propaganda to get all adolescents to identify with prescribed values and attitudes.

Erikson proposed that, in our culture, adolescence is a period of psychosocial moratorium—a "time-out" during which adolescents experiment with a variety of identities, yet experience no responsibility for the consequences. Erikson stated that indecision—and tolerance of it—and idealism are essential in the identity-seeking process. Some youths, however, commit themselves to an identity too early, without adequately considering all choices. As youths search for truth, they are building commitments to people, belief systems, and institutions that help unite their personal values.

MARCIA'S IDENTITY STATUS

Elaborating on Erikson's ideas, James Marcia (Berzonsky & Kuk, 2000; Marcia, 2002) stresses two vital factors in the attainment of a mature identity: crisis and commitment. First, the person must undergo several crises relating to choice, such as deciding whether to hold or to give up one's religious beliefs. Second, the person must commit to these choices. A person may or may not have gone through a crisis of choice and may or may not have made a commitment to choices. Thus, four **identity statuses** are possible (see Table 8.1):

Identity confusion: No crisis has been experienced and no commitments have been made.

Identity foreclosure: No crisis has been experienced, but commitments have been made, usually forced on the person by the parent.

Identity moratorium: A number of crises have been experienced, but no commitments are made.

Identity achievement: Numerous crises have been experienced and resolved, and relatively permanent commitments have been made.

Research indicates that Marcia's identity statuses tend to progress in a linear fashion. The college years, for example, are known to be a time when adolescents make great strides in their identity development. As they are exposed to new information that presents alternate positions on numerous issues, they are forced to experience psychological and social conflicts that contribute to their sense of self and overall identity. Carol Gilligan and others (1982, 1990) have focused on gender differences in identity formation. They have concluded that women are less concerned than men with achieving an independent identity status and more likely to define themselves by their relationships and responsibilities to others.

HILL'S BIOPSYCHOSOCIAL THEORY

Relationships factor into the theory of psychologist John Hill (1987), whose biopsychosocial theory of adolescence has led to current research on a wide range of adolescent issues (Collins et al., 2001; Keel et al., 2001; Meschke et al.,

identity crisis Erikson's term for a time of analyzing and making major decisions about one's identity

identity statuses Marcia's categories that depict levels of crisis and commitment that contribute to a sense of identity.

TABLE 8.1

Marcia's Four Identity Statuses

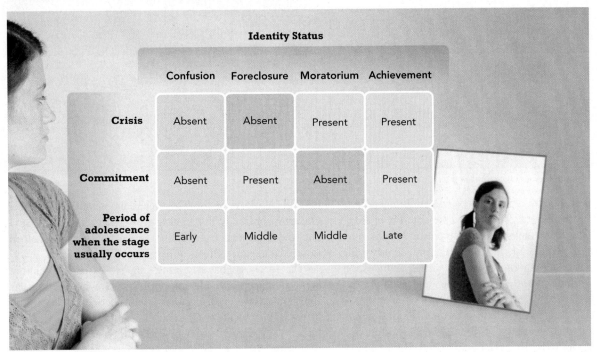

	Identity Status			
	Confusion	**Foreclosure**	**Moratorium**	**Achievement**
Crisis	Absent	Absent	Present	Present
Commitment	Absent	Present	Absent	Present
Period of adolescence when the stage usually occurs	Early	Middle	Middle	Late

2000). In Hill's theory, biological factors are central because they are present at birth. However, psychological and social factors begin playing a part immediately after birth. Each factor is embedded in the other two, and the meanings of each are tightly woven. A fourth factor running through the others is time—the aging process from early to late adolescence as well as events during a particular historical period.

Hill's ideas about psychological factors in adolescence are important to note. Hill (1973) discussed "detachment" as a matter of growing "independence in decision making and feelings of confidence in personal goals and standards of behavior" (p. 37). Hill disagreed with the psychoanalytic view of sexuality—that change in one's sense of a sexual self follows a gradual, continuous pattern. He argued that puberty is brought on by abrupt physiological changes. The social changes involved in acquiring the new self-concept of adolescence force teens to view themselves in a whole new light, potentially influencing intimacy and relationships.

Social Development

As relationships with others assume a prominent position in adolescents' developing identity, the nature of close relationships changes. The changing roles of family and peers are noticeable as teens shift qualities of their intimate relationships from their family to their friends.

THE ROLE OF FAMILY

The report *Changing Rhythms of American Family Life* (Bianchi, Robinson, & Milkie, 2006) states that although mothers today spend more time in the workplace than in previous decades, they spend as much time interacting with their children as mothers did decades ago—perhaps even more. While adolescents' relationships with both parents remain significant, mothers are generally perceived as more supportive than fathers. As adolescents begin to spend less time at home and more time with peers, conflicts with parents can help solidify peer relationships. As they strive for identity and greater independence, adolescents exert greater authority over their lives, but must also accept more responsibility for their choices. Conflict forces adolescents to consider positions with which they may initially disagree. Sometimes, conflicts within the home translate into a difficult environment for adolescents.

Divorce tends to occur most often in families with a newborn, and second most often in families with an adolescent present. Estimates suggest that divorce affects as much as one half of the adolescent population. The family undergoing divorce clearly contributes additional stress to a developing adolescent. One obvious effect is economic. The increased living expenses that result from the need to pay for two homes most often leads to a significant decrease in the standard of living for the children. Young adolescents may resent being unable to keep up with their peers in terms of material goods (e.g., clothes, computer accessories). Older adolescents are better equipped to cope with this type of additional stress psychologically and financially, because they can enter the workforce.

THE ROLE OF PEERS

Although it is clear that friendships are vital throughout life, there seems to be something special about the role of the peer group during adolescence. Related to the quest for

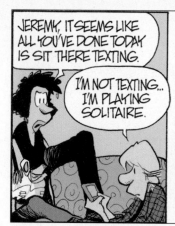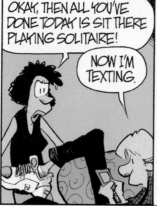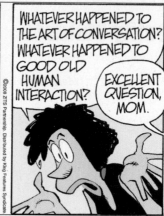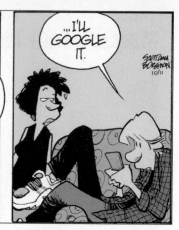

ZITS © 2008 ZITS Partnership, King Features Syndicate.

identity, adolescents are attracted to qualities in others that they aspire to themselves. They also take comfort in finding others who share their personal interests, beliefs, and understandings about the world. They therefore identify with groups that have a reputation for certain values, attitudes, or activities. Common crowd labels among high school students include "jocks," "geeks," "pot-heads," "popular kids," and "burnouts." Interestingly, although the distinct adolescent groups change over time, these crowds seem to exist in some form across all periods in which adolescence has been studied. Brown and associates (1997) made an important distinction between cliques (subgroups within crowds) and crowds: a **clique** is a group of close friends who share similar interests and activities, whereas a **crowd** is a larger, reputation-based group whose members may or may not spend time with one another.

The formation of peer friendships is an important adolescent achievement that supports an individual's developing sense of self and the desire to form relationships with others.

tions to people of the same sex in childhood and adolescence. Growing sensitivity to the struggles that lesbian, gay, bisexual, and transgender (**LGBT**) youth experience has helped lessen the negative effects of perceived societal norms.

The process of accepting one's sexual orientation is particularly difficult for adolescents who identify as LGBT and face a society that is not necessarily accepting of anything outside traditional expectations for males and females. "Coming out"—proclaiming one's homosexuality to others—is a significant and often painful process for adolescents, whose family and friends may not be supportive. As a result, many LGBT teens often suffer in school, resort to alcohol or drugs to cope with emotional pain, or contemplate or even commit suicide (Russell, 2006).

SEXUAL BEHAVIOR

Masturbation is the most common sexual outlet in adolescence. Although most people still consider it an embarrassing topic, it has always been a recognized aspect of

Sexual Identity

Sexual identity is linked to other aspects of identity, to an individual's interests, lifestyle and behavior, and evolving sexual orientation. Whereas some adolescents are comfortable with the physical and emotional sensations that accompany sexuality, others are not. Cognitive and social factors strongly influence how adolescents view their sexuality. Attractions to individuals of the same or opposite sex may be purely physical or emotional, and do not necessarily involve deeper intimacy or love.

Most people identify as **heterosexual**—attracted to members of the opposite sex—but some people experience this attraction to members of the same sex and identify as **homosexual.** Many homosexual adults recall personal struggles with attrac-

clique Group of friends who share similar interests and activities.

crowd Reputation-based group whose members may or may not spend time with one another.

heterosexual Sexual attraction to members of the opposite sex.

homosexual Sexual attraction to members of the same sex.

LGBT An acronym referring to lesbian (female), gay (male), bisexual, and transgender individuals; it can include a Q for queer or questioning (LGBTQ).

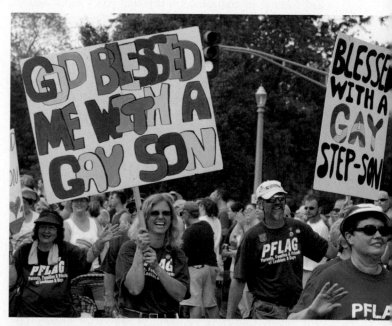

Organizations such as Parents, Families, and Friends of Lesbians and Gays (PFLAG) promote the well-being of teens and their families.

sexuality. Masturbation is a normal, healthy way for people to discharge their sexual drive, but some teens feel a sense of shame, guilt, and fear about it.

The decision to engage in sexual behavior with others depends on many factors, and the timing of such decisions varies by culture, gender, and geographic location. Some adolescents are not emotionally prepared to handle sexual behaviors, which contributes to other risk-taking behaviors. For example, risk behaviors such as drug and alcohol abuse and juvenile delinquency are often associated with intercourse during adolescence (Ngai, Ngai, & Cheung, 2006). Interestingly, Schwartz (2002) found that males and females have considerable levels of sexual exploration before intercourse. Many adolescents do not think they are having sex if their physical acts stop short of actual intercourse.

Many adolescents are sexually active, although available data show that sexual activity among United States adolescents appears to have declined in the past 15 years, likely the result of a growing concern about AIDS and other sexually transmitted infections. Results of studies indicate that the percentage of college sophomores who are sexually active is about 75% for both males and females. In their comparison of the sexual risk-taking behaviors of 9th- through 12th-grade female athletes and their non-athletic counterparts, Savage and Holcomb (1999) found that athletes were less likely to have engaged in risk-taking behaviors as well as less likely to be sexually active, and concluded that participation in sports is positively associated with reduced sexual risk-taking behaviors. Other factors that contribute to adolescents' sexual risk-taking are less parental supervision, a family's low socioeconomic status, and sexually active older siblings (Miller et al., 2002).

When do most Americans first experience intercourse? The statistics vary, but all research confirms that adolescents are indeed sexually active (Gebhardt, Kuyper, & Dusseldorp, 2006). In 2009, the Centers for Disease Control and Prevention published the findings of the national Youth Risk Behavior Survey (YRBS) 1991–2007, which monitored major health risk behaviors that contribute to the leading causes of death, disability, and social problems among youths and adults in the United States. The national YRBS is conducted every 2 years during the spring semester and provides data representative of 9th- through 12th-grade students in public and private schools throughout the United States. Table 8.2 features two of the most relevant of the study's findings on teen sex: The incidence of adolescents who have ever had sex has decreased in the last decade, as has the number of adolescents with multiple sex partners.

How to Talk to Teens About Sex (or Anything Else)

Adolescents are more likely to talk to adults who know how to listen—about sex, alcohol, and other important issues. But certain kinds of responses, such as giving too much advice or pretending to have all the answers, have been shown to block the lines of communication.

Effective listening is more than just "not talking." It takes concentration and practice. Following are five communication skills that are useful to anyone who wants to reach adolescents. (These skills can also enhance communication with other adults.)

1. Rephrase the teen's comments to show you understand. This is sometimes called *reflective listening*. Reflective listening serves these purposes:

   - It assures the teenager you hear what he or she is saying.

   - It persuades the teen that you correctly understand what is being said (it is sometimes a good idea to ask if your rephrasing is correct).

   - It allows you a chance to reword the teen's statements in ways that are less self-destructive.

   - It allows the teen to "rehear" and reconsider what was said.

2. Watch the teen's face and body language. Often a person will assure you that he or she does not feel sad, but a quivering chin or watery eyes will tell you otherwise. When words and body language say two different things, always consider the body language.

3. Give nonverbal support. This may include a smile, a hug, a wink, a pat on the shoulder, eye contact, or holding the person's hand (or wrist).

4. Use the right tone of voice for what you are saying. Remember that your tone communicates as clearly as your words. Make sure your tone does not come across as sarcastic or all-knowing.

5. Use encouraging phrases to show your interest and to keep the conversation going. Helpful phrases such as "Tell me more about that," spoken appropriately during pauses in the conversation, can communicate how much you care.

TABLE 8.2

Trends in Prevalence of Sexual Behavior, 1991–2007

	1991	1995	1999	2003	2007	Changes from 1991 to 2007
Ever had sex	54%	53%	50%	47%	48%	Down 6%
4 or more partners, lifetime	19%	18%	16%	14.5%	15%	Down 6%

Source: Adapted from Centers for Disease Control and Prevention, National YRBS: 1991–2007.

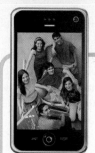
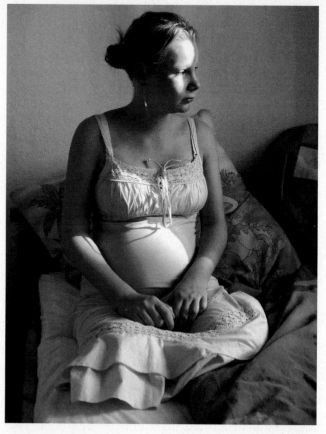

Remember, if you are judgmental or critical, the teen may decide that you just don't understand. You cannot be a good influence on someone who won't talk to you.

TEENAGE PREGNANCY

Each year, about 1 million teenage girls in the United States become pregnant. About half of those pregnancies result in live births, one third result in abortions, and one sixth result in miscarriages. In 2007, most births to teenagers (86%) were to unmarried mothers. Miller and associates (2001) report a series of factors that place some teens at greater risk for pregnancy: poverty, unsafe communities, a single-parent household, a history of sexual abuse, and teenage siblings who are sexually active or are parents.

There are many reasons that teenage girls get pregnant. One of the most serious reasons is the lack of accurate information that teens receive about sex and contraception, as illustrated in the example of Wendla in *Spring Awakening,* who is given insufficient facts about how babies are conceived and born. Without accurate information, adolescents are less likely to make informed decisions or recognize the consequences of their actions. Some girls desire pregnancy for social or psychological reasons, such as feeling accepted in society as a mother, a caregiver, or, ironically, a responsible adult. Some adolescent girls get pregnant by sheer accident. Figure 8.7 illustrates the rate of teen pregnancy in the United States.

Efforts at educating teenagers about pregnancy and contraception have become more widespread, and many families want to have their adolescents informed about the risks involved in sexual activity. Whether or not sex education deters teens from engaging in sexual activity is not certain, but it is acknowledged to impact teens' choices to use contraception.

FIGURE 8.7

Teen Pregnancy in the United States

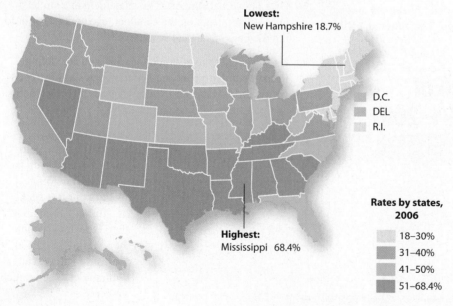

Lowest:
New Hampshire 18.7%

D.C.
DEL
R.I.

Highest:
Mississippi 68.4%

Rates by states, 2006

18–30%
31–40%
41–50%
51–68.4%

SEXUAL ABUSE

When adolescents are abused, it's typically by someone they know and trust. It is often a continuation of abuse that started during childhood. The most common type of serious sexual abuse is incest between father and daughter. This type of relationship may last for several years. The daughter is often manipulated into believing it is all her fault and that, if she says anything to anyone, she'll be a bad person—even be arrested and jailed—or else the father threatens to hurt the mother or a sibling. The outcome is an adolescent at greater risk for running away, having eating disorders, being a sexual victim, and engaging in substance abuse (Conners, 2001; Whitbeck et al., 2001; Yoder et al., 2002).

Adolescents who have been abused tend to discuss their abuse with a friend or with no one. Very seldom do they report it to parents, police, social workers, or other authorities. Research has also found that the effects of abuse may influence a youth's future relationships. Directly following the experience, children may engage in "acting out" behaviors (for example, truancy, running away, sexual promiscuity), but symptoms may persist for years and into adulthood (Deblinger et al., 2006; Hussey, Chang, & Kotch, 2006).

Adolescents are not only the victims of sexual abuse; they also are perpetrators of it (Murphy et al., 2001). Male adolescents and adults are most often behind reported abuses (Salter et al., 2003). Abusive acts also include sexual coercion, in which both males and females bear responsibility (Oswald & Russell, 2006).

Research has led to increased awareness of how to support victims of sexual abuse, including reporting systems, legal definitions, and treatment of victims (Malloy, Lyon, & Quos, 2007). These may help us better understand and intervene so that victims can receive professional attention earlier, which may reduce the long-term effects of abuse or unwanted pregnancy.

Mental Health Issues

Several psychologists and psychoanalysts (most notably Freud) have suggested that the distressing, turbulent, unpredictable thoughts deemed normal in adolescence would be considered pathological in an adult. This disruptive state is partly characteristic of the identity stages of confusion and moratorium. Identity confusion is sometimes marked by withdrawal from reality. Researchers propose that true psychopathology (mental illness) is relatively rare during adolescence. It is impossible to determine the frequency of mental illness, however, because of current disagreements over its definition. Studies do indicate that when adolescents become seriously disturbed and do not receive appropriate treatment right away, their chances of "growing out" of their problems are slim (Dacey, Kenny, & Margolis, 2006; Findling et al., 2001; Woodward, 2001).

The National Institute of Mental Health has reported that the incidence of mental health problems among adolescents is about 1 in 10 youths and rising (Child and Adolescent Mental Health Government Guide, 2002; Haliburn, 2000). Adolescents suffer from a wide range of mental health disorders that affect their normal development and functioning. The most common of these are anxiety disorders (13% of children 9 to 17), depression (8% of adolescents), and attention deficit hyperactivity (3–5% of school-age children) (Child and Adolescent Mental Health Government Guide, 2002). Other disorders adolescents may experience include eating disorders, autism and other pervasive developmental disorders, conduct disorders, and substance abuse. Many teens are not treated for mental disorders, because some parents and doctors believe that the problem the teen is experiencing is just part of adolescence and he or she will grow out of it. Since a number of factors may affect adolescent mental health, such as age, gender, culture, socioeconomic status, and genetics, the diagnosis and treatment of an adolescent's mental health disorder are therefore crucial for the long-term development of the youth.

It is especially important for adults to recognize the warning signs of mental health disorders in adolescents so that they may receive the support they need. Some adolescents may resist help at first for reasons of pride, embarrassment, or sheer will, but most come to appreciate the persistence of caring friends and family.

SUICIDE

Adolescent suicide represents the third leading cause of death among teenagers (Shaffer & Pfeffer, 2001). Approximately 2 million U.S. adolescents attempt suicide each year, with nearly 700,000 receiving medical treatment for the attempt (Shaffer & Pfeffer, 2001). Adolescent males are five times as likely to commit suicide as adolescent females. In addition, Native American, Native Alaskan, and Hispanic teens have higher rates of suicides than do White teens, while African Americans have lower rates of suicide than do Whites.

A number of factors increase the likelihood of a suicide attempt (Shaffer & Pfeffer, 2001). The majority of adolescents who commit suicide suffer from some associated psychiatric disorder. These teens may have poor communication with their parents, have experienced a recent stressful life event, and/or have a history of suicide attempts, substance abuse, abnormal behavior, or self-destructive behavior. Teens who attempt and/or achieve suicide are more likely to be friends with peers who have attempted suicide, use drugs, or have psychiatric problems (Ho et al., 2000). LGBT teens and teen survivors of childhood sexual or physical abuse are also at higher risk because of factors such as family conflict and harassment at school.

King (2000) suggests the following warning signs for adolescent suicide:

- Depressed mood
- Substance abuse

- Loss of interest in once-pleasurable activities
- Decreased activity and attention levels
- Distractibility
- Withdrawal from others
- Sleep or appetite changes
- Morbid ideation (for example, thinking about death)
- Verbal cues ("I wish I were dead") or written cues (notes, poems)
- Giving possessions away
- A previous suicide attempt
- Low self-esteem or a recent relationship breakup
- Being homosexual
- Coming from an abusive home
- Easy access to a firearm
- Low grades
- Exposure to suicide or suicidal behavior by another person

SUBSTANCE ABUSE

Table 8.3 highlights some results about substance abuse presented in a study conducted by the National Center for Health Statistics (2009). As these data indicate, use of alcohol, amphetamines, and tobacco is dropping significantly. These welcome trends are probably the result of many educational efforts by the government, schools, and social service agencies.

Nevertheless, recent research points to some alarming evidence that excessive alcohol use during one's teen years can impair later brain functioning (Cleveland & Wiebe, 2003). Because teenagers' brains continue to develop throughout adolescence, the toxic effects of alcohol abuse can damage their memories, learning abilities, and language skills. According to one study, teenagers who begin drinking before 14 are three times more likely to injure themselves while drinking than those who begin drinking after 21. These injuries include falls, burns, unintentional wounds, and automobile accidents (Hingson et al., 2000).

Not surprisingly, school context influences the prevalence of smoking and drinking among adolescents (Cleveland & Wiebe, 2003). If a school has many substance-using students, then other students are more likely to imitate the negative actions of their peers. Use of tobacco products such as kreteks (clove cigarettes) and bidis (hand-rolled cigarettes primarily made in India) has become popular among high school students. In 2008, the overall prevalence of tobacco use was 27.2% among high schoolers, with males using all forms of tobacco more than females.

STRESS

The relationship between stress and emotional illness is well established. Therefore, it is important to know to what extent adolescents feel that their lives are stressful. The most reliable source for this information is the Higher Education Research Institute, which has been studying this question for the past 35 years (Reisberg, 2000). Of the more than 260,000 students interviewed at 462 colleges by the institute in 2000, 30% say they feel "overwhelmed by all I have to do." This is up from 16% in 1985. The concern is almost twice as great among women (39%) than among men (20%). A significant part of this pressure comes from the need to work. In 1982, 16% of entering freshmen felt they would have to get a full-time job while attending college; in 1999, that figure had risen to 25%.

TABLE 8.3

Substance Abuse Trends, 1991–2007

	1991	1995	1999	2003	2007	Changes from 1991 to 2007
Smoked at least once/month	28%	35%	35%	22%	20%	Drop of 8%
Drank at least once/month	51%	52%	50%	45%	45%	Drop of 6%
Meth-amphetamine used at least once/month	N/A	N/A	9%	8%	4%	Drop of 5%

Source: Adapted from NCHS Data Brief, 2009.

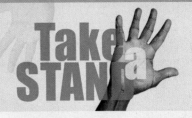

John Forte, a hip-hop artist who co-wrote and produced songs on The Fugees' Grammy-winning album
The Score, was arrested for possession of and intent
to distribute cocaine in 2000. In 2008, Forte was par-
doned by President George W. Bush and released
from jail. Three months later, he began working with
In Arms Reach, Inc., a nonprofit community-based
program that uses art and music to create a positive
environment for at-risk teens and children who have a
parent in jail. As part of the program, Forte will teach
a music therapy class geared to 12- to 15-year-olds.

Hip-hop is already a controversial music genre.
Some studies suggest that adolescents who prefer
hip-hop music have more behavior problems than
those who prefer other types of music (Selfout et
al., 2008). Other studies argue that hip-hop music
opens lines of communication between children and

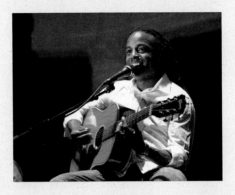

adults, and does not lead to dangerous or undesirable
behavior (Stephens et al., 2000).

Is John Forte a role model or a negative influence?
How should the media portray key figures, with
whom adolescents may identify, who display less-
than-perfect moral conduct?

Adolescents who are not attending college are turning
to long hours at work, not always with positive results.
Because they are working long hours, they are getting
injured more frequently on the job. Over 40% of their
occupational fatalities occur when they are engaged in
work prohibited by child labor laws (Wright, 2000).
National laws prohibit children under 18 from many
work-specific tasks, such as meatpacking or slaughtering
or operating power equipment. Children under 16 are even
more restricted.

CRIMINAL BEHAVIOR

Although the national crime rate for individuals has remained
fairly stable, the amount of gang violence has increased, as
evidenced in the rise of law enforcement agencies reporting
gang activity between 2004 and 2008 (National Gang Intelligence Center, 2009). With the decline in gang prevention and
enforcement programs, today's youth may view the elements
of gang life as attractive, without knowing about the bloodshed that occurred when gang participation peaked in the
1990s. Furthermore, the level of gang violence may increase
as more influential gang leaders return from prison sentences
and reestablish their power. To stop the resurgence of gang
violence, many criminologists propose that cities must rein-
vest in prevention programs such as boys and girls clubs and
youth athletic leagues, as well as to restore the strength of
police anti-gang units.

Numerous studies aimed at identifying the causes behind
gang popularity have pointed to factors such as financial
trouble, family involvement in a gang, drug and alcohol
use, and social pressures (Lauber, Marshall, & Myers,
2005). Violence has also been attributed to neglect and
lack of physical affection in the home environment (Field,
2002). Fortunately, research shows parenting practices can
reduce children's involvement with gangs (Walker-Barnes
& Mason, 2004). In addition, programs and interventions
help reduce violence and raise awareness in schools and
communities (Wright & Fitzpatrick, 2006).

Increasing attention has been paid to youth violence
over the past several years. Specifically, two major paths
of youth violence have been identified, known as early-
onset and late-onset trajectories. The **early-onset trajectory** refers to children who commit their first violent crime
before puberty (about age 13), and the **late-onset trajectory** refers to children whose criminal activity begins after
puberty. Early-onset youths generally commit more serious crimes for a longer time than do late-onset individuals,
often continuing this pattern into adulthood. However, the
majority of youth violence is late onset and stops before
adulthood.

Many factors affect how likely a
young person is to engage in violent
acts. These risk factors are found
in family interactions as well as in
peer and school influences. During

early-onset trajectory
Criminal behavior that begins
before puberty.

late-onset trajectory
Criminal behavior that begins
after puberty.

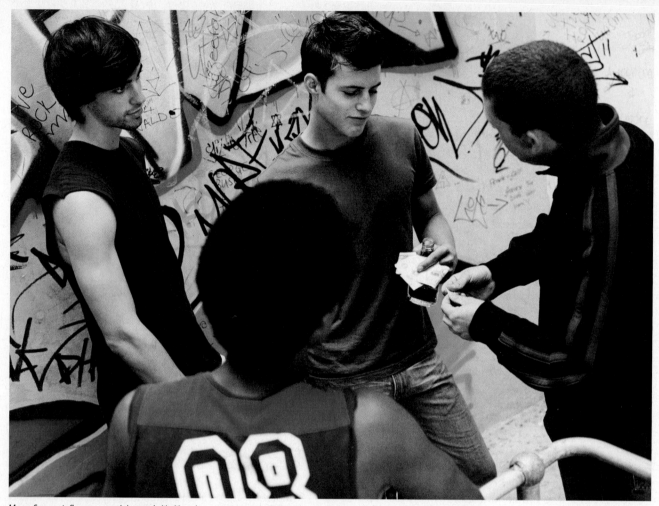

Many factors influence an adolescent's likelihood to engage in risky behaviors.

childhood, risk factors include family and individual characteristics, such as poverty, antisocial parents, and aggressive behavior. During adolescence, however, these risk factors become more peer-oriented, including associations with delinquent friends or gang membership.

As you might expect, researchers are also concerned with finding out which factors might protect young people from becoming perpetrators of violent crime. Again, these factors exist across a number of different areas, such as individual characteristics, family, and peer groups. Examples of these protective factors include an outgoing personality, high IQ, and commitment to achievement in school.

Many researchers are quick to blame the occurrence of youth violence on the changing American family, including working mothers and nontraditional households. Others might say that youth aggression results from increased portrayals of violence in the media, such as on television, in movies, and in song lyrics. Social changes have augmented the number of intervention programs aimed at adolescents. In particular, programs designed to address the complex relationships between teens' problem behaviors have been proven effective.

Resiliency is a characteristic that can be attributed to biopsychosocial factors. Some teens may be born with a temperament that helps them recognize dangerous choices and make wise decisions. Other teens have the support of one person in their lives who buoys their spirits and gives them the strength and guidance their own developmental needs require—emotional support, academic assistance, career advice, or even the most basic needs as outlined in Maslow's hierarchy of needs, discussed in Chapter 2. When a community effort is made to support local teens, as is the case with the Harlem Children's Zone discussed in Chapter 6, it is more likely that adolescence will be less a time of storm and stress, and more a time to lay the groundwork for the next phase of the lifespan—adulthood.

Career Apps

As a social worker at a local Boys and Girls Club, how could you assist teens and their families in developing successful conflict resolution skills?

CONCLUSIONS & SUMMARY

Defining adolescence is a complex task. Any explanation must be biopsychosocial in order to be comprehensive. In terms of biology, there is a marked increase in the flow of sex-related hormones, as well as a maximum growth spurt and the appearance of secondary sex characteristics. Psychologically, the formation of the identity is a prominent process woven throughout adolescence, and cognitive changes such as formal operations, the personal fable, and the imaginary audience occur. The social world of the teen undergoes many changes, including the inauguration of new privileges and new responsibilities.

The good news is that most adolescents develop improved mental abilities that enable them to get a more realistic view of themselves. Evidence suggests that adolescents' cognitive development evolves in stages. Contrary to earlier beliefs, thinking is qualitatively different in childhood, adolescence, and adulthood.

How should we define adolescence?

- Most experts state that the majority of adolescents are happy and productive members of their families and communities.
- Hall's interpretation of adolescent development was greatly influenced by his observation that it is a period of storm and stress.

What are the leading theories that attempt to explain adolescence?

- According to Erik Erikson, human life progresses through eight psychosocial stages, each of which is marked by a crisis and its resolution. The fifth stage—identity versus identity confusion—applies to adolescence.
- John Hill's biopsychosocial theory, with its emphasis on the six factors of dependence, autonomy, sexuality, intimacy, achievement, and identity, offers the most inclusive theory of adolescence.

What are the key factors of physical development in adolescence?

- Theories of adolescence in the early 20th century were largely based on personal bias, because little empirical data existed.
- Those who work with adolescents need complete knowledge of the reproductive systems of both sexes.
- The order of physical changes in puberty is largely predictable, but the timing and duration of these changes are not.
- The normal range in pubertal development is very broad and includes early, average, and late maturers.
- Maturity of appearance affects whether adolescents are treated appropriately for their age.
- Early maturing is usually a positive experience for boys but may be negative for girls.
- Late maturing is often difficult for both boys and girls.

What are some challenges to physical development in adolescence?

- Two of the most disruptive problems for adolescents are the eating disorders known as anorexia and bulimia nervosa.
- Adolescent girls develop eating disorders more often than any other group.
- Developmental, cultural, individual, and familial factors are associated with the development of eating disorders.
- Teens are working longer and longer hours, and this has resulted in a serious increase in injuries on the job.

How does cognition develop during the adolescent years?

- Piaget focused on the development of the cognitive structures of the intellect during childhood and adolescence.
- Piaget's highest stage of cognitive development, formal operations, begins to develop in early adolescence.
- Adolescents focus much attention on themselves and tend to believe that everybody is looking at them. This phenomenon is called the imaginary audience.
- Many adolescents also hold beliefs about their own uniqueness and invulnerability. This is known as the personal fable.

How do critical and creative thinking impact cognitive development?

- Critical thinking combines both convergent thinking, in which there is only one correct answer to a problem, and divergent thinking, in which there are many possible answers to a problem.
- Effective decision making, a formal operational process, is a part of critical thinking.

- Creative thinking includes divergent thinking, fluency, flexibility, originality, and remote associations.
- Conventional schooling often has a dampening effect on students' willingness to risk doing creative, metaphorical thinking.
- The idea that those who develop mental illness during adolescence will "grow out of it" is not supported by research. Depression can be an especially dangerous illness at this age.
- Adolescence is not a time of turmoil and distress for most teens. Rates of mental disturbance among teens are very similar to rates of disturbance among adults.

What changes have occurred in American families and their roles in adolescent life in recent years?

- American families have lost many traditional functions; the only remaining one is providing affection for family members.
- A number of effects of divorce pertain only to adolescents.

What is the nature of peer relations during the teen years?

- Peer groups provide adolescents with a source of social activities and support, as well as an easy entry into opposite-sex friendships.
- The biological, psychological, cognitive, and social changes of adolescence affect the development of a teenager's peer relationships.
- Peer groups serve to control aggressive impulses, encourage independence, improve social skills, develop reasoning abilities, and form attitudes toward sexuality and sexual behavior. They may also strengthen moral judgment and values and improve self-esteem.
- Peer groups also aid in the development of self-concept and allow an adolescent to try out a new identity.

How do teens deal with sexual relations?

- Many teenagers are sexually active.
- Homosexuality poses specific challenges for adolescents.
- Masturbation is believed to be a developmental, universal form of human sexual expression.
- Many teens still obtain a great deal of information and misinformation about sex from their peers.
- Effective listening skills are essential for parents who wish to maintain good communication with their adolescents.
- Many adolescent runaways and prostitutes are the products of sexual abuse, often by someone they know, a family member, or a parent.

What factors contribute to a teen becoming a parent?

- It has been found that teens are at a greater risk of becoming a teenage parent if they live in poverty, unsafe communities, a single-parent household, or have a history of sexual abuse.

What recent information do we have on adolescent illegal behavior?

- Drug, alcohol, and tobacco abuse are still a problem among teens, though less so than in previous years.
- Gangs typically have a high degree of cohesion and organization, a consistent set of norms, clearly defined leaders, and coherent organization for warfare.

KEY TERMS

adolescent egocentrism *192*
anorexia nervosa *190*
bulimia nervosa *191*
clique *196*
convergent thinking *193*
crowd *196*
divergent thinking *193*

early-onset trajectory *201*
executive functioning *193*
formal operational stage *191*
heterosexual *196*
homosexual *196*
hormonal balance *187*
identity crisis *194*

identity statuses *194*
imaginary audience *192*
late-onset trajectory *201*
LGBT *196*
menarche *187*
personal fable *192*
puberty *187*

reticular activation system (RAS) *192*
secular trend *189*
spindle cells *192*

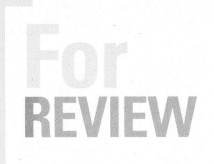

1. Should children be taught about their bodily functions in school, and should this teaching include information about sexuality? How might you design a program to teach adolescents about potentially awkward, socially charged topics that are based in biology but have extreme social relevance?

2. Describe family life in the United States 50 years from today. What biological, psychological, and social factors are at the core of your ideas, and why?

3. You are the mayor of a medium-size city. What actions would you take to try to reduce adolescents' high-risk behaviors and promote and sustain healthy alternatives? Who would you need to involve as partners in your efforts?

Chapter Review Test

1. What marks the onset of puberty?
   a. menarche for females; first ejaculation for males
   b. the growth spurt for females and males
   c. the beginning of breast development for females; the enlargement of the genitals for males
   d. No single event marks the onset of puberty.

2. The identity status in which numerous crises have been experienced and resolved and relatively permanent commitments have been made is called
   a. identity moratorium.
   b. identity achievement.
   c. foreclosed identity.
   d. confused identity.

3. To think of oneself in heroic or mythical terms is known as
   a. egocentrism.
   b. imaginary audience.
   c. the personal fable.
   d. invincibility.

4. What occurs during Piaget's formal operational stage?
   a. Concrete operations combine to become formal operations.
   b. Preoperations turn into formal operations.
   c. Parts of the sensorimotor stage turn into formal operations.
   d. The preoperational stage and the sensorimotor stage combine to become formal operations.

5. To solve problems that have only one correct answer, we are using _____ thinking.
   a. divergent
   b. convergent
   c. creative
   d. critical

6. The process of declaring one's homosexuality to others is called
   a. identification.
   b. individuation.
   c. coming out.
   d. walkabout.

7. What reason is cited in the text for why there may be a decline in early sexual activity?
   a. concern about AIDS and other sexually transmitted infections
   b. prevailing conservative attitudes
   c. more people devoting time to making money
   d. increasing influence of religion

8. Risk factors that predict teenage pregnancy are
   a. early school failure.
   b. early behavior problems.
   c. both a and b
   d. neither a nor b

9. John joins a gang because it serves as a pseudo-family for him. Most likely, John has strong ____ needs that are being displaced onto the peer group.
   a. dependency
   b. friendship
   c. financial
   d. All of the answers are correct.

10. Recent research indicates that gangs have which of these characteristics?
    a. They possess a consistent set of norms and expectations that are understood by all gang members.
    b. Members have lower expectations of success than do nonmembers.
    c. Members are as likely to have divorced parents as are nonmembers.
    d. Members are more likely to score high on IQ tests than are nonmembers.

EARLY ADULTHOOD

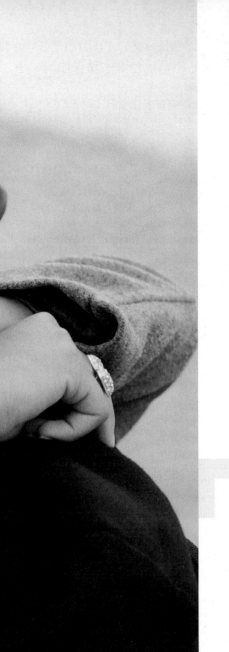

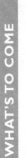
As You READ

After reading this chapter, you should be able to answer the following questions:

- How are American youths being initiated into adulthood today?

- What are the significant factors affecting physical development in early adulthood?

- How does cognition change during the early adult years?

- What factors affect American marriages and families?

- What are the relationships between sexual identity and gender roles?

- How do young adults deal with the interpersonal relationships of sexuality and love?

- What patterns of work typify young adults today?

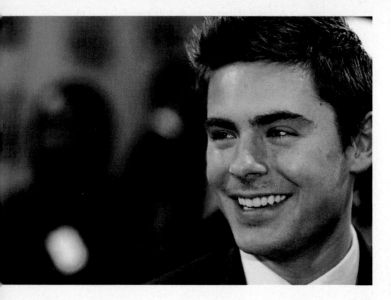

emerging adulthood Transition from adolescence to adulthood (approximately ages 18 to 25 years) that includes exploration and experimentation.

hazing The practice of initiating individuals into group membership through arduous and demeaning tasks.

When does adolescence end and adulthood begin? Is the transition the same around the world? Whereas adolescence is often distinguished by physical changes and capabilities, adulthood is marked more by social and cultural experiences. Many different factors contribute to the transition from adolescence into adulthood and are considered more or less appropriate by society's standards.

Initiation into Adulthood

Virtually all cultures value some form of rite of passage, such as hazing, and many adolescents—highly intelligent and reasonable—are willing and eager to endure pain and humiliation to make it through. Is it simply because they want to join the group, to feel that they belong? There is more to it than that. Throughout the world, adolescents readily engage in such activities because they want (or are forced) to be tested, to prove to themselves and society that they have achieved such adult virtues as courage, independence, and self-control. Adults seem to agree that adolescents should prove they have attained these traits before being admitted to the "club of maturity."

EMERGING ADULTHOOD IN THE UNITED STATES

The transition into adulthood in the United States has become more complicated as expectations for education and skills have changed over centuries. Western initiation rites have generally become social or secular in nature, and there is less clarity for young adults (approximately 18 to 25 years old), who are adults in terms of biology and physical ability, but are perhaps less equipped intellectually and emotionally for the challenges of adulthood. The term **emerging adulthood** is commonly used to identify the transition into adulthood. Young adults tend to engage in exploration and experimentation as they attempt to navigate their life paths, often with little structure to guide them.

This is not to say that Americans have no activities that signal the passage to maturity. We have a number of types of activities, which usually happen at various ages and signal the onset of adulthood in symbolic as well as practical terms and responsibilities (see Table 9.1).

Most people have heard about accidents and even deaths of young men and women who have been put through **hazing,** the initiation rite that precedes full acceptance into fraternity and sorority membership. The tragic mistakes of college social club initiations have decreased due to legal restrictions on hazing and more humane ways to initiate new members. Yet hazing continues to exist in fraternities and sororities, and among athletes and school leaders (Campos, Poulos, & Sipple, 2005).

Traditional initiation rites are inappropriate for today's American emerging adults. For example, in preindustrial societies, the tribe determined individual status, and success or failure for the tribe determined the prestige of its

TABLE 9.1

American Rites of Passage

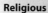

Religious
- Bar/bat mitzvah
- Confirmation
- Participating in a ceremony, such as a year-long spiritual study

Physical
- Menarche (first menstruation)
- Nocturnal emissions (male "wet dreams")
- First sexual encounter
- Beginning to shave

Educational
- Getting a driver's license
- Graduating from high school
- Going away to college

Social
- "Sweet Sixteen" or debutante parties, such as Quinceañera
- Going to the senior prom
- Joining a gang, fraternity, or sorority (hazing)
- Moving away from one's family and relatives
- Joining the armed forces
- Getting married
- Becoming a parent
- Voting for the first time

Economic
- Getting a checking or credit card account
- Buying a first car
- Getting a first job

Initiation Rites Around the World

There is no one way to cross from childhood into adulthood, and many rituals have existed for thousands of years—attesting to the importance of such acts in societies around the world. Some rites involve physical acts, whereas others are social or introspective. Despite variations, there appears to be a human need to mark the transition into adulthood.

Maasai (Kenya/Tanzania). The Maasai people believe that boys should demonstrate their bravery and skill by hunting lions with spears. In a society that values warrior-like abilities, surviving such a hunting experience demonstrates competence and signals the male's ability to protect the group, ensuring its survival.

Bar/Bat Mitzvah (Israel/worldwide). The Jewish people have been following the tradition of a boy's bar mitzvah for thousands of years and, more recently, a girl's bat mitzvah. In this ceremony, the 13-year-old chants memorized passages of Torah and leads a portion of a religious service, after which he/she is deemed a responsible adult member of the group. In today's society, when life expectancy is much longer than it was thousands of years ago, 13-year-olds are hardly considered adults. When the ceremony originated (over 5,000 years ago), however, 13 years may have been one third of a person's life.

Walkabout (Australia). The Aborigines have a tradition of sending their adolescent males into the bush for approximately 6 months, where they are expected to fend for themselves. Upon their return, they are respected for their

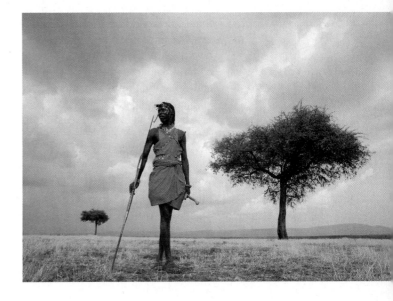

ability to survive and contemplate their roles as members of the group. They have proven themselves capable of survival, which makes them capable of contributing to the group's survival.

Vision Quest (Native American). According to the ancient tradition of vision quest, young boys, typically in late childhood or puberty, leave their community for a period of time, similar to a walkabout. On this journey, the boy (often under the influence of a hallucinogenic substance) experiences an internal search for meaning and purpose, and becomes more in tune with the natural world that he is already so familiar with, but now with a different relationship to it.

Ritual circumcision (Africa). In many African countries, there is a practice of circumcising young men and women as a sign of their eligibility for marriage and adulthood. There has been a growing movement to raise awareness of female genital cutting (FGC), a practice that in some countries is done without the woman's consent and can result in lack of sensation during intercourse and severe mental and physical damage.

Considering these practices as a whole, what general ideas do you have about transitions into adulthood? Which activities help in the passage from adolescence to adulthood? How might we improve this passage?

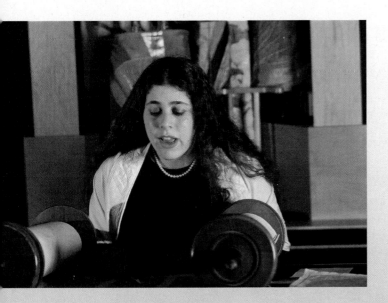

members. Family background and individual effort usually made little difference. Social scientists call this an **ascribed identity.**

In earlier times in the United States, few children from poor families became merchants, doctors, or lawyers. Today, personal effort and commitment, coupled with family and community support, play a far greater role in an individual's economic and social success. This is called an **achieved identity.** Achieved identity plays a larger role in one's early adulthood than ascribed identity because of an individual's investment in her life course, even though the values of certain cultures continue to dictate roles based on sex and gender. Physical development, however, provides clear evidence of a person's markedly different appearance and abilities in adulthood, and transcends cultural boundaries.

Physical Development

Psychologist Malcolm Knowles (1989) defined the biopsychosocial facets of adulthood as (1) biological—when we reach the age at which we can reproduce, (2) psychological—when we arrive at a self-concept of being responsible for our own lives, and (3) social—when we start to take on adult roles and responsibilities. Let's consider Knowles's first defined area—physical development.

THE PEAK IS REACHED

Early adulthood is the life period during which physical changes slow down after the dramatic changes that occur in adolescence (see Table 9.2).

In terms of speed and strength, young adults are in peak condition. A healthy young adult can participate in

relatively strenuous activity for years without concern for injury due to age-related restrictions. As the aging process continues, however, the individual will notice a decline in energy and strength. Although early adulthood also marks the beginning of a time when many bodily functions are less efficient, most young adults tend to rate their health as "good" or even better, and tend to report few limitations due to chronic illness (see Figure 9.1).

> *Carpe, carpe diem.* Seize the day, boys—make your lives **extraordinary.**

JOHN KEATING, *DEAD POETS SOCIETY* (1989)

ORGAN RESERVE

Organ reserve refers to the part of the total capacity of our body's organs that we do not normally need to use. Our bodies are designed to do much more than they are usually called upon to do. Much of our functional capacity is thus held on reserve. As we get older, these extra resources grow smaller. The peak performance capacity of each of our organs, muscles, and bones declines approximately 1% per year after age 30, and it varies from person to person. The most significant decreases in organ reserve occur in the heart, lungs, and kidneys. A 50-year-old man might fish all day with his 25-year-old son and take a long walk with him without becoming exhausted, but has little chance of winning a footrace against him.

Of course, some individuals regularly try to use the total capacity of their organ reserves. Professional athletes are an example. Here again we see evidence of biopsychosocial interactions: Biology sets the limits, but psychological

TABLE 9.2

Physical Development in Early Adulthood

Height
Female: maximum height reached at age 18.
Male: maximum height reached at age 20.

Weight
Female: 14-pound weight gain and increase in body fat.
Male: 15-pound weight gain.

Muscle Structure and Internal Organs
From age 19-26: Internal organs attain greatest physical potential. The young adult is in prime condition as far as speed and strength are concerned.
After age 26: Body slowing process begins. Spinal disks settle, causing decrease in height.

Fatty tissue increases, causing increase in weight. Muscle strength decreases. Reaction times level off and stabilize. Cardiac output declines.

Sensory Function Changes
The process of losing eye lens flexibility begins as early as age 10. This loss results in difficulty focusing on close objects. During early adulthood, women can detect higher-pitched sounds than men.

Nervous System
The brain continues to increase in weight and reaches its maximum potential by the adult years.

Source: U.S. Census Bureau, 2006.

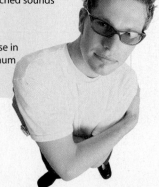

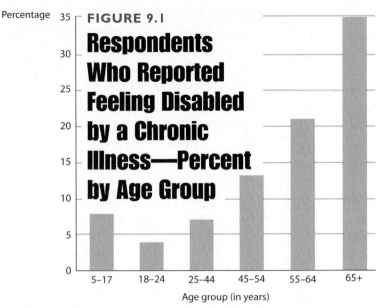

FIGURE 9.1

Respondents Who Reported Feeling Disabled by a Chronic Illness—Percent by Age Group

Percentage

Age group (in years): 5–17, 18–24, 25–44, 45–54, 55–64, 65+

Source: National Center for Health Statistics, 2006.

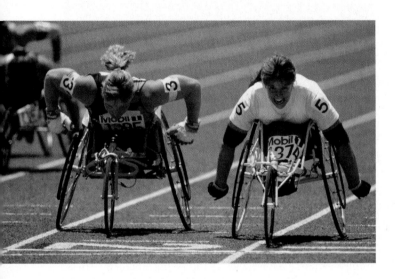

factors (such as the perseverance to train) and social factors (such as the cheering crowd) determine whether the person can push the limits.

THE EFFECT OF LIFESTYLE ON HEALTH

Young adults are healthier than older adults in just about every way. Good health is clearly related to influences such as genetics, a factor that is beyond a person's control. Increasingly, however, people are beginning to realize that their lifestyle plays an enormous role in their own health.

Diet and Nutrition

Nutrition plays an important role throughout human development. In early adulthood, however, increasing evidence demonstrates the influence of nutrition on two major health concerns, heart disease and cancer. Medical science has established a link between heart disease and **cholesterol,** a natural substance in the blood. Cholesterol, specifically low-density lipoprotein (LDL), has been found to leave deposits on the walls of blood vessels, blocking the flow of blood to the heart and brain. The main culprit in high levels of LDL cholesterol is diets high in fat. Changes to the typical American diet, which contains 40% fat, such as eating fish and poultry instead of red meat, choosing low-fat yogurt and cheese, drinking skim milk instead of whole milk, and avoiding trans fats (for example, hydrogenated oils used to cook fried chicken and French fries), will help lower cholesterol in the body.

Although young adults tend to feel healthy and fit, the nutrition choices they make are not always healthy. Building on the foundation laid in earlier years, young adults who make poor nutrition choices over time compound the results of earlier nutrition, which might lead to later health problems. In the film *Super Size Me,* filmmaker Morgan Spurlock documented the unwelcome effects that a month of eating only at McDonald's had on his biological, psychological, and social well-being. It is an eye-opening film, and facts presented have had a life-changing impact on many who have watched the documentary.

The American Cancer Society (2008) has a set of recommendations for an improved, healthy diet. The organization also recommends lowering fat intake to no more than 30% of the daily caloric total and following a diet that is high in fiber, which helps the digestive process. High-fiber foods include leafy green vegetables and cruciferous vegetables such as cauliflower, broccoli, and brussels sprouts, as well as whole-grain cereals and breads. Although these foods are not as readily available for young adults "on the go" compared to fast-food options, they are increasingly available and fairly inexpensive at farm stands, health food markets, and community-supported agriculture (CSA) farms, and can even be delivered farm-to-door through food cooperatives that allow people to order and manage their accounts online.

Experts argue that our current society has become "obesogenic," meaning that we live in an environment that promotes increased food intake, unhealthy foods, and a sedentary lifestyle (see Figure 9.2). The Centers for Disease Control and Prevention (CDC) has stated that the most effective measures to combat the rise in obesity will be those policy and environmental changes that make healthier choices readily available (CDC, 2009). Recent decisions such as the one to eliminate trans fats from many foods, and media attention to the dangers of trans fats in films such as *Food Inc.* (2008), have had a strong influence on the food choices made by young adults, as well as the aging parents and children that young adults care about.

cholesterol Substance in the blood that can adhere to the walls of the blood vessels, restricting blood flow and causing strokes and heart attacks.

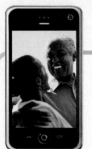

Mindful Living

Many experts in a variety of fields are emphasizing the importance of being in touch with our thoughts and feelings—and the connections between these and our bodies—for healthy living. This is especially important for young adults, who are beginning to take on more responsibilities and become less dependent on others for financial and emotional support. During these years, there is often an increase in stress in the course of everyday life experiences. Mindfulness is defined as a calm awareness of one's feelings, one's body, and one's consciousness, and is linked to Buddhist and other teachings. Growing interest in Eastern practices such as yoga and tai chi has brought about an interest in meditation practice as a way to incorporate mindfulness into everyday living.

Among young adults, the growing use of iPods, iPhones, and other portable electronic devices makes a tranquil meditation setting as close as a click away. Popular apps can be found on iTunes and other sites, and include the following:

Mindfulness Meditation is guided meditations written and spoken by the author of *Meditation for Dummies*, Stephan Bodian.

Meditation Timer is a simple application that provides users with a timer to prepare for meditation, a timer for the actual meditation, and a bell to begin the meditation.

Bubbles provides visuals and sounds of delicate bubbles floating and popping in a relaxing format that lends itself to focusing on thoughts and feelings.

iZen Garden provides a daily inspirational quote, and then a simple tap takes you to a Zen garden of your own design; you choose from stones, shells, sands, rakes, and background sounds.

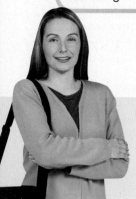

Career Apps

As a registered dietician, how would you work with college students to increase their awareness about healthy eating and overall lifestyle choices?

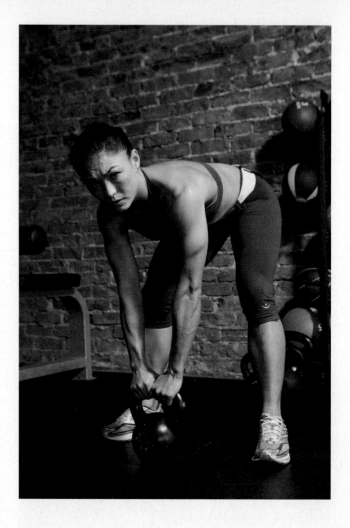

Physical Fitness

Popular exercise trends in recent years include activities as diverse as Pilates, spinning, Zumba, and boot camp classes. Health benefits are an obvious reason for this enthusiasm for exercise, but among young adults, the social aspects of working out add to the benefits of the physical activity. One of the challenges in early adulthood is finding time for work, exercise, and social activities, so workouts can potentially help balance the busy lives of young adults along with providing real health boosts. Studies have shown that women who increase their physical activity by 2½ hours a week can add months to their lives (Fitzpatrick, 2003). Moderately intense exercise, such as brisk walking, also reduces the risk of stroke, osteoporosis, some types of cancer, and diabetes.

Many corporations are now providing the time and facilities for employees to build regular exercise into their workday, which is much appreciated by young adults who may have been used to flexible daily schedules in earlier years. Health insurance programs often offer reduced rates to exercise facilities or rebates for membership, looking at the long-term gain of having healthier members of all ages. In early adulthood, when people typically are no longer considered dependents on their parents' health-care plans, such benefits are quite attractive.

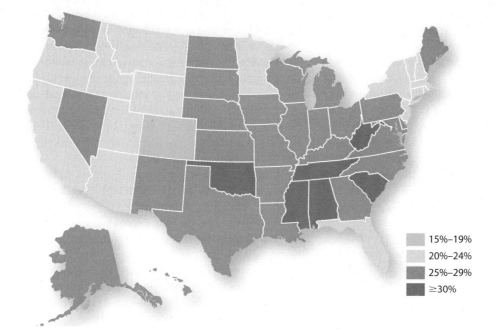

FIGURE 9.2

U.S. Obesity, 2008

In 2008, only one state (Colorado) had a prevalence of obesity less than 20% for adults aged 20 and older. Thirty-two states had a prevalence equal to or greater than 25%; six of these states (Alabama, Mississippi, Oklahoma, South Carolina, Tennessee, and West Virginia) had a prevalence of obesity equal to or greater than 30%.

Source: http://www.cdc.gov/obesity/data/trends.html

15%–19%
20%–24%
25%–29%
≥30%

Use of Alcohol

Most people consume alcohol to attain the relaxed, uninhibited feeling that alcohol tends to produce. In fact, alcohol dulls the senses. Specifically, it decreases reaction times in the brain and nervous system, and inhibits the immune system. Despite education efforts showing the association of alcohol use and driving fatalities, violent crimes, birth defects, and health problems, binge drinking (defined as 5 or more drinks in a row for men and 4 or more for women) among young adults remains at a high level (see Figure 9.3). The National Household Survey on Drug Abuse (NHSDA) reports that the highest prevalence of both binge and heavy drinking is among young adults aged 18 to 25, with the peak rate occurring at age 21. Rates of binge alcohol use in 2008 were 33.7% among persons aged 18 to 20 and 46% among those aged 21 to 25.

FIGURE 9.3

Binge Drinking

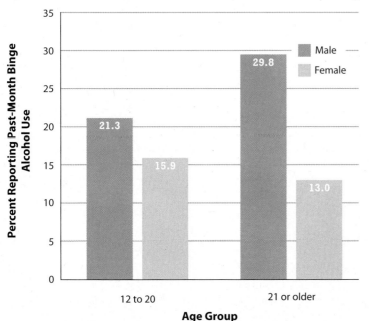

This graph shows the percent reporting past-month binge alcohol use by age and gender.

Source: NHSDA Report, 2002.

Use of Tobacco

To some people, smoking is considered a rite of passage, much like those presented earlier. Although the use of tobacco has been falling rapidly, at about 1% per year since 1987, it continues to attract people because of the images associated with smoking that are perpetuated in movies, advertisements, and the behavior of celebrities who are role models for young adults.

Smoking continues to be the leading preventable cause of death in the United States. Every year, more people die from smoking than from alcohol, AIDS, drug abuse, murder, car accidents, suicide, and fires combined (CDC, 2006a). Cigarette smoke—a combination of tar, nicotine, carbon monoxide, and various other chemicals—has been proven to cause lung and esophageal cancer, heart disease, and chronic lung disease. It also increases heart rate and blood pressure, constricts blood vessels, and reduces oxygen supply to tissue, thereby straining the heart. However, these sobering facts are not enough to convince many young adults to avoid or quit smoking.

In fact, more exotic forms of smoking tobacco have risen in popularity among young adults. Hookahs, for example, are waterpipes used to smoke

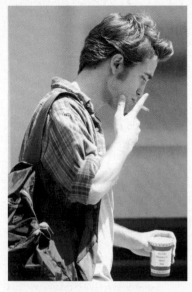

flavored tobacco and can be found in trendy bars and restaurants. Many people think this type of tobacco contains fewer toxic products than cigarettes, but it actually contains more toxins and is equally addictive.

Peer pressure from friends is the major reason that young adults smoke. Some see smoking as a way of appearing more mature. Others, especially females, believe that smoking will either help them lose weight or keep them from gaining weight. Among young women, smoking is associated with being less athletic and more social, studying less, getting lower grades, and generally disliking school more than nonsmoking females do (Colditz & Stein, 2005).

RAPE AND SEXUAL HARASSMENT

Women are often the victims of unwanted sexual acts—forcible sex and inappropriate sexual remarks and/or contact. College-age women are four times more likely than women of other ages to be raped, which makes this issue quite relevant for young adults (Humphrey & Kahn, 2000). **Rape** is forced sexual intercourse when a person does not consent, and legal definitions vary in the United States. Although approximately 1 in 4 college women has been a victim of rape or attempted rape at some point during her life, many victims do not report the crime, so actual numbers may be higher. A report by the U.S. Department of Justice states that over one third of rapes occur in the victim's residence and that over two thirds occur between 6 p.m. and 6 a.m.

A form of rape, **date rape,** is coercive sexual activity between a victim and an offender who is known or an acquaintance. It is generally considered as criminal a behavior as a rape perpetrated by a stranger. In many cases, drugs and/or alcohol are involved in cases of date rape, on the part of the victim and the perpetrator. In two related studies, male undergraduates identified what they felt were circumstances that would contribute to rape: (1) if a couple went to the man's apartment, (2) if the woman initiated the date, and (3) if the man paid for the date expenses (Muehlenhard, Friedman, & Thomas, 2006). Victims of date rape often do not perceive the event as rape

rape Forced sexual intercourse when a person does not consent.

date rape Coercive sexual activity between a victim and an offender who is known or an acquaintance.

sexual harassment Unwelcome sexual advances, such as repeated requests for sexual favors, or other comments or physical contact that lead to a very difficult work or other environment for the victim.

and hence may be reluctant to report the incident to authorities. Reporting date rape can be emotionally difficult, and victims of date rape are encouraged to get help from support groups for those who have been victims of violence.

Whereas rape refers to forced sexual intercourse, **sexual harassment** refers to a broader range of unwelcome sexual advances, such as repeated requests for sexual favors, or other comments or physical contact that lead to a very difficult work or other environment for the victim. People tend to associate sexual harassment with the workplace, but it can occur in any setting.

Rape and sexual harassment involve a person exerting power over another person. Men and women of all sexual orientations can be victims of such behavior, but heterosexual women are the most frequent victims. It is critical that the environments young adults are in—including home, school, and the workplace—support safe, healthy, zero tolerance policies to ensure the comfort and well-being of people in that setting. The impact of sexual assault—physical and verbal—can have long-term effects on the victim, including substance abuse, depression, and anxiety. Indeed, all lifestyle choices have the potential to affect development, particularly the many facets of cognitive development.

Cognitive Development

Young adults' ability to confront challenges is in part due to cognitive changes that occur in early adulthood. In early adulthood, people are able to capitalize on the life experience they've gained prior to and during adolescence, as seen in their ability to focus on a specific area of knowledge and apply information to a specific task. For example, at this time of life, people are able to identify an area of interest or something that they are curious about, and then pursue that topic with formal and informal research. A stu-

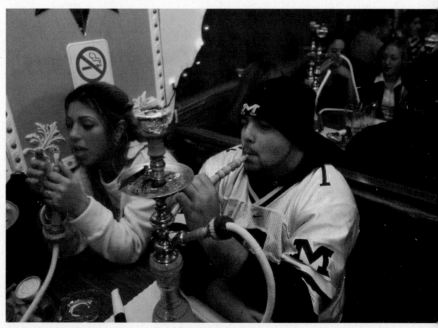

dent curious about American history and indigenous people can develop a research plan to answer questions relating to politics and other forces that contributed to socioeconomic inequities.

PIAGET AND EARLY ADULTHOOD

Although both adolescents and adults fall into Piaget's formal operational stage of cognitive development, Piaget argued that young adults generally possess more knowledge than adolescents, especially in specific areas of interest. This is not surprising, given that young adults are older than adolescents and have therefore amassed more everyday life experiences than adolescents. Over the course of cognitive development through the lifespan, some people develop successful strategies for planning and testing ideas, whereas others may never demonstrate the level of thinking and action of which they are capable.

Some theorists have argued for another stage of cognitive development, known as **postformal thought.** Postformal thought is more flexible and less absolute than formal operational thought. It takes into account the relativistic nature of problems and answers, and acknowledges that the answers to big questions may never be found. In early adulthood, such questions might involve religion, politics, love, and feelings about home and work.

INTELLECTUAL/ETHICAL DEVELOPMENT

In the 1950s and 1960s, William Perry (1968a, 1968b, 1981) studied the intellectual and ethical development of several hundred Harvard University students, a group of males aged 17 to 22. The results of these studies led Perry to suggest a sequence of intellectual and ethical development that typically occurs during early adulthood. This sequence consists of nine positions grouped into three broader categories that show progress from belief in the absolute authority of experts to the recognition that one must make commitments and be responsible for one's own beliefs, and from a simple right versus wrong mentality to one that considers multiple perspectives on an issue:

I. Dualism (Things are either absolutely right or absolutely wrong.)

- *Position 1:* The world is viewed in terms of right versus wrong, good versus bad. If an answer is right, it is absolutely right. Authorities have absolute knowledge.

- *Position 2:* Uncertainty exists due to poorly qualified authorities. Individuals can learn the truth for themselves.

- *Position 3:* Diversity and uncertainty are acceptable but temporary; authorities do not know the answers yet.

II. Relativism (Anything can be right or wrong depending on the situation; all views are equally right.)

- *Position 4a:* Uncertainty and diversity of opinion are often extensive. Two authorities may disagree without either of them being wrong.

- *Position 4b:* Sometimes, authorities (such as college professors) are not talking about right answers. Rather, they want students to think for themselves, supporting their opinions with data.

- *Position 5:* All knowledge and values, including those of an authority, exist in some specific context. Right and wrong are relatively rare, and they exist in a specific context.

- *Position 6:* Because we live in a relativistic world, we must make some sort of personal commitment to an idea or a concept, as opposed to looking for an authority to follow.

III. Commitment (Because of available evidence and my understanding of my own values, I have come to new beliefs.)

- *Position 7:* Commitments are made in specific areas.

- *Position 8:* Implications of commitments are experienced, and various issues of responsibility are explored.

- *Position 9:* One's identity is affirmed through the various commitments made. There is recognition of the necessity for balancing commitments and the understanding that one can have responsibilities that are expressed through daily life.

Perry's theory has been criticized because all the subjects of his research were male. However, his work has sparked additional research. Individual differences and cultural complexities have been suggested as important influences on how a person views the world. Labouvie-Vief (2006) argues that as knowledge and challenges change in the world, reflection and more multifaceted thinking will be required for people to form their own perspectives. Both Perry and Labouvie-Vief emphasize the impact of education on thinking, especially its influence on helping people reach their thinking potential.

Gender and Sexuality

Betty Friedan's 1963 book, *The Feminine Mystique,* marked the beginning of a worldwide reexamination of the female gender role and identity. Sparked in part by Friedan's book, the **feminist movement,** defined broadly as a social and political movement that seeks to establish equality for women in all aspects of life, has fostered a new commitment to women's issues and to studies of women themselves. We are still undergoing societal inquiry into the appropriate gender roles of both sexes. As men and women enter early adulthood, confusion about

postformal thought A proposed cognitive development stage after Piaget's formal operations in which people acknowledge the relativistic nature of problems and answers.

feminist movement A social and political movement that seeks to establish equality for women in all aspects of life.

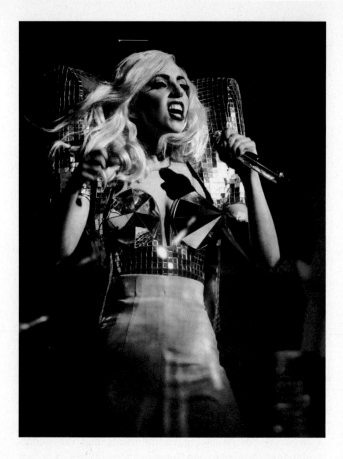

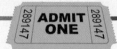

FEATURED MEDIA

Women's Thinking Portrayed in Films

The Color Purple (1985) – Can the bonds of friendship give women the strength to accept the hands they've been dealt, or to take control of their own lives despite societal obstacles posed by race and gender?

North Country (2005) – How are some people able to find courage to fight for justice in the face of danger and humiliation?

The Sisterhood of the Traveling Pants (2005) – As their life paths lead them in different directions, how can four friends maintain their close connection and still develop their own unique identities in early adulthood?

Sophie's Choice (1982) – How does a woman define herself in the face of tragedy and love? How does she live with decisions that she is forced to make that involve those she loves most?

---

sexual identity How one thinks of oneself in terms of sexual and romantic attraction, linked to genetic traits/physical characteristics of male and female.

gender role Expected behavioral traits associated with men and women in a given society.

gender roles may compound confusion about their identity. Images in the media and among celebrities present ideas about what is desirable for each sex and their behavior in society.

First, we need to distinguish between sexual identity and gender role. **Sexual identity** refers to those physical characteristics that are part of our biological inheritance—genetic traits that make us males or females. This relates to how one thinks of oneself in terms of sexual and romantic attraction. **Gender role,** in contrast, is a set of expected behavioral traits associated with men and women in a given social system at any one time—how one is supposed or not supposed to dress, act, behave, think of oneself, and so on. For example, it is still expected that men will be the primary breadwinners in a household, but no known physical cause accounts for this difference. People may accept or reject their sexual identity, their gender role, or both.

ASPECTS OF GENDER ROLE

Some people accept their sexual identity but reject their gender role. Gender role itself has two aspects:

- *Gender-role orientation.* Individuals differ in how comfortable they feel about their gender role. Some young adults don't want to characterize themselves according to strict definitions relating to male versus female or het-

erosexuality versus homosexuality, and prefer to belong to the categories in varying degrees.

- *Gender-role expectations.* Some individuals feel unhappy about their gender role and want society's expectations to change. The feminist movement has had a major impact on many of the world's societies in this regard.

Some research indicates that people's gender roles evolve, in part, because of relationships with important individuals. Some research suggests that mothers influence the development of their daughters' gender-role attitudes in early life, whereas daughters may influence the development of their mothers' gender-role attitudes as they both mature (Balsam & Fischer, 2006).

EVOLUTIONARY PSYCHOLOGY

A more recent theory about gender roles that also reflects the biological viewpoint is known as evolutionary psychology. Proponents of this view hold that our evolutionary history has biologically predisposed men and women to act in certain ways and constrained us from acting in others (Bjorklund & Pellegrini, 2002; Buss, 2001; Grossman & Kaufman, 2002). Gender-bound behaviors are thought to have evolved over time because they serve some useful purpose.

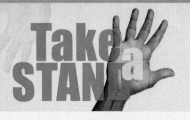

Gender Differences and Conflict Resolution

Researchers Toussaint and Webb (2005) surveyed 127 individuals, 45 men and 82 women, and found that while women showed higher levels of empathy than men did, empathy was more important for men in terms of forgiveness and resolving conflicts. Such gender differences, however, are not cast in stone. Despite new understandings of the differences in male and female biology, society is clearly guiding the sexes toward less rigid gender roles. As a result, developmental theorists tend to agree on a view of identity that holds men and women are really more similar, especially in our need to interrelate, than we have realized.

Are there gender differences in empathy and forgiveness when men and women engage in conflicts? Do men and women seem different only because we have been taught to think so?

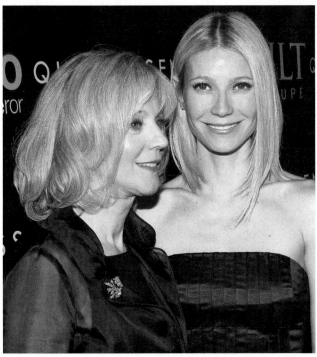

Mother-daughter pair Blythe Danner and Gwyneth Paltrow are one example of women whose relationship influences many aspects of their identity.

Over the many centuries of human development, males and females have developed expectations about gender that are linked to biological abilities. For example, many women in early adulthood think about motherhood, which includes the physical act of conceiving and delivering a baby as well as the emotional issues relating to choices about partner, career, and identity. Many males of this age begin to think about their responsibility for protecting and providing for a family, as well as issues relating to partner, career, and identity. For example, current advances in assisted reproduction technologies (as discussed in Chapter 3) have added a new dimension to the previously accepted limits on men and women as determined by biology, affording more flexibility in gender roles and responsibilities.

> **androgyny** Gender-role identification that allows expression of both male and female gender roles.

ANDROGYNY

One gender-role researcher, Sandra Bem (1999), argues that stereotypical American gender roles are unhealthy. She has posited that highly masculine males tend to have better psychological adjustment than other males during adolescence, but as adults they tend to become highly anxious and neurotic and often experience low self-acceptance. Highly feminine females suffer in similar ways. Bem believes we would all be much better off if most behaviors were viewed as appropriate to both sexes. **Androgyny** is not merely the midpoint between two poles of masculinity and femininity. Rather, it is a level of gender-role identification that allows expression of both masculine and feminine gender roles.

Identity precedes intimacy for men.... For women, intimacy goes with **identity,** *as the female comes to know herself as she is known, through her* **relationships** *with others.*

CAROL GILLIGAN

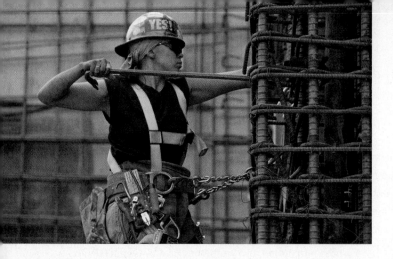

or less dangerous depending on the infection. Chlamydia, for example, is a bacterial infection that occurs most often among young adults, primarily because the symptoms are virtually invisible. At its worst, chlamydia can cause damage to a woman's reproductive organs and can cause blindness in men and women.

The practice of "pack dating"—going out in groups rather than dating one-on-one with a romantic partner—may be an attempt, in part, to lessen the risk of contracting an STI. Choosing a sex partner from a small circle of friends allows a person to know the histories and habits of the potential partners, which could possibly reduce the risk. Another explanation for pack dating is that young adults simply don't have time for relationships. Many young adults hold at least one job while carrying a full course load in school, and others are focused on earning grades that will help get them into graduate school or land a desirable job. After graduation, young adults tend to push themselves to achieve career status, which can be consuming in terms of time and energy.

Social Development

Forming a secure sense of self and being able to successfully relate to others are two of the most important human conditions in early adulthood. The models of development presented by Levinson and Erikson offer insights into the adult personality and ability to form lasting, mutually rewarding relationships in early adulthood.

LEVINSON'S CONCEPT OF INDIVIDUATION

Developmental psychologist Daniel Levinson (1978, 1990a, 1990b) believed that "even the most disparate lives are governed by the same underlying order—a sequence of eras and developmental periods" (1978, p. 64). During some of these periods, people go through crises. The purpose of these developmental transitions is to cause greater individuation.

Individuation refers to how we develop a separate and special personality, derived less and less from our parents and teachers and more from our own behavior. This idea is reinforced by research suggesting that problems in earlier stages of development can affect ego and status attainment in adulthood (Chen & Kaplan, 2003; Krettenauer et al., 2003). For example, adolescents who struggle in school because of academic or behavior problems may tend to struggle with self-esteem and achievement in adulthood. The fact that Levinson conducted his initial research with only male participants raised questions by many critical thinkers, who argued that the male perspective is not representative of an entire world population. This prompted Levinson to conduct subsequent research focusing on women's experiences.

Although Levinson hypothesized more than 10 substages in the course of a man's life, the relevant phase in

individuation Refers to our developing a separate and special personality, derived less and less from our parents and teachers and more from our own behavior.

Androgyny refers to the ability to behave in a way appropriate to a situation, regardless of one's sex. For example, when a male coworker takes credit for a successful marketing campaign, the traditional female role calls for a woman to look disapproving but to say nothing. The androgynous female would correct the interpretation of the situation and give credit where credit is due. When an unattended baby starts to cry, the traditional male response is to look slightly uncomfortable and find the nearest woman to comfort the baby. The androgynous male would pick up the infant and attempt to soothe him. Not surprising, Joensson and Carlsson (2000) found that people who were more androgynous were rated as more creative than people who were either strongly masculine or strongly feminine. Unhindered by restrictive stereotypes, they were able to act according to their instincts.

SEXUAL BEHAVIOR

In Chapter 8, we noted that in recent years sexual activity among U.S. adolescents appears to have declined recently. This holds true for young adults as well. According to a study by the Kaiser Family Foundation (2008), young people are having sex less frequently and with fewer partners than they did in previous years. Figure 9.4 illustrates the typical number of sex partners young adults have in a given year. Adults also report using contraception, such as condoms, more often than ever. Researchers think that this may be due to increases in sex education across the country, particularly with regard to contraceptive use and abstinence, as well as knowledge about sexually transmitted infections.

SEXUALLY TRANSMITTED INFECTIONS (STIs)

Although HIV infection rates appear to be relatively low on campuses, rates of other sexually transmitted infections (STIs), such as venereal warts and chlamydia, are soaring. Millions of young adults contract an STI each year, transmitted through sexual activity, and these can be more

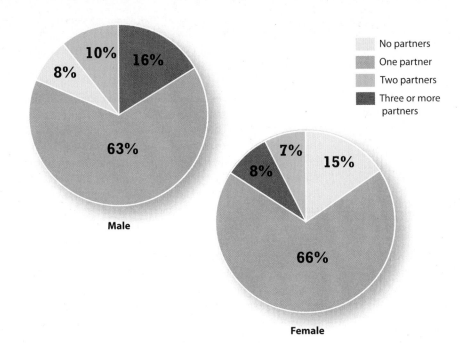

FIGURE 9.4

Number of Sex Partners by Age

This graph shows the percentage of males and females 15–44 years of age, by number of opposite-sex partners in the last 12 months in 2002.

Source: Mosher, Chandra, & Jones, 2005.

Legend:
- No partners
- One partner
- Two partners
- Three or more partners

Male: 16%, 63%, 8%, 10%

Female: 7%, 15%, 66%, 8%

---

early adult development is referred to as the novice phase. The **novice phase** of human development extends from age 17 to 33 and includes the early adult transition, entering the adult world, and the age 30 transition. In this phase of life, hopes and dreams are established that motivate decisions related to work and relationships (see Figure 9.5).

Levinson found that age 30 (plus or minus 2 years) is a common time for people to reexamine their feelings about major life tasks. Important decisions are made at this time, such as modifying hopes and dreams, seeking a mentor, changing jobs, and even getting married or divorced. For some, this transitional period proves to be very smooth. In most cases, however, it challenges the very foundations of life itself. Many people, especially men, experience a serious period of self-doubt. Fortunately, most transition from the age 30 transition to Levinson's Settling Down phase with a clearer understanding of their strengths and weaknesses and a clearer view of what they wish to make of themselves in middle adulthood.

MALE AND FEMALE IDENTITIES

Recent research has noted gender differences in identity development (Bergh & Erling, 2005). For the young adult male, identity formation involves establishing himself as an independent, self-sufficient adult who can compete and succeed in the world. For the young adult female, career and self-sufficiency may not be emphasized to the same degree. Gaining the attention and commitment of a man is often viewed as a more important aspect of a woman's identity, and intimacy is the major goal. According to Carol Gilligan and others (1982, 1990), male development is defined by separation and individuation, whereas female development is defined through attachment and relationship. In Gilligan's view, because females believe in the necessity of maintaining relationships within the family, and because this role often involves self-sacrifice, women find it harder to individuate. As a result of their research on the female perspective, Gilligan and others (1982, 1990) have proposed that feminine identity doesn't depend on separation or on the progress of individuation.

novice phase Levinson's phase of human development that captures the early adult transition, entering the adult world, and the age 30 transition.

intimacy Erikson's stage that represents the ability to relate one's deepest hopes and fears to another person and to accept another's need for intimacy in turn.

ERIKSON'S THEORY: INTIMACY VERSUS ISOLATION

Erikson offered his own views on this time of life, particularly emphasizing young adults' relationships with others and the impact of these relationships on one's self. In his psychosocial theory of development, the sixth stage is described as one of **intimacy** versus isolation. This stage covers the ages of approximately 18 to 35. In his definition of intimacy, Erikson (1963) described this stage as follows:

> The young adult, emerging from the search for and the insistence on identity, is eager and willing to fuse his identity with others. He is ready for intimacy, that is, the capacity to commit himself to concrete affiliations and partnerships and to develop the ethical strength to abide by such commitments, even though they call for significant sacrifices and compromises. (p. 263)

Erikson pointed out, however, that sexual intercourse should not be assumed to be the most important aspect of intimacy between individuals. By intimacy, he meant the ability to relate one's deepest hopes and fears to another person and to accept another's need for intimacy in turn.

FIGURE 9.5

Levinson's Phases and Transitions

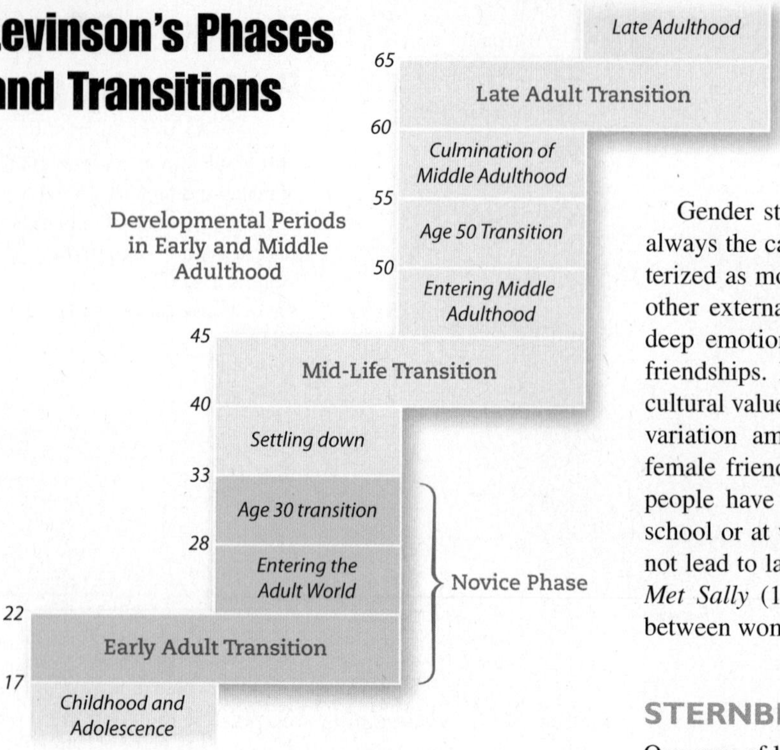

Age	Period
	Late Adulthood
65	
	Late Adult Transition
60	
	Culmination of Middle Adulthood
55	
	Age 50 Transition
50	
	Entering Middle Adulthood
45	
	Mid-Life Transition
40	
	Settling down
33	
	Age 30 transition
28	
	Entering the Adult World
22	
	Early Adult Transition
17	
	Childhood and Adolescence

Developmental Periods in Early and Middle Adulthood

Novice Phase

Those who have achieved the stage of intimacy are able to commit themselves to concrete affiliations and partnerships with others and have developed the "ethical strength to abide by such commitments, even though they may call for significant sacrifices and compromises" (Erickson 1963, p. 262).

A tension that people experience related to intimacy is isolation—the readiness people have to isolate or distance themselves from others when feeling threatened by their behavior. Most young adults vacillate between their desires for intimacy and their need for isolation. They need social distance because they are not yet sure of their identity. They are vulnerable to criticism, and because they can't be sure whether the criticisms are true or not, they protect themselves by a "lone wolf" stance.

FRIENDSHIP

Young people seek intimacy in other close relationships that are vital to personal development on many levels. Friendships in early adulthood are especially important as people generally leave the relatively safe environments of home or school to pursue their dreams. Friends provide a source of support, and because they are chosen rather than thrust upon us, as is the case with family, the mutually satisfying benefits of friendships can sustain these relationships for decades.

Although friendships are important throughout the lifespan, more friendships tend to be formed in early adulthood than in other life stages. Because this is also the stage of life when people commonly find their life partners, challenges and balancing acts are required that cause friendships to go through periods of change as friends readjust their relationship when one person finds love with someone outside the friendship bond.

Gender stereotypes exist about friendships, but are not always the case. For instance, male friendships are characterized as more superficial, focusing on sports, politics, or other external interests, as opposed to the more intimate, deep emotional sharing that tends to characterize female friendships. Ideas about friendships tend to be rooted in cultural values and expectations, and there is actually much variation among behaviors of same-sex friends. Male–female friendships tend to be less stereotyped, and many people have several close friends of the opposite sex in school or at work. Friendships between sexes may or may not lead to later romance. The popular movie *When Harry Met Sally* (1989) captures the importance of friendships between women and men in numerous pairings.

STERNBERG: LOVE STORIES

One way of looking at love is offered by Robert Sternberg. He suggests (2000) that, throughout early adulthood, everyone develops a personal "love story." He has identified a number of these love stories:

- The travel story ("I believe that beginning a relationship is like starting a journey that promises to be both exciting and challenging.")

- The gardening story ("I believe any relationship that is left unattended will not survive.")

- The horror story ("I find it exciting when I feel my partner to be somewhat frightened of me.")

- The business story ("I believe close relationships are like good partnerships.")

- The pornography story ("It is very important to be able to satisfy all my partner's sexual desires and whims.")

Sternberg argues that, even when couples have similar values and interests, they may still have problems in their love relationship because they are operating from significantly different love stories.

I pretty much try to stay in a constant state of confusion *just because of the expression it leaves on my* face.

JOHNNY DEPP

Sternberg also developed a theory about love known as a triangular theory of love. It is represented visually and conceptually by a triangle with three components—passion, intimacy, and commitment. Passion consists of physical and sexual attraction. Intimacy refers to feelings of closeness and sharing with another person. Commitment means that one is willing to endure challenges and tensions in a relationship because the investment is so rewarding. Consummate love, according to Sternberg, is the fullest form of love an individual can experience and involves all three aspects of the triangular theory of love. Sternberg described other forms of love that reflect lesser degrees of passion, intimacy, and commitment (see Figure 9.6).

FROMM: VALIDATION

In a classic book on this subject, *The Art of Loving* (1956), Erich Fromm provided a highly respected understanding of the meaning of love. He argued we must first recognize that we are prisoners in our own bodies. Although we assume that we perceive the world around us in much the same way as others do, we cannot really be sure. We are the only ones who truly know what our own perceptions are, and we cannot be certain they are the same as those of others. In fact, most of us are aware of times when we have misperceived something, such as hearing a phrase differently than everyone else. Thus, we must constantly check on the reality our senses give us.

Fromm argues that as important as these "reality checks" on our physical environment are, checks on our innermost state—our deepest and most important feelings and thoughts—are much more important. To check on the reality of these, we must get the honest reactions of someone we can trust. Such a person tells us, "You're not alone—I feel the same way, too." Even more important, these individuals prove their insight and honesty by sharing with us their own secret thoughts and feelings. In Fromm's words, others give us **validation.**

Validation is essential to our sanity. We are social animals, and we need to know that others approve of us (or, for that matter, when they don't). When someone regularly makes you feel validated, you come to love him or her. This is the essence of what Erikson has called intimacy—the primary focus in the early adulthood period. Intimacy fulfills what Maslow calls the need for self-esteem (see Maslow's hierarchy of needs in Chapter 2), so in the process of achieving intimacy and experiencing love, young adults are validating their own identities.

There is, however, great risk in receiving validation. The person who gives it to you is able to do so only because you have revealed your deepest secrets to him or her. This gives the person great power. Because that individual knows you and your imperfections so well, he or she has the capability to hurt you. This is why many break-ups and divorces are so painful. No one knows how to hurt you better than someone with whom you have shared so many intimacies.

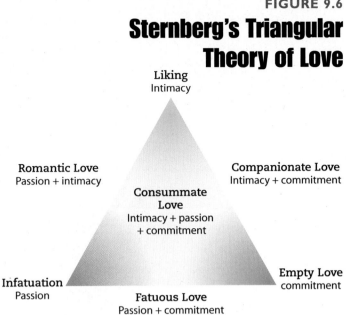

FIGURE 9.6

Sternberg's Triangular Theory of Love

Liking
Intimacy

Romantic Love
Passion + intimacy

Companionate Love
Intimacy + commitment

Consummate Love
Intimacy + passion + commitment

Empty Love
commitment

Infatuation
Passion

Fatuous Love
Passion + commitment

Marriage and the Family

Unlike the early years in the 20th century, when marriage was viewed as the final step in adult development, young adults who choose to marry in the early 21st century view that step as the beginning of their development together and as individuals in a long-term relationship. The goal is not simply to achieve a marriage, but is also to maintain satisfaction outside the marriage.

MARITAL PRACTICES

Although marriage rates have declined in recent years, more than 95% of people marry at some point in their lives, most commonly during early adulthood. The average age for women to marry is 25 years old, and the average age for men is 27. Over several decades, the average age for first marriage has been rising (see Figure 9.7). Some people argue that those young adults who marry early (mid-20s or younger) can look forward to a lifetime of growing old together. Others take a different stance, arguing that marrying later means that the partners are more mature and financially stable, which lessens the likelihood of divorce or separation. The amount of happiness felt by partners at the time of marriage is no guarantee, however, of the strength or resilience of their love for each other and their union.

Increasing numbers of people are choosing to live together without getting married, a practice called **cohabitation.** Cohabitation involves sharing a residence and personal assets, and sometimes having a child, without being married. Since 1960, there has been a dramatic increase in numbers of unmarried partners living together—from less than half a million to more

validation Fromm's term for the reciprocal sharing of deep secrets and feelings that allows people to feel loved and accepted.

cohabitation A living arrangement in which unmarried partners share a residence and personal assets and sometimes have a child.

> *When two people are under the influence of the most* **violent,** *most divisive, and most transient of* **passions,** *they are required to swear that they will remain in that excited, abnormal, and exhausting condition continuously until* **death** *do them part.*

GEORGE BERNARD SHAW

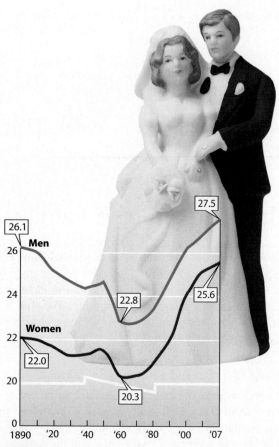

FIGURE 9.7

Median Age for First Marriage in the United States

Source: U.S. Census Bureau, 2008.

than 5 million couples (Whitehead & Popenoe, 2006). This includes both heterosexual and homosexual domestic partners.

CHANGING AMERICAN MARRIAGES AND FAMILIES

The U.S. Census Bureau defines a family as "a group of two or more people (one of whom is the householder, the person in whose name the housing unit is owned or rented) who reside together and who are related by birth, marriage, or adoption." The average U.S. family consists of 3.2 people, down from 3.6 in 1970. Latino families are larger, with

an average of 3.9 members, than either African-American (3.4) or non-Latino white families (3.0).

About 54 percent of all American adults (about 11 million people) are married and living with their spouses, according to the U.S. Department of Commerce (2005). One of the major changes in the families of young adults is that the number of single parents has increased. Nearly 30% of all children under 18 years of age live with just one parent, and of this group, 84% live with their mother.

Parenthood

Becoming a parent is a life-altering event that impacts every facet of a person's life. Whereas historically children may have been desired for religious or economic reasons (such as working to sustain a farm), many contemporary U.S. couples do not consider parenthood an essential part of their marriage. Many couples choose to delay parenthood until their careers and marriage have achieved a desired level of security. In situations where parenthood is a conscious choice, rather than an accident, couples tend to consider having children as a goal for their personal happiness. Despite the stresses that accompany parenting, couples that have realistic expectations for their new roles and responsibilities find the adjustment to parenthood manageable. As indicated in Table 9.3, the number of births in the United States is growing steadily. The birthrate for married women has declined somewhat, but for unmarried women, it has nearly doubled in the past 25 years.

Divorce

Divorce rates almost tripled from 1960 to 1980, before flattening out and even declining in recent years. Generally speaking, the increase in divorce rates was likely influenced by four factors:

Career Apps

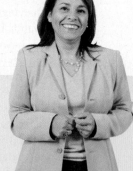

As a marriage and family counselor, how might you help a young adult couple face obstacles in their daily lives that can feel devastating or insurmountable at times?

TABLE 9.3

Number and Rate* of Births to Unmarried Women and Married Women in the United States (1980-2006)

Year	Number	Births to unmarried women	Births to married women
		Rate	Rate
2006	1,641,946	50.6	88.0
2000	1,347,043	44.1	87.4
1995	1,253,976	44.3	82.6
1990	1,165,384	43.8	93.2
1985	828,174	32.8	93.3
1980	665,747	29.4	97.0

*Rate refers to births per 1,000 women aged 15-44.

A major goal of civil rights groups in recent years has been the recognition and legalization of same-sex marriages. LGBT activists around the nation are challenging state legislation that prohibits same-sex marriage. Social networking sites such as Facebook and Twitter make it possible to enter the conversations in a variety of ways. People can learn about legislation and advocacy efforts with the click of a mouse, or join groups that provide updates on key issues.

Just as attitudes toward marriage vary greatly throughout the United States, attitudes toward same-sex marriage also vary. At the time of the writing of this book, there is great division of opinion as to what constitutes marriage and who should be allowed to marry on a state and national level. A stark example of the dissonance is seen in Figure 9.8, which indicates that more states accept marriage between cousins than accept marriage between same-sex individuals. This map has been referenced on several social networking sites and blogs.

- Liberalization of divorce laws
- Growing societal acceptance of divorce and of remaining single
- Reduction in the cost of divorces, largely through no-fault divorce laws
- Broadening educational and work experience of women, which has contributed to their increased economic and social independence

However, the often quoted "50% of all marriages end in divorce" doesn't account for many complicating factors, such as age of partners at marriage; whether it is the first or subsequent marriage for the partners; whether the partners are the same race, sex, ethnicity, and/or religion; and whether or not the couple has children. All of these factors have an effect on the success of a marriage.

SAME-SEX RELATIONSHIPS

Defining relationships, whether we're talking about family or marriage, involves a degree of subjectivity that implies judgment, values, and even politics. At the center of the controversy over homosexuality is same-sex marriage, specifically the question of whether gays and lesbians should be allowed to marry. Some states have passed laws to allow same-sex unions, but others have passed legislation barring recognition of same-sex marriages. In some states, same-sex marriage is not legal, but civil unions afford same-sex couples many of the same advantages as heterosexual couples.

Patterns of Work

Changes in the world of work are occurring more rapidly than ever before. Working in the U.S. today is complicated because of competing pressures (such as family, technology, education), and the recent economic crisis only adds to the complexity. As young adults develop their worldviews, their choices about work often relate to their goals and values. A look at some of the major trends in the area of work, the causes of these trends, and their likely results helps illustrate some of the issues facing young adults today.

One of the most stressful aspects of one's college experience is career planning. Though a daunting task if left until the spring semester of senior year, it can be a time of exploration, reflection, and excitement if the pursuit is spread out over 4 years of school. In Kim Hays's "Coping with College" series (2004), she gives a general timeline for career planning during the college years.

- Freshman and sophomore years are most conducive to exploration of major and career choices. Hays says that "even students who begin college knowing what they want to major in may question their choice at one point." Questioning at this early stage is normal and even advisable; committing to a major without exploration of other options often leads to regret later on.

- By the end of sophomore year, exploration should be coming to a close as the student begins to feel more committed to a major and career path. Failure to choose a focus at this time makes it difficult for the student to pursue in-depth his or her chosen path.

FIGURE 9.8
States' Attitudes Toward Marriage in the United States

States that allow same sex marriage.

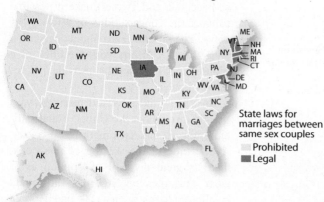

State laws for marriages between same sex couples
- Prohibited
- Legal

States that allow marriage between first cousins.

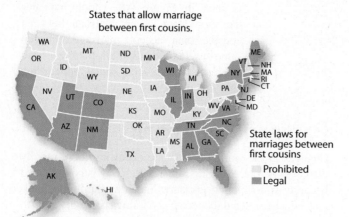

State laws for marriages between first cousins
- Prohibited
- Legal

More states accept marriage between cousins than between same-sex partners, according to current legislation.

Source: New York Times : http://thenewcivilrightsmovement.com/wp-content/uploads/2009/12/nyt.jpg

FIGURE 9.9
Men and Women in the Workplace

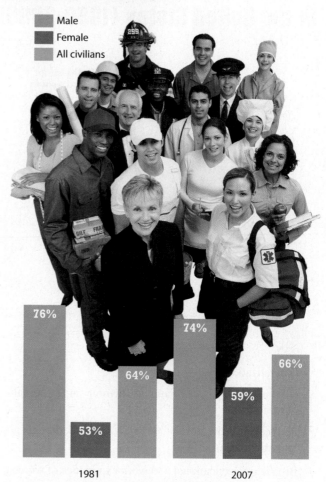

- Male
- Female
- All civilians

76%
53%
64%
74%
59%
66%

1981   2007

More opportunities for women has translated into a greater number of women in the workplace.

Source: U.S. Department of Labor, Bureau of Labor Statistics.

- Junior year should be used to solidify choices and begin taking advantage of opportunities in the student's chosen field. Hays suggests that juniors develop career-related experience to help bridge the gap between college and that first job. The best way to do this is through summer jobs, internships, and co-op placements in a specific field related to one's major.

mentoring The act of assisting another, usually younger, person with his or her work or life tasks.

If these preliminary exploratory steps have been completed, beginning a formal job search is no longer as intimidating.

CAREER DEVELOPMENT AND WORK IDENTITY

In early adulthood, people begin to form patterns that affect their future lifestyle, and work, in turn, begins to shape a person's identity. For some, years spent in formal education were leading up to the ultimate goal of attaining a job. A person's work situation has direct impact on her financial opportunities, peers, leisure time, and living arrangements. Although an individual can find satisfaction setting career goals and climbing the career ladder to achieve them, there is also the risk when identity is so tightly woven with career that failure to achieve those goals will lead to emotional distress or depression. One way to frame one's work identity is to separate financial hopes and needs from creative and/or intellectual needs. Over time, the pace that is set with career and workload impacts later decisions about self and family.

The concept of **mentoring**—an individual helping another, often younger, person with work or other tasks—has received considerable attention in recent years (B. Johnson, 2002; Thompson & Kelly-Vance, 2001). A mentor provides each individual with guidance around life and/

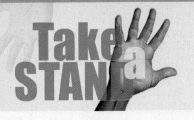
And Tango Makes Three

Challenging traditional views of many topics, including love, parenting, and family, this children's story caused quite a stir. It is a story, based on an actual event that occurred at the Central Park Zoo in New York, beginning in 1998, about the relationship between two male penguins that form a couple and eventually raise a baby penguin. The book has won many awards, but has also been banned by organizations that don't agree with the themes presented in the story. The American Library Association reported that it was the most challenged book for three consecutive years (2006–2008) and the most banned book of 2009.

Given the current social and political climate, what is your reaction to the idea that same-sex parents can create a loving family unit in ways that challenge expectations related to gender roles and sexual behavior? What argument(s) can you make to support views that are in opposition to your own?

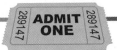

ADMIT ONE   289147   289147

FEATURED MEDIA

Films About Relationships

Casablanca (1942) – Can love be so deep that you can give up the person you love most?

Harold and Maude (1971) – What are the limits on age difference in a loving relationship?

Milk (2008) and ***Monster (2003)*** – How can personal beliefs about sexual preference and lifestyle choices breed hatred so vicious as to provoke one person to murder another?

Normal (2003) – How can love support the partners in a marriage when one partner decides that she can no longer live trapped in a man's body?

or work issues in a way that friends and family cannot. A true mentor relationship offers each person wisdom and mutually rewarding exchange over time. More and more occupations are formally instituting mentor positions, but people can seek out a mentor from any aspect of their lives—hobbies, career, religion, and so on.

I know the price of SUCCESS: *dedication, hard work, and an unremitting* **devotion** *to the things you want to see happen.*

FRANK LLOYD WRIGHT

THE DUAL-CAREER FAMILY

The family pattern of the husband who goes off to work to provide for his family and the wife who stays home and manages that family is much less common than it was 50 years ago, although stereotypes remain, as discussed previously. It has been replaced by the family dynamic known as the **dual-career family,** in which both husband and wife work, typically full time. In 2008, 60% of women were in the labor force, a number that has been relatively stable over the past several years (see Figure 9.9). Women are choosing and succeeding in careers once considered men's fields, such as finance and medicine. Increased career opportunities for women have led to higher stress levels for some women, while increasing their personal satisfaction (Rosser, 2004; Schmader, Johns, & Barquissau, 2004).

Despite their increased presence in the workforce, most women are still considered responsible for the maintenance of the family. As a result, they often choose jobs that meet family needs and demands and tend to work

dual-career family Family in which both partners work, usually full time.

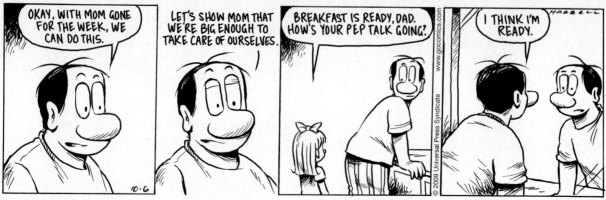

shorter hours than men do. In addition, women change the nature of their work more often than men do.

Another changing aspect of the American family is the increasingly active role of fathers in the raising of the children. Paternal child care—the father cares for children while the mother works outside the home—is receiving more attention in the field because of the changing role of fathers and the implications of father involvement for child development, marital relations, and the family's economic situation. Organizations such as the Father Involvement Research Alliance (FIRA) recognize that society as a whole, and policies specifically, must be examined to gain an appreciation of what fathers' roles in parenting and child care can and should be.

Paternal child care in the United States occurs most often in families where a mother's salary is high or when the cost of nonmaternal child care is comparatively high. The occurrence of paternal child care also strongly depends on factors such as the father's work schedule in a dual-career family, the number of opportunities for the father's employment outside the home, and the extent to which both fathers and mothers identify with traditional gender roles.

CONCLUSIONS & SUMMARY

Youths are initiated into adulthood in preindustrial societies. The transition into adulthood in the United States is much more complex, and clear initiation rites are for the most part absent.

Early adulthood is a period during which many changes are taking place. The peak of physical development is reached, and the decline of certain abilities begins. Lifestyle has a powerful effect on this development, including diet, physical fitness, and use of alcohol, drugs and tobacco.

The major change in the area of cognitive development involves progress from dualistic thinking through relativism to the ethical/intellectual stage of commitment. Research also suggests that there are distinctive "women's ways of knowing."

How are American youths being initiated into adulthood today?

- Initiation rites in other cultures offer a formal ceremony marking the transition from child to adult.

- The purpose of initiation rites in preindustrial societies is to cushion the emotional disruption arising from the transition from one life status to another.

- Entry into adulthood is far more complex for adolescents today, largely due to the increase of sophisticated technologies and the need for many more years of formal education.

- Five types of activities signal the passage to maturity in America today: religious, physical, social, educational, and economic.

What are the significant factors affecting physical development in early adulthood?

- Young adults experience a peak in energy and strength.

- Lifestyle patterns (exercise, diet) affect current and future health.

- Perry suggested three categories of intellectual and ethical development that typify transition from late adolescence to early adulthood: dualism, relativism, and commitment.

- Distinct life cycles apparently exist, the goals of which are individuation and maturity.

- As we do more research, more similarities between male and female development are becoming apparent.
- Levinson suggested that adults develop according to a general pattern known as the life cycle.
- According to Erikson's theory, early adulthood is defined in terms of intimacy and solidarity versus isolation.

What are the relationships between sexual identity and gender roles?

- Sexual identity results from those physical characteristics and behaviors that are part of our biological inheritance.
- Gender role, on the other hand, results partly from genetic makeup and partly from the specific traits in fashion at any one time and in any one culture.
- Views of acceptable gender role behaviors have changed considerably during the past 20 years. Androgyny is now considered an acceptable alternative to masculine and feminine gender roles.
- Dating trends include group dating as well as the tendency to pair off for social events.
- Pack dating is an important change in the interpersonal relationship patterns among young adults.
- It is difficult to categorize the current sexual practices of young adults because their partnerships tend to change more than previously. Love, too, may be variously explained—for example, with the theories of Sternberg and Fromm.

How do young adults deal with the interpersonal relationships of sexuality and love?

- Sternberg argues that love involves developing a story.
- Fromm states that people need to have their deepest and most important thoughts and feelings "validated" by others who are significant to them.

What patterns of work typify young adults today?

- Women often choose jobs that fit in well with the needs of their family. Women tend to work shorter hours and change the nature of their work more often than men do.
- Economic realities and the feminist movement have given rise to dual-career families, in which both husband and wife work.

KEY TERMS

achieved identity *210*
androgyny *217*
ascribed identity *210*
cholesterol *211*
cohabitation *221*
date rape *214*

dual-career family *225*
emerging adulthood *208*
feminist movement *215*
gender role *216*
hazing *208*
individuation *218*

intimacy *219*
mentoring *224*
novice phase *219*
organ reserve *210*
postformal thought *215*
rape *214*

sexual harassment *214*
sexual identity *216*
validation *221*

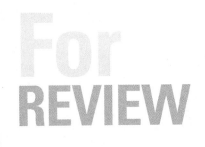

1. Societal changes have led to a change in the nature of initiation rites into adulthood. Are young adults better off today as a result, or should we try to return to the societal structures of the past?

2. The media offer countless advertisements to help a person look younger, feel better, be better. Why are these ads so effective? What do they say about Western society?

3. Levinson believed that forming a mentor relationship is an essential part of the novice phase. Have you formed such a relationship? If so, what are its characteristics?

Chapter Review Test

1. A bar mitzvah or bat mitzvah is an example of a(n) _____ rite of passage.
   a. religious
   b. physical
   c. social
   d. educational

2. Because we seldom call on its total capacity, people often are not aware of the decline of their _____ during early adulthood.
   a. aerobic capacity
   b. blood pressure
   c. heart rate
   d. organ reserve

3. Cigarettes, cigars, and trendy pipes called _____ are equally addictive and contain nicotine that is toxic to the human body.
   a. hookahs
   b. tubas
   c. poppers
   d. None of these is correct.

4. Perry's stages of dualism, relativism, and commitment refer to a person's
   a. relationship development.
   b. intellectual and ethical development.
   c. ability to make moral decisions.
   d. interpersonal relationships.

5. In terms of young adults' dating behaviors, pack dating is
   a. a group of young adults going out together, rather than one-on-one.
   b. a form of dating that involves cigarettes.
   c. more common in warm climates.
   d. for people who have a habit of dependency in relationships.

6. The role of a _____, according to some theorists, is to provide an individual with guidance during life transitions, assistance with decision making, and a clearer view of what the individual wishes to make of himself or herself.
   a. teacher
   b. mentor
   c. partner
   d. sibling

7. *Androgyny* refers to
   a. people who are more likely to behave in a way appropriate to a situation, regardless of their sex.
   b. women who have higher-than-average male elements in their personalities.
   c. men who have higher-than-average female elements in their personalities.
   d. the midpoint between the two poles of masculinity and femininity.

8. Researcher Carol Gilligan states that femininity is defined through
   a. work.
   b. personality.
   c. attachment.
   d. separation.

9. Over the last two decades, one reason for the increase in the age of people at first marriage may be higher numbers of women
   a. entering the workforce.
   b. traveling alone.
   c. afraid of divorce.
   d. having children.

10. The person who used the term *validation* to describe our need, as humans, to feel loved and accepted is
    a. Fromm.
    b. Levinson.
    c. Bem.
    d. Erikson.

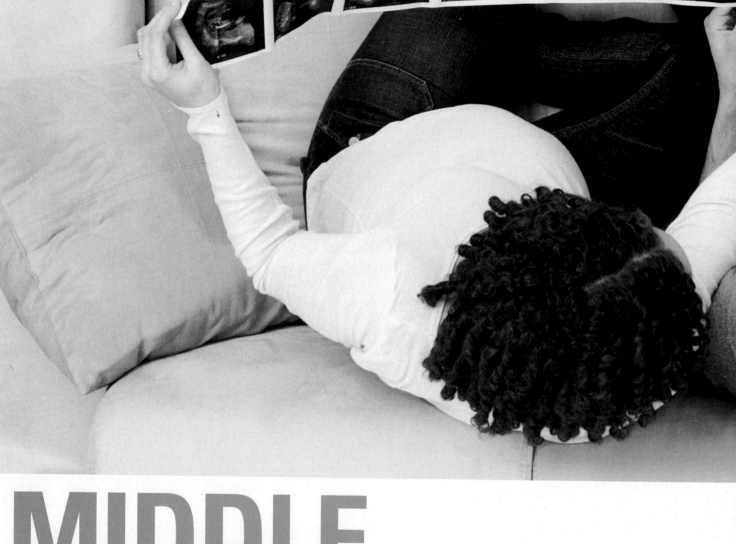

MIDDLE
ADULTHOOD

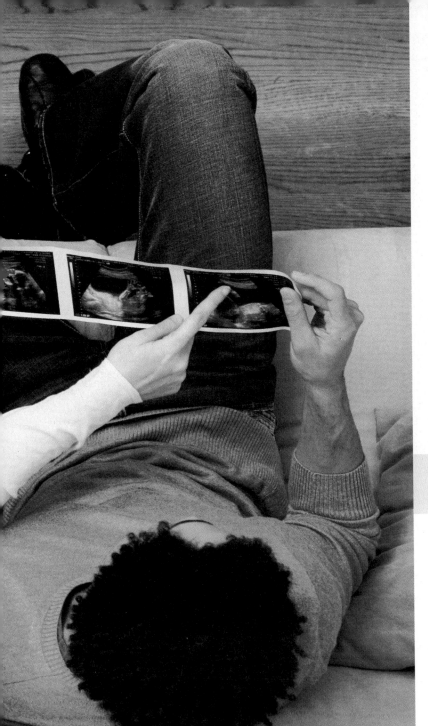

As You READ

After reading this chapter, you should be able to answer the following questions:

- What kinds of physical changes affect people in middle adulthood?

- What are the main factors affecting a person's intellectual development in middle adulthood?

- What are the patterns of work that we most often see in this life stage?

- How do adults deal with stress?

- What are the typical patterns of marriage during middle adulthood?

- What are the main factors that affect sex and love among middle-aged people?

- What happens to personality during the adult years: Does it typically change or remain constant?

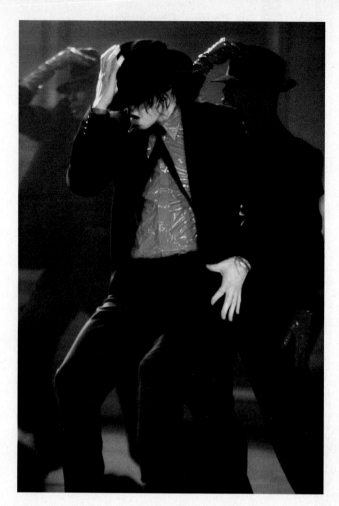

I was a **veteran** before
I was a **teenager.**

MICHAEL JACKSON

their stride. In fact, development continues in significant ways. As with all life stages, how one navigates this stage varies considerably from person to person.

Physical Development

"Aged to perfection" is how one T-shirt says it. While physical systems do change with age, decline in middle adulthood is not inevitable and is highly individual. As you will see, biological forces greatly influence physical development, but psychological and social forces are important factors too.

OVERALL HEALTH

Concerns about health tend to increase in middle adulthood. A person's image of the future becomes increasingly health-related in midlife, because of more firsthand experiences with illnesses and deaths among friends and loved ones than in earlier stages of life. Also beginning in middle adulthood, it is recommended that people begin getting tested for serious conditions that can occur past a certain age. These preventive measures force people to become mindful of potential threats to their health that they had been unaware of before. Campaigns about specific threats, such as colon cancer and breast cancer, aim to raise awareness about prevention and therefore reduce incidence and terminal cases of those conditions.

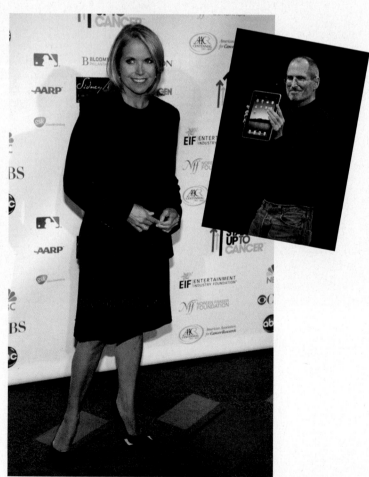

The shocking reports of Michael Jackson's death in June 2009 spread with amazing speed and impact around the world. At 50 years old, Michael was a true superstar, rehearsing for a series of 50 concerts one month away from kickoff. One reason his death came as such a surprise is that people don't associate death with a man considered to be in the prime of life. As the baby boom generation ages, in particular, middle age is becoming much more distinct from old age in public perception.

The Japanese use several words for middle age: *sonen,* which refers to the "prime of life"; *hataraki-zakari,* which means the "full bloom of one's working ability"; and *kan-roku,* which means "weightiness" or "fullness," as in both bearing a heavy load of authority and being overweight. In the United States, our perception of middle adulthood also takes many forms. While it is a period in which there can be physical and cognitive changes due to aging, these do not decline as much as people once thought. Middle adulthood also can be a period in which individuals are just hitting

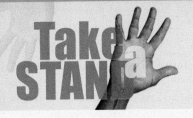
A statement by the U.S. Preventive Services Task Force in 2009 featured new recommendations for women regarding mammograms, contradicting the long-standing position of the American Cancer Society that women begin getting annual screenings at age 40. The new recommendations suggest age 50 as the date of a woman's first mammogram, followed by a mammogram every 2 years.

Many women are concerned that the risk of missing cancer in a woman's younger years outweighs the small risk of radiation involved in mammograms. Others are also concerned that insurance companies will adopt these new recommendations, making it more difficult for a woman to have such a screening exam at a younger age, thus leading to more cases of serious cancer caught when it's too late to save the woman's life.

How should the government address women's fears about breast cancer risks? Who should decide whether the number of women identified with breast cancer at younger ages justifies the risks of having mammograms in their younger years?

VISIBLE SIGNS OF AGING

It doesn't take a screening exam to detect typical signs of middle age. In fact, changes in physical appearance are usually visible in a person's 30s and 40s, and become more apparent in the 50s. Skin tone and texture and hair color undergo visible changes. The pigment in skin changes, so that a person might see new areas of pigment on the hands and face (commonly called age spots) while noticing a lack of pigment in hair. Other changes occur, such as fingernails becoming thicker and teeth becoming slightly yellow. Each person experiences visible signs of aging in an individual way, and some people are more bothered by these changes in appearance. Numerous products and services are available to help people look younger, such as hair coloring, Botox injections, and teeth whitening. The psychological effects of such treatments may help some people deal with the obvious signs of aging.

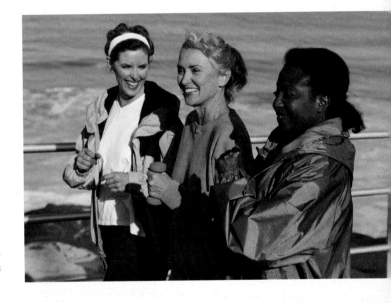

CARDIOVASCULAR HEALTH

In middle adulthood, changes in the cardiovascular system sometimes result in heart disease, which is typically linked to high blood pressure and high cholesterol levels. A report by the World Health Organization estimated that in 2005, 30% of all deaths around the world were the result of heart disease (http://www.who.int/mediacentre/factsheets/fs317/en/print.html). Heart disease commonly results from the buildup of fat in the lining of blood vessels, which reduces the flow of blood to the heart and brain. Eating habits from earlier periods in life influence cardiovascular health in middle adulthood, as the blood vessels have experienced years of effects from the two kinds of cholesterol—LDL (low-density lipoprotein) and HDL (high-density lipoprotein). LDL is commonly known as "bad" cholesterol, because it sticks to artery walls when the concentration is too high. Fortunately, HDL can lessen the risk of heart disease, because it counters the threat posed by LDL.

Both high blood pressure and cholesterol levels are affected by diet and exercise. It may be difficult for some adults to change their lifestyle when in middle adulthood, but doing so can literally save, or at the very least extend, their lives. Researchers have found that middle-aged men and women who had moderate to high levels of physical activity lived 1.3 to 3.7 years longer than those who got little exercise, largely because this kept them from developing heart disease (Franco et al., 2005).

SENSORY ABILITIES—VISION AND HEARING

Everyday experiences depend on one or more of the five physical senses—vision, hearing, smell, taste, and touch. Although the gradual loss of function in the senses is most pronounced in late adulthood, it can become a serious concern in middle age.

In middle adulthood, changes in vision and hearing are most noticeable. Beginning in the early to middle 40s, most individuals will start to experience difficulties with the ability to see clearly at close distances. This normal aging change continues to progress over time. To compensate for these changes in the eye's focusing ability, people begin to wear reading glasses or bifocals. Another age-related change in vision is that our eyes don't adapt to sudden, intense light or darkness as effectively as they once did. For most people, these changes in visual ability pose a problem only when reading fine print or when lighting is reduced, such as in night driving.

Age-related hearing loss is very common and begins at around age 40 (see Figure 10.1). Individuals begin to lose the ability to detect certain tones, particularly high pitches. To compensate for these changes, individuals may begin to use hearing aids, which can greatly improve hearing ability. The Centers for Disease Control (2001b) reported that noise-induced hearing loss is the second most reported occupational illness or injury. The use of headphones, such as ear buds with iPods and MP3 players, can impact hearing over time. Small changes in lifestyle early in life, such as listening for no more than about an hour a day and at levels below 60% of maximum volume, can mean no noise-related hearing loss in middle adulthood.

basal metabolism rate (BMR) The minimum amount of energy a person uses when in a resting state.

FIGURE 10.1
Hearing Loss

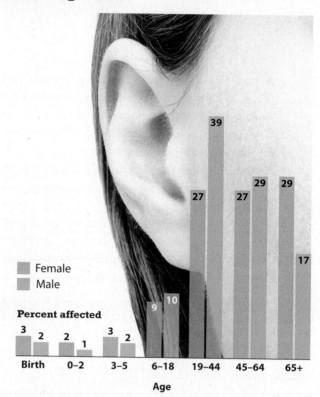

This graph shows the percentage of individuals in different age groups who have experienced hearing loss.

Source: http://www.nidcd.nih.gov/health/statistics/begins.htm

EFFECTS OF HEALTH HABITS

In middle age, habits that formed in earlier life stages can start to have consequences that affect health and well-being (see Figure 10.2). Binge drinking (more than five drinks in one sitting) is more prevalent among middle-aged adults over 50 than previously thought, with research showing that 22% of individuals between the ages of 50 and 64 had consumed at least five alcoholic beverages in the same day within the past month (Blazer & Wu, 2009). (See Table 10.1 for details.) Binge drinking was associated with the use of tobacco and illicit drugs and, among men, with being separated, divorced, or widowed.

In middle age, as true in earlier life stages, overweight is a matter of concern. The difference is that older individuals do not often have the same time or energy to sustain exercise plans and practices they made in younger years (see Figure 10.3). Obesity in middle age—even without established cardiovascular disease risk factors such as high blood pressure or high cholesterol levels—greatly increases risk of hospitalization and is linked to generally worse outcomes in many cancers, including breast and prostate cancer (sciencedaily.com, 2009). For some, the influences of heredity and environment result in obesity—about 40% of the people with one obese parent become obese, as compared with only 10% of those whose parents are not obese (CDC, 2000b). Others become overweight simply because they do not compensate for their lower **basal metabolism rate (BMR),** the minimum amount of energy an individual tends to use when in a resting state. Therefore, if you continue to consume the same number of calories throughout your life, and do not increase exercise, you will definitely gain weight as you age.

Muscle growth is complete in the average person by age 17, but in middle adulthood there is a common but unnecessary decline in muscular ability. Aerobic activities such as swimming and brisk walking appear to help maintain general health and counter the trend toward middle-adulthood weight gain and muscle loss.

The results of poor health habits can ultimately take a serious toll in the form of illness or death during the middle years. Chronic diseases, such as heart or lung disease, are the main causes of death in middle age. Heredity, independent of or combined with choosing to drink alcoholic beverages, smoke cigarettes, overeat, and not getting enough exercise, increases the likelihood that a chronic condition can contribute to death in this period of life.

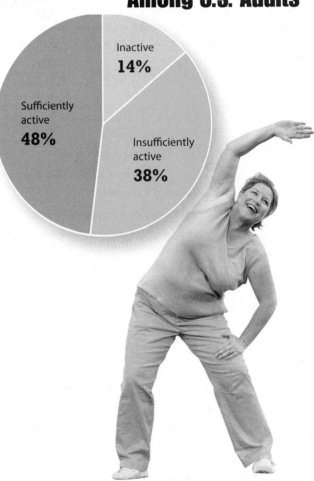

TABLE 10.1

The Face of Binge Drinking

- 20% of men and 6% of women aged 50–64 reported binge drinking within the last month.

- 17% of men and 11% of women reported drinking two or more drinks *a day*.

- Those with *higher* income reported more binge drinking.

- Those who used tobacco and illegal drugs reported more binge drinking.

- Being separated, divorced, or widowed was associated with binge drinking in men.

- Nonmedical use of prescription drugs was associated with binge drinking in women.

FIGURE 10.3

Physical Activity Among U.S. Adults

Inactive **14%**

Sufficiently active **48%**

Insufficiently active **38%**

FIGURE 10.2

Alcohol Use in Older Adults

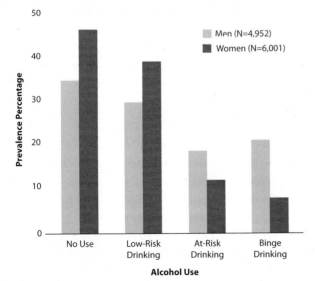

This graph depicts patterns of alcohol use among middle-aged and elderly men and women.

Approximately half of U.S. adults do not meet recommended levels of physical activity.

Source: http://www.cdc.gov/datastatistics/archive/physical-activity.html

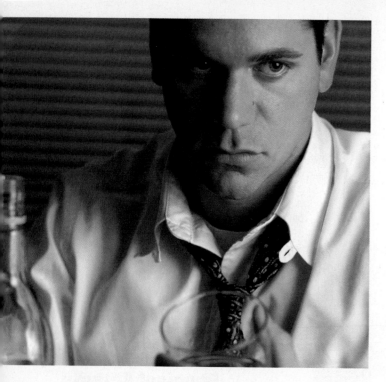

Many conditions are preventable, however, and lifestyle choices within a person's control can greatly alter the likelihood that someone in middle age will suffer from a chronic condition. The availability and utilization of health-care resources also plays a role. For example, a recent report from the CDC stated that 75% of adults aged 50–64 do not get recommended screening exams and immunizations, such as breast and other cancer screenings, flu shots, and even behavioral screenings that could help identify risk of potential problems and negative health behaviors (CDC, 2009). Table 10.2 shows the percentages of middle-aged adults in various age groups who have had recommended screenings and immunizations.

SEXUALITY

As men and women go through middle age, physiological changes occur in both males and females, affecting their sexuality in ways that are distinct to this particular time of life. Such changes are often related to hormone levels that influence fertility and reproduction. Changes in sexuality for women and men occur gradually, and while sexual activity declines in middle adulthood, the decline is gradual as well. According to the 2005 Durex Global Sex Survey, Americans aged 16 to 55+ engage in sex an average of 113 times a year, which ranks the United States 11th of 41 countries in that category (see Figure 10.4).

Changes in sexuality differ between men and women and between any two individuals. Men do not lose their fertility in the same way that a woman's ability to conceive and carry a healthy baby ends, for example, and the timing of a woman's changes varies from person to person and can involve very different experiences and symptoms.

TECH TRENDS

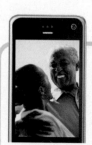

Virtual Fitness

One of the main obstacles to maintaining a healthy weight is the lack of time to exercise. Middle-aged adults are often juggling caregiving responsibilities and career, leaving less time ... period. Thanks to new innovations in the digital age, adults can use computers, phones or portable media players (such as iPhone or iPod Touch), and videogame consoles (Nintendo Wii) to fit exercise into their daily routine without leaving home or the workplace. The following are some examples of technology geared toward a healthier adulthood:

RunKeeper Free – This application for iPhone or iPod Touch tracks all personal statistics for walking or running, and allows people to see a map of their activities on the iPhone and the Web. It's integrated with Facebook and Twitter, so people can connect with friends and help share the motivation.

Six Pack App – This comprehensive fitness application for the iPhone or iPod touch provides a library with pictures and text describing hundreds of exercise techniques. Divided into different sections to focus on different parts of the body, yoga, and stretching, there are exercise sections utilizing equipment (weights, exercise ball) and exercises focusing on core muscles.

Wii Fit – This videogame system by Nintendo is a bestselling product designed to help keep people fit in four categories: yoga, strength training, aerobics, and balance. Using the key component—a balance board—users create a profile, enter height and weight, and perform a few tests that calculate their body mass index (BMI) and assess their basic balance. Based on these scores, people are assigned a Wii Fit age. The game has about 50 different activities to exercise and entertain those who use it.

TABLE 10.2

Screenings and Immunizations—Practices in Middle Age

	Indicators	All Adults Ages 50–64	Ages 50–54	Ages 55–59	Ages 60–64
Screenings	Mammogram within past 2 years	80.3%	78.7%	81.4%	81.4%
	Pap test within past 3 years	85.5%	86.8%	85.3%	83.6%
	Colorectal cancer screening	53.3%	43.9%	56.9%	63.1%
	Cholesterol screening within past 5 years	89.7%	87.3%	90.6%	92.2%
Immunizations	Flu vaccine within past year	42.3%	35.4%	43.1%	51.6%

Source: Adapted from Behavioral Risk Factor Surveillance System (BRFSS) data—CDC, 2009.

FIGURE 10.4

Top 10 Countries by Sexual Activity

Average number of times having sex per year

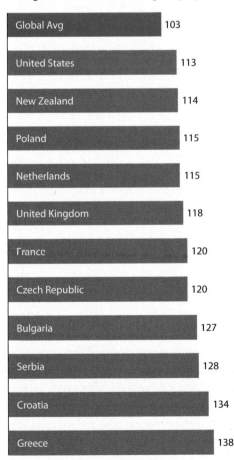

Global Avg	103
United States	113
New Zealand	114
Poland	115
Netherlands	115
United Kingdom	118
France	120
Czech Republic	120
Bulgaria	127
Serbia	128
Croatia	134
Greece	138

Source: http://rankingamerica.files.wordpress.com/2009/01/chart-of-sexual-activityxls.jpg

These changes can be summed up in the word **climacteric,** which refers to a relatively abrupt change in the body, brought about by changes in hormonal balances. In women, this is called **menopause,** which typically occurs over several years during a woman's late 40s or early 50s, and refers to the cessation of menstruation. On average, women experience their last periods around age 51, but the transition from regular periods to no periods can span an entire decade.

> **climacteric** The midlife change in hormone levels that affects fertility.
>
> **menopause** Cessation of women's menstruation, typically occurring in the late 40s or early 50s.

The main physical change in menopause is that the ovaries cease to produce the hormones estrogen and progesterone. The symptoms related to such reduced hormone production can be vary widely among women. Some experience discomfort in the form of stomachaches or queasiness, exhaustion, mood swings, and hot flashes—periods of elevated body temperature that cause a woman to sweat and feel feverish. Lower levels of estrogen can cause less vaginal lubrication, which can make intercourse uncomfortable. Sexual arousal may be somewhat slower, and women may need extra stimulation to attain and sustain orgasm. Some studies have found a reduction of female interest and desire during menopause (Burgess, 2004).

One of the big misperceptions about menopause is that it is a very distressing time for women. An online article about menopause listed readers' responses to the question "What are women's top concerns?" "Truth #1: Your Vagina is *Not* Going to Shrivel Up Like a Prune" (Jio, 2009). Most women, however, do not experience a reduction in sexual activity or satisfaction, during menopause, and many women are quite relieved to no longer menstruate.

Women do often grapple with some effects of menopause related to hot flashes or other symptoms, and strategies for treating women have been somewhat controversial. **Hormone replacement therapy (HRT)** is a common treatment for the unpleasant side effects of menopause. Supplementing women's reduced supply of estrogen and progesterone seems to help with some symptoms, such as vaginal dryness, hot flashes, and night sweats. In the short-term, hormone therapy can reduce a woman's risk of heart disease, colorectal cancer, and osteoporosis (bone loss), but studies in the 2000s showed that hormone therapy increased the risk of blood clots, stroke, breast cancer, and heart disease. Data support the initiation of hormone therapy close to menopause, but the risks increase for older women. The balance of benefits and risks for a woman will be influenced by her personal preferences, risks for specific diseases, and the degree of menopausal symptoms.

The male climacteric refers to the male change of life, typically related to sexual performance and sperm production. At one time, it was thought that the male hormone balance parallels that of the female, but most men are still able to father children even into old age. Men's sperm count may drop a bit, but not significantly in middle adulthood. Men also experience less of a decline in hormone levels and sexual desire than women. There may be lower levels of testosterone, fewer viable sperm, and changes in the testes and prostate gland (Beutel, Weidner, & Brahler, 2006). There is usually a need for more direct stimulation to the penis to attain and sustain erection, and men have a longer refractory period between ejaculations. Erectile dysfunction (ED) can be a problem impacting middle-aged men. Besides aging, risk factors for ED include conditions such as hypertension and diabetes and lifestyle habits such as smoking.

Drugs such as Viagra and Levitra are used to reduce erectile problems, and have become household names, owing to marketing campaigns. These drugs primarily work by increasing blood flow to the penis (Wright, 2006). Side effects of drug treatment may include headaches,

hormone replacement therapy (HRT) Menopause treatment whereby women receive hormone supplements.

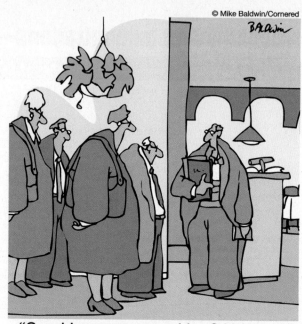

© Mike Baldwin/Cornered

"Smoking or nonsmoking? Hormone therapy or nonhormone therapy section?"

Source: www.CartoonStock.com

Middle age is the awkward period when Father Time *starts catching up with* Mother Nature.

HAROLD COFFIN, FORMER HUMOR COLUMNIST FOR *THE ASSOCIATED PRESS*

sudden drop in blood pressure, and vision problems. Men who are considering drug treatment for ED should tell their doctors about any medications they are taking for routine health problems. Certain drug combinations can have dangerous effects.

perspectives on **Diversity**

Menopause in the United States and Japan

Women in the United States tend to experience hot flashes as the most common symptom of menopause, whereas women in Japan experience it so infrequently that there is no word in the Japanese language to describe it. Menopausal Japanese women, however, tend to experience symptoms known as "frozen shoulders," which refers to painful, limited shoulder movement. Nigerian women also experience shoulder discomfort during menopause.

Experts have determined that differences in symptoms are related to a woman's diet, as well as genetic and environmental factors. Psychological factors, such as how a woman's aging is perceived in her culture (a place of honor versus a place of loneliness and isolation), impact a woman's personal experience of this life transition.

Cognitive Development

Middle adulthood is a time of physical changes. Can we assume that cognitive abilities change too? The question of how our cognitive abilities change has been the focus of much research, which has largely focused on intelligence and creativity.

INTELLIGENCE

No aspect of adult functioning has received more research than intelligence. Most efforts have examined whether intelligence declines with age, and if so, how much and in what ways. Theorist J. L. Horn (1978) described two dimensions of intelligence: fluid and crystallized. **Fluid intelligence** refers to the ability to think and act quickly and solve problems, as well as the ability to use abstract thinking.

Crystallized intelligence refers to accumulated information and verbal skills over time, reflecting the effect of culture and learning. More specifically, crystallized intelligence allows a person to make connections between information and/or objects. As a person develops over time and comes across new information, that person increases the crystallized intelligence that may be accessed in future experiences. Horn hypothesized that while crystallized intelligence does not decline and may even increase with age, fluid intelligence does deteriorate to some degree, since it relies on an efficient nervous system (see Figure 10.5).

FIGURE 10.5

Fluid and Crystallized Intellectual Development Across the Lifespan

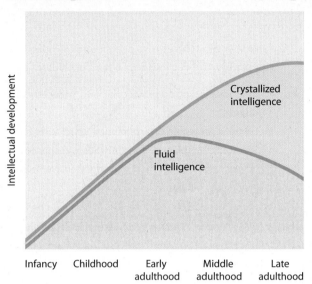

According to Horn, crystallized intelligence increases throughout the lifespan, but fluid intelligence steadily declines from middle adulthood.

NEW VIEWS OF INTELLIGENCE

In a noteworthy attempt to understand the adult range of intellectual abilities, psychologists K. Warner Schaie and Sherry Willis (Schaie, 2005) have been conducting a longitudinal study known as the Seattle Longitudinal Study. Recall from Chapter 1 that a longitudinal study looks at the same individuals over a period of time. The Seattle Longitudinal Study has focused on the question of individual change versus stability in intelligence: Do our abilities change over time, or are we consistent in our abilities according to intelligence tests? More than 500 participants were initially tested in 1956 on a variety of abilities including vocabulary, verbal memory, number (math calculations), spatial orientation, perceptual speed, and inductive reasoning. Schaie and Willis concluded that people reach a peak in many cognitive skills during middle adulthood. Perceptual speed—the ability to compare symbols and objects quickly and accurately—is the one area that declines most noticeably throughout adulthood (see Figure 10.6).

In middle adulthood, measures of intelligence are not as pertinent as they may have been in earlier stages of life, because the information gained from such measures is not as influential during the middle years. Most middle-aged adults are not in school, and are often settled in their careers and family lives, so learning new information and developing new skills is not expected in the same way, although it is certainly valued highly. In fact, most commonly used intelligence tests measure only a few of the cognitive abilities that could be considered factors in intelligence, such as memory and perception. Horn believed that intelligence is not the result of one general factor but, rather, a combination of many abilities working in different ways and that different people display intelligence in different ways.

fluid intelligence The ability to think and act quickly and solve problems, as well as the ability to use abstract thinking.

crystallized intelligence Accumulated information and verbal skills over time, reflecting the effect of culture and learning; allows a person to make connections between information and/or objects.

It is a little bit surreal. *I never could have anticipated finding myself back playing that same* character *after time had passed. It is sort of surreal and* cool.

**LAURA LEIGHTON, TELEVISION ACTRESS WHO REPRISED HER ROLE AS
SYDNEY ANDREWS ON THE REMAKE OF *MELROSE PLACE***

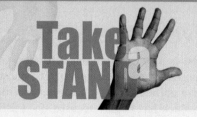

Socioeconomic Bias and Cognitive Decline

A number of variables have been found to reduce the risk of cognitive decline (Schaie & Elder, 2005):

- The absence of cardiovascular and other chronic diseases
- Living in favorable environmental conditions
- Substantial involvement in activities and stimulating environments, such as travel and extensive reading
- Having a flexible personality style
- Being married to a spouse who has a high cognitive functioning level
- Engaging in activities that require quick perception and thinking

- Being satisfied with one's life accomplishments through midlife

The variables listed above are biopsychosocial in nature and therefore the result of many influences. Using an example from above, how could you argue that socioeconomic status impacts intelligence? For example, which variables become less risky if a person has more money and more options for lifestyle adjustments? Using an example from above, how could you argue that biology trumps environment and determines a person's cognitive path?

FIGURE 10.6
Changes in Intellectual Abilities

This graph illustrates changes in six intellectual abilities in middle adulthood.

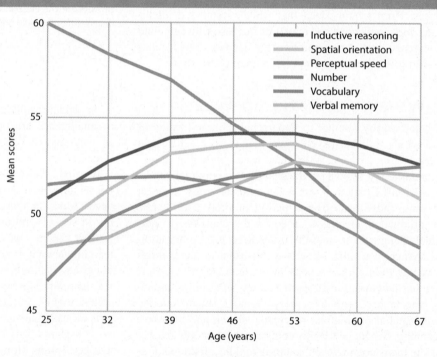

analytic intelligence
Sternberg's term to describe a person's ability to break down a problem or situation into the smaller parts of the whole.

creative intelligence
Sternberg's term to describe a person's ability to solve problems in unique ways and to feel comfortable with new or different situations and ideas.

practical intelligence
Sternberg's term to describe "common sense"—a simple, logical understanding of a situation and how to work through a problem.

Individuals in middle adulthood may utilize and display several distinct cognitive abilities. For example, the eight types of intelligences in Howard Gardner's (1983) theory of multiple intelligences, presented in Chapter 7, are becoming more widely recognized as a measure of intelligence in middle-aged adults. Although not a formal assessment tool, the recognition of intelligence and ability in specific domains (as proposed by Gardner) is a way to assess intelligence and ability in middle-aged individuals.

Robert Sternberg has also challenged traditional views of intelligence tests on the grounds that they measure only crystallized intelligence. He suggests that intelligence isn't as much about quantity as balance—knowing when and how to use analytic, creative, and practical intelligence components. **Analytic intelligence** refers to the ability to break down a problem or situation into the smaller parts of the whole. **Creative intelligence** refers to the ability to solve problems in unique ways and to feel comfortable with new or different situations and ideas. **Practical intelligence** refers to the

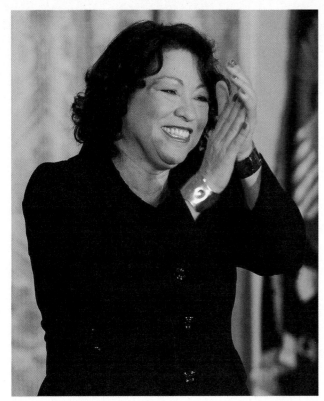

Supreme Court Justice Sonia Sotomayor

quality people might call "common sense"—a simple, logical understanding of a situation and how to work through a problem. The abilities Sternberg describes peak in the middle adult years. Because middle-aged adults have a better understanding of their own limits, they can more easily capitalize on their strengths and compensate for their weaknesses.

INFORMATION PROCESSING AND EXPERTISE

As described in previous chapters with regard to earlier life periods, our ability to process information is related to cognitive development. Aspects of information-processing theory, such as expertise, speed of processing, and memory, are especially relevant in middle adulthood. Generally speaking, someone who is new to a task or situation requires more effort, attention, and energy to complete the task than an expert—someone who possesses skills or experience in a specific task or activity.

Over time, as people have more life experiences and acquire more knowledge, they are able to transfer that knowledge into novel situations. This allows people to solve some problems more readily in middle adulthood than at earlier ages because they have more information to draw upon and more resources to refer to when making decisions. Examples can range from knowing how to whip up a delicious dinner when the only food in the refrigerator is eggs and potatoes to knowing what to do when the IRS calls for an audit. However, people experience a gradual decline in the ability to process information quickly. This

mild decline is noticeable, for example, when a middle-aged adult attempts to retrieve information quickly or participate in an activity that requires him to use quick reflexes, such as retrieving a new name or phone number.

Related to the ability to retrieve information is memory. In the early middle-age years, there is not much difference in memory speed and capacity than in early adulthood. However, as a person approaches late adulthood, a lifetime's accumulated knowledge takes up memory space that can interfere with the acquisition of new knowledge and retrieval of older, previously stored information.

THE ROLE OF CREATIVITY

A key factor in the ability to continue to be productive well into the later years is creativity. Research shows that creativity does not decline with age and that, on the contrary, middle adulthood is one of the peak periods of creativity. As the world changes more and more rapidly, the role of creativity has become an important aspect of cognitive functioning. People live with innovations in all aspects of life (think of iPads, hybrid cars, and robotic surgery) and need to respond to the challenges new ideas bring.

Creativity studies have found that highly creative adults

- like to do their own planning, make their own decisions, and need the least training and experience in self-guidance;

- do not like to work with others and prefer their own judgment of their work to the judgment of others;

- take a hopeful outlook when presented with complex, difficult tasks;

- have the most ideas when a chance to express individual opinion is presented, even at the risk of incurring ridicule;

- are most likely to stand their ground in the face of criticism;

- are the most resourceful when unusual circumstances arise; and

- are not necessarily the "smartest" or "best" in competitions.

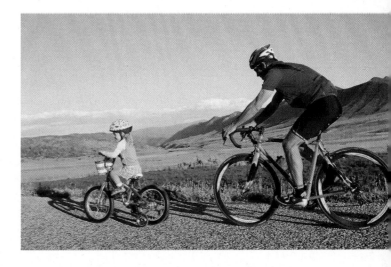

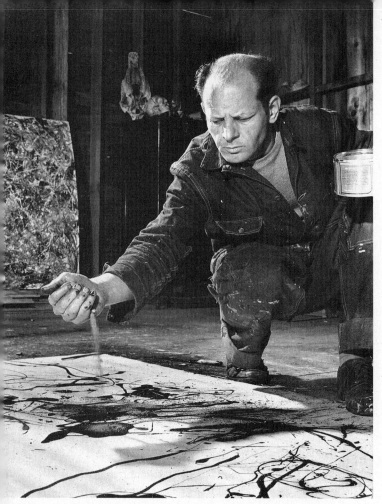

Jackson Pollock was famous for making paintings by splattering paint over a large canvas, then cutting out sections he considered to be artistic.

> *People* **underestimate** *how remarkable it is to create something that no one has ever seen or done before. It's like* **discovering** *the vaccine for polio.*
>
> **SHERYL CROW**

Their ideas are qualitatively different from those of the average person.

Classic research has looked at the lives of creative people and their contributions, revealing that the period between 40 and 60 years of age can be a peak period for creative output (Dennis, 1966; Lehman, 1953). (See Figure 10.7.) For example, most scientists and scholars tend to peak in their 40s to 60s, while artists peak in their 40s.

While creativity is easily noticed in famous people, all people have the capacity for creative output in middle

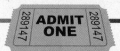
adulthood. One of the biggest factors relates to motivation—how much a person cares to create, dares to take risks, and works to learn and refine new ideas and skills.

LEARNING ABILITY

It has been suggested that people in middle adulthood are less motivated to learn than are younger people. The meaningfulness of a task affects motivation, and the decline in cognitive ability due to aging can often be countered by motivation and new learning experiences. The rate of change and innovation is currently so rapid that learning new skills is a necessity both on the job and off. Routinely asked to use computers and related technology at work, people often take classes to gain the technological and other skills needed in order to advance or even maintain their career.

Career Apps

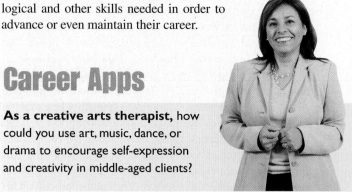

As a creative arts therapist, how could you use art, music, dance, or drama to encourage self-expression and creativity in middle-aged clients?

FIGURE 10.7
Creative Output through the Years

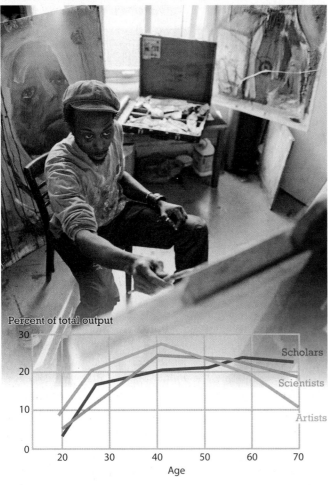

Percent of total output

This graph depicts creative activity at different ages.

Source: Dennis, W. (1966). Creative Productivity between 20 and 80 Years, in Journal of Gerontology, *21, pp. 1–8.*

Social Development

Individuals experience life events and crises differently, depending on many factors rooted in heredity and the environment, such as temperament or political realities (e.g., affordable health care). Whether or not a person experiences middle adulthood as a period of crisis or opportunity varies greatly.

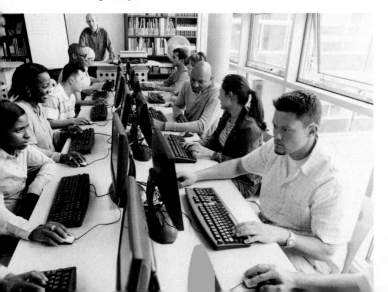

FIGURE 10.8
Levinson's Middle Adulthood

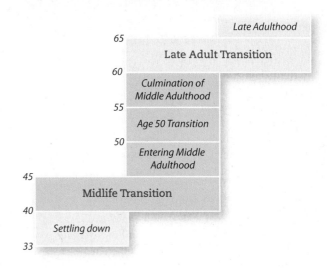

LEVINSON'S SEASONS OF LIFE

Levinson interviewed groups of men initially, and women later in a separate investigation, and analyzed the findings in relation to how life experiences result in a change in personality.

The Midlife Transition

Middle adulthood corresponds to five of Levinson's stages (see Figure 10.8). Beginning with the settling-down stage, an individual establishes a role in society in the central part of their life, whether in their career or their family life. The final stage applicable to middle adulthood is the culmination of middle adulthood, but between those two periods adults undergo many changes that include a specific transition at age 50. For the purposes of this chapter, Levinson's **midlife transition**—a period that lasts from approximately age 40 to 45—is highlighted. Levinson identified this time as a crucial point in adult development, one that bridges early adulthood and middle adulthood. Because people today are expected to live well into their 70s and 80s, the midlife transition does indeed capture the feeling of hitting the middle of one's life, which some encounter as a crisis.

This stage involves three developmental tasks:

- Review, reappraisal, and termination of the early adult period.

- Decisions on how middle adulthood should be conducted.

- Dealing with the polarities that are the source of division in life at this stage. These polarities are being young versus being old, being destructive versus being creative, being masculine versus being feminine, and being attached to others versus being separate from others.

During the midlife transition, individuals question their past life deci-

> **midlife transition** Levinson's term to describe the period of life that bridges early and middle adulthood, approximately ages 40 to 45.

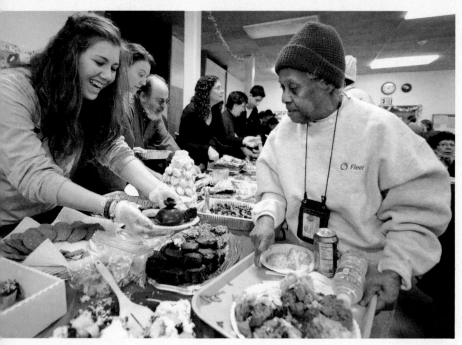
Generativity can take many forms.

generativity Erikson's term for the ability to be useful to self and to society.

stagnation Erikson's term for boredom, self-absorption, and the inability to contribute to society.

sions and accomplishments, and reevaluate where they are going. The process of the midlife transition can result in a different life structure and goals. According to Levinson, even if individuals do not change their life structure during the midlife transition, they still need to reappraise their life and come to terms with choices they made earlier in life.

Most people want to feel that their life has made some difference, and they want to leave something behind them that can be remembered. Therefore, it is typical at this time that the person becomes more creative and often works harder than in the past to make a contribution considered worthwhile by those who follow him or her.

Levinson's research revealed that both men and women experience a similar midlife transition. Members of each sex go through an alternating series of structure-building and structure-changing stages. The old division of female homemakers and male providers feels quite outdated today, and members of both sexes experience challenges throughout their lifetimes that affect their development. Individual differences in personality make these experiences unique and compelling in the study of human development.

ERIKSON'S THEORY: GENERATIVITY VERSUS STAGNATION

Erikson described the seventh stage of psychosocial development, covering 25 to 65 years of age, as generativity versus stagnation.

Generativity means the ability to be useful to self and to society, with the goal of being productive and creative. In the generativity stage, one's productivity is aimed at guiding the next generation. The act of being productive is itself rewarding, regardless of recognition or reward.

Although Erikson certainly believed that the procreation of children was an important part of generativity, he did not believe people must become parents in order to achieve generativity. Some people apply this drive to other forms of altruistic concern and creativity, such as socially valued work (Erikson, 1968).

At this stage of adulthood, some people can become bored, self-absorbed, and unable to contribute to society's welfare; they fall prey to **stagnation.** People who have given birth to children may fail to be generative in their parenthood and come to resent the neediness of their offspring.

Research examining generativity has found that adults in midlife may be more psychologically mature and happier than younger people. Sheldon and Kasser (2001) report that as adults age, their level of psychological maturity influences their level of well-being. Adults in midlife with higher levels of maturity report higher levels of well-being than younger adults. Ackerman and associates (2000) found that higher levels of generativity for middle-aged adults were associated with greater feelings of satisfaction with work and life. In addition, differences in the level of generativity for middle-aged adults were associated with the social support they receive from friends and family and their involvement in religious and political activities.

In Erikson's theory, generativity depends on the successful resolution of the six preceding psychosocial crises that define the human life cycle. People who are able to achieve generativity have a chance to reach the highest level of resolution in Erikson's stage theory: integrity.

Age is an issue of mind *over matter: if you don't mind, it* **doesn't matter.**

MARK TWAIN

STABILITY VERSUS CHANGE

You've probably heard someone say, "Oh, he's been like that ever since he was a baby!" Such a comment doesn't sound like a philosophical statement, but think about what it implies: that individuals' personalities can remain basically the same throughout their lifespan. Whether they do or not is a fundamental question asked by adult development researchers. Do human beings really change very much over the course of their lives, or do we all stay pretty much the same? If we assume that people remain the same regardless of what happens to them as their life continues, then the period of early childhood takes on great meaning. Several of the developmental theorists this book has discussed (for example, Freud and Piaget) have focused much of their attention on the early years of childhood in the belief that what happens to a person during childhood determines much of what will happen to him or her in the future.

Conversely, theorists such as Erikson and Maslow believe that because people are constantly changing and developing, all life experiences must be considered important. In that case, early childhood becomes a somewhat less significant period in the whole of development, and adolescence and adulthood take on more significance. It also implies that getting children "off on the right foot" is not enough to ensure positive development.

In just the same way, some theorists feel that adults remain basically the same throughout adulthood—that the adult personality remains stable. This is termed *continuity* in adult development. Such researchers look at pieces of the personality (personality traits) as measured by detailed questionnaires. They argue that the answers to such questionnaires assess adult personality. These researchers are known as **trait theorists.** Trait theorists (e.g., McCrae & Costa, 2004; McCrae et al., 2000) might say: "If nothing unusual happens, then the adult personality will stay relatively the same. Normal adult personality development is really the maintenance of personality."

Other theorists consider adults in a consistent process of change and evolution. That is what the position of *change* refers to. These theorists argue that adult personality is quite complicated—more so than a list of personality traits. What is interesting to them is how those traits fit with the whole of the person and how an adult's personality interacts with the world around her or him. They believe that research based on personality traits is too narrow in focus and that we must also look at the stages of change each person goes through. These researchers are known as **stage theorists.** Stage theorists Levinson, Vaillant, and Erikson, looking at the whole of the adult, might say: "The adult personality naturally and normally develops through change. Normal adult personality development is a continual process of growth and change."

Which theory explains personality development best? Let's start with the position that the adult personality is made up of traits that remain continuously stable, in most cases, throughout adulthood.

CONTINUOUS TRAITS THEORY

An individual trait can be thought of as an individual's tendency to have consistent patterns of thoughts, feelings, and behaviors (McCrae & Costa, 1990). In the **five factor model (FFM) of personality,** McCrae and Costa describe five traits or dimensions of personality: **o**penness to experience, **c**onscientiousness, **e**xtraversion, **a**greeableness, and **n**euroticism, or OCEAN (McCrae & Costa, 2004). Each of these five traits consists of a cluster of qualities (see Figure 10.9). For example, agreeableness includes qualities such as a tendency to be trusting and cooperative rather than suspicious and critical toward others. People vary continuously on the traits, with most people falling in between the extremes.

An extensive body of research has used the five factor model in an effort to understand the influence of personality traits on a wide range of issues. Research has found that the five traits remain stable throughout adulthood even though a person's habits, life events, opinions, and relationships may change over the course of their life.

VAILLANT'S PREDICTIVE POWER

The work of George Vaillant focuses on the future, rather than the present, for middle-aged adults in his efforts to

trait theorists Researchers who look at pieces of the personality (personality traits), as measured by detailed questionnaires.

stage theorists Theorists who consider stages of change across the lifespan and how one's personality interacts with the world.

five factor model (FFM) of personality McCrae and Costa's theory that there are five major personality traits, which they believe govern the adult personality.

FIGURE 10.9

The Big 5 Factors of Personality

Openness	**C**onscientiousness	**E**xtraversion	**A**greeableness	**N**euroticism (emotional stability)
• Imaginative or practical	• Organized or disorganized	• Sociable or retiring	• Softhearted or ruthless	• Calm or anxious
• Interested in variety or routine	• Careful or careless	• Fun-loving or somber	• Trusting or suspicious	• Secure or insecure
• Independent or conforming	• Disciplined or impulsive	• Affectionate or reserved	• Helpful or uncooperative	• Self-satisfied or self-pitying

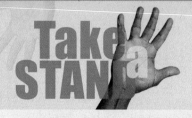

A national organization that puts family and friends at the heart of its mission is PFLAG—Parents, Families, and Friends of Lesbians and Gays. The group aims to provide "opportunity for dialogue about sexual orientation and gender identity, and acts to create a society that is healthy and respectful of human diversity" (http://www.pflag.org). The organization also supports bisexual and transgender individuals.

In middle adulthood, many parents choose to support their LBGT children, friends, and others even as issues such as gay marriage and gays in the military remain deeply divisive. Supporters and opponents argue over human rights, faith, and basic freedoms.

Who should decide who may marry, adopt children, or serve in the military? Do people need to agree on controversial topics in order for society to function? Why or why not? How do controversies over

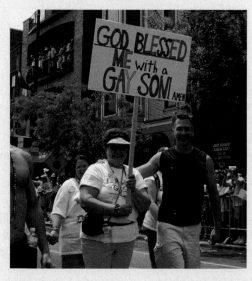

gay marriage and gays serving openly in the military affect people's lives?

---

understand successful aging. Vaillant has spent the last 35 years as director of the Study of Adult Development at the Harvard University Health Service. As we saw in Chapter 1, Vaillant has overseen longitudinal studies spanning over 70 years, with an emphasis on exploring the components of happiness and successful aging. Vaillant identified seven major factors that predict healthy aging, both physically and psychologically:

- employing mature adaptations
- education
- stable marriage
- not smoking
- not abusing alcohol
- exercise
- healthy weight

Vaillant concluded that in order to reach the age of 80 in a good place, an individual had to have five or six of these factors in place at age 50. Of the men in his study who had only 3 or fewer of these protective factors in place at age 50, none reached the age of 80 in good health. Surprisingly, money and overall income were not related to happiness. When asked what he had learned from the men in the Harvard study, Vaillant responded: "The only thing that really matters in life are your relationships to other people."

FRIENDSHIPS

Middle adulthood is typically a time when close friendships become fewer and more precious. The findings of Fung and associates (2001) suggest that people begin narrowing their range of social partners long before middle age. In early adulthood, interaction frequency with acquaintances and close friends begins to decline, while it increases with spouses and siblings. It would seem that, at about age 30, individuals choose a select few relationships from which to derive support, self-definition, and a sense of stability. These relationships with a select few become increasingly close and satisfying during middle adulthood. The idea that face-to-face contact is necessary for closeness is no longer true, thanks to technological advances with cell phones, email, social networking, and programs such as Skype that allow people to communicate instantly despite geographic or other constraints.

Marriage and the Family

Interpersonal relationships in middle adulthood tend to revolve around family. Although individuals may reside under one roof, family members each bring their individual personalities and experiences outside the home into the home environment over a period of many years. What a parent experienced as a teenager is vastly different from what his 16-year-old experiences today. Likewise, a couple's relationship undergoes significant changes before and after parenting roles and responsibilities emerge, regardless of how much the partners love each other. This means that the complex family relationship involves specific factors that grow and change within a family, just as each individual grows and changes over time.

MARRIAGE AT MIDDLE AGE

Middle age is often a time when husbands and wives reappraise their marriage. Often, marriages that were challenging in early adulthood grow better with time, as couples learn to communicate and negotiate successfully. A reduction in the stresses relating to money, children, and career achievement can allow couples to rediscover the positive aspects of their relationship. For example, the period after the children leave home can be like a second honeymoon for many couples. After the initial feelings of sadness and loss that result when the last child leaves the home (often called the **empty nest syndrome**), married couples can evaluate the job they have done with their children and focus future plans on their own interests and needs. Because life expectancy is now longer than in years past, the period after children leave home is longer than it used to be, and couples can typically look forward to spending another 30 or more years together.

FIGURE 10.10

Duration of Marriages That Ended in Divorce

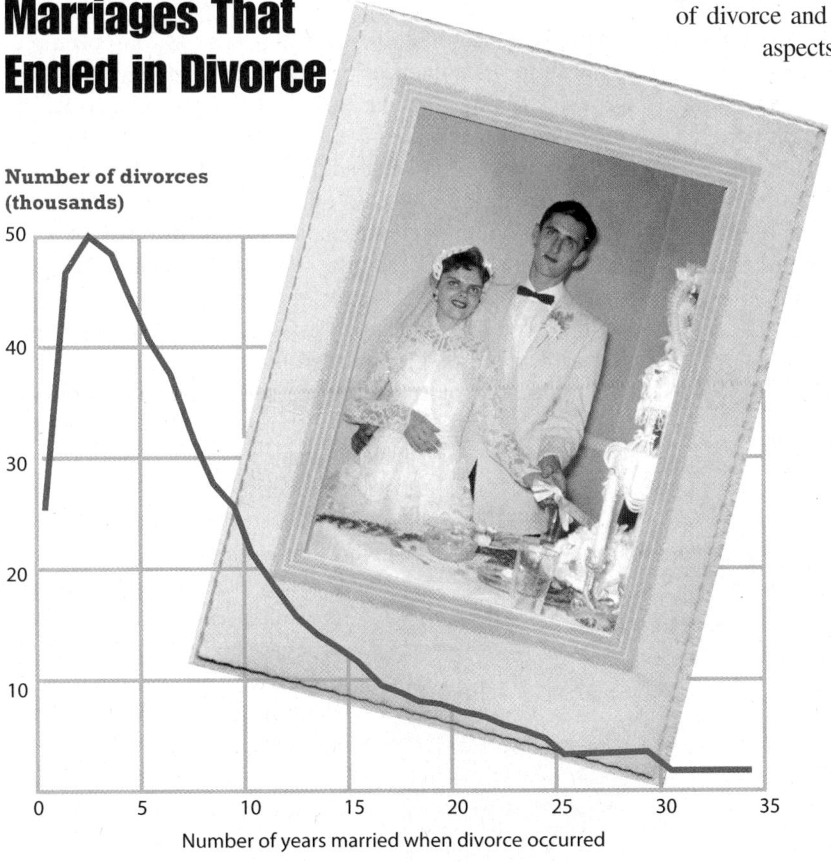

Number of divorces (thousands)

Number of years married when divorce occurred

On the other hand, marital tension is sometimes suppressed while young children live at home. As children leave home to go to college or to start families of their own, these tensions may be more openly expressed. Sometimes partners learn to "withstand" each other, and the only activities and interests they share are ones that revolve around the children—they engage in **emotional divorce.** When the children leave home, the partners realize how far apart they have drifted and are able to recall many small incidents that led up to the larger decision to end the marriage.

empty nest syndrome
The feelings parents may have as a result of their last child leaving home.

emotional divorce
Sometimes partners learn to "withstand" each other. The only activities and interests they share are ones that revolve around the children.

sandwich generation
Term used to describe adults who are simultaneously caring for their children and their aging parents.

DIVORCE IN MIDDLE ADULTHOOD

Although most divorces take place during the first 5 years of marriage and the number tapers off rapidly after that, the proportion of divorced people in middle adulthood is relatively high, because many who divorced earlier have never remarried. Figure 10.10 shows the duration of marriages that ended in divorce.

Divorce in middle adulthood can have positive and negative aspects, as it does in other life periods. Some of the positive aspects of later divorce are that the adults are typically more financially stable, their children are older and less reliant on them for support, and the partners may have a stronger sense of self that will help them cope with the trauma of divorce and the prospect of living alone. Some negative aspects are that older adults' finances are often more complicated than in early marriage. They may own property together and share investments, and if one partner earns substantially more than the other, this can greatly impact the divorce negotiations. Older adults have more-established social networks than younger adults, and friends are sometimes forced to choose their loyalties. The divorcing couple may feel like they have failed at a major part of life and have let down their families. Table 10.3 provides data about the divorce rate in the United States.

RELATIONSHIPS WITH AGING PARENTS

A reality that complicates the lives of many couples in middle adulthood involves relationships with aging parents. Often, the time previously spent caring for young children is filled with concerns and efforts to care for elderly parents. The term **sandwich generation** describes the one in eight adults who gets squeezed between simultaneous responsibilities caring for their children and their parents. Many adults, however, avoid the complications of being squeezed because of timing or financial resources that allow them to hire additional help in the care of either the children or the aging parents.

As parents grow older, they sometimes become as dependent on their middle-aged children as those children once were on them. Most people fail to anticipate the costs and emotional strains that the aging of their parents can engender. The most frequently cited problem of middle-aged women is not menopause or aging, but caring for aging parents or parents-in-law (Singleton, 2000). Daughters, often the oldest or the one living the closest with the fewest demands on her, are most likely going to be the primary caregiver of aging parents. These caregivers sometimes face a number of issues in balancing work and family, but siblings often recognize the stresses they have, and those without children to care for tend to pick up the slack in caring for aging parents.

In some cases, caring for a family member who is very sick can have negative effects on the psychological health of the caregiver. For example, Beeson and colleagues (2000) found that caregivers for relatives with Alzheimer's disease were at high risk for feelings of loneliness, because the disease causes the ailing relative to withdraw psychologically and emotionally from any relationship with the caregiver. The loneliness that results from the loss of companionship between the caregiver and the patient has been linked to higher levels of depression among caregiving wives, husbands, and daughters. The researchers also found that female caregivers experienced more depression than male caregivers, with caregiving wives experiencing the highest levels of depression. The support of siblings and friends greatly helps reduce the negative effects of caring for elderly parents.

In fact, many middle-aged adults enjoy closer relationships with their aging parents at this time. Adult children recognize strengths in their parents that they hadn't before, as they experience some challenges of adulthood that they couldn't appreciate when they were younger. They also tend to see eye-to-eye on issues they'd clashed over previously, such as politics, religion, and child rearing.

TABLE 10.3
Age at Marriage and Subsequent Divorce Rate for Americans

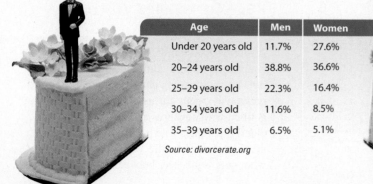

Age	Men	Women
Under 20 years old	11.7%	27.6%
20–24 years old	38.8%	36.6%
25–29 years old	22.3%	16.4%
30–34 years old	11.6%	8.5%
35–39 years old	6.5%	5.1%

Source: divorcerate.org

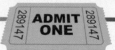

RELATIONSHIPS WITH SIBLINGS

The importance of sibling relationships has long been recognized for its influences on a person's cognitive and social growth. Sibling relationships have the potential to be the most enduring that a person has. People don't usually meet their spouses until young adulthood or at least adolescence. Most parents usually pass away before their children do. Yet most sibling relationships last the lifespan of most adults; and can be very close, somewhat distant, or rife with rivalry.

One would hope that the passage of time and growing maturity would lessen sibling rivalry. Certainly adult siblings are faced with more serious tasks than are childhood siblings. For example, most middle-aged siblings must make mutual decisions concerning the care of their elderly parents and eventually deal with the aftermath of parents' deaths. Changing family patterns raise questions about sibling relationships, as couples more often choose to have fewer or even no children. Children who have few or no siblings to turn to for companionship and psychological support may become adults who consider work and career very important in their lives.

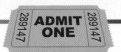
Patterns of Work

Work issues that arise during middle adulthood include challenges involved with working from home, nontraditional work schedules, caring for ill or aging family members, and the rising cost of health insurance. Whereas employers used to focus most human resources on younger employees, a trend has emerged among employers to acknowledge some concerns of middle-aged employees, such as

- advancing age and death,
- bodily changes related to aging,
- adjusting and attaining career goals, and
- change in family and work relationships.

Businesses have responded to these issues and others with continuing education, workshops, and other forms of professional development. As the demand for new skills grows, training in emerging technologies is common, and employees are often reimbursed if they enroll in degree programs that will make them more valuable contributors in the workplace. A greater appreciation for the contribution of older workers is important. As the labor pool shrinks, the welfare of the older, established workforce becomes more valuable. Employees who feel valued and respected by their employers find their jobs more meaningful and feel more empowered (Gomez & Rosen, 2001; Thompson & Bunderson, 2001).

WORK–FAMILY CONFLICT

Work–family conflict is defined as the phenomenon that occurs when demands of a person's role as a caregiver conflicts or spills over into demands of his/her role as a worker. When this type of role overload or role conflict occurs, it often causes stress for the adult and the family. The role of family emotional support, the quality of the employee–supervisor relationship, and the personality of the individual all influence feelings of work–family conflict. For example, Bernas and Major (2000) found that higher levels of emotional support from a woman's family were associated with less work–family conflict, and decreased reports of stress. Somewhat paradoxically, although a positive employee–supervisor relationship at work often resulted in lower feelings of stress in women studied, it also resulted in the women feeling that their work was spilling over into family life. Men and women often compensate by bringing work home or working from home in order to care for younger family members or aging parents.

work–family conflict Phenomenon that occurs when a person's roles as caregiver and worker conflict or overlap.

globalization The outsourcing of much work to a less expensive labor supply in foreign countries.

downsizing A reduction in a company's workforce to improve its total revenue.

MIDCAREER CHALLENGES

Considerable attention is now being given to the career challenges people face in middle adulthood. For some it is a problem of **globalization,** in which much work is outsourced to a less expensive labor supply in foreign countries, while for others **downsizing** is a reality that threatens their lives and livelihood, with layoffs and decreased benefits. Many employers attempt to motivate employees to retire early by promising financial rewards.

By the time a person reaches the age of 40 in a professional or managerial career, it is typically clear whether he or she will make it to the top of the field. If people haven't reached their goals by this time, most adjust their goals or, if possible, begin a new career. Some middle-aged adults take a mentoring attitude toward younger employees.

Middle adulthood is also a time when family expenses, such as college education or elder care, can become great. If family income is threatened or insufficient, this obviously can create stress, especially if only one partner is employed. If the nonworking spouse decides to get a job, other types of stress can sometimes occur. At other times, this is a period of renewed spirit as individuals rise to the challenges and one partner feels a sense of pride in contributing to the welfare of the other partner in a new way.

Coping with Stress

The stresses of middle adulthood are unique in one important way: Adults are usually expected to deal with stress entirely on their own. Their children and aging parents (if

TABLE 10.4
Proactive Stress Reduction

Dr. John Dacey (2000) created a simple four-step program, called COPE, for people to use to recognize and reduce anxiety:

1. Calm your nervous system. This step relates to the innate human tendency to either attack or run away when threatened. Calming the stress response enables people to think clearly about situations and actions.

2. Originate a plan. The second step helps people to think of a creative plan for dealing with their stress. Plans vary from person to person and interest to interest.

3. Persist with your plan. Most people start out well but then lose faith in their plans. Persistence is almost always needed to succeed in the face of adversity.

4. Evaluate your progress. Although having faith in your plan is important, evaluations must be performed while the plan is in operation, as well as after it has been carried out, to ensure success.

Lisa: *Look on the bright side, Dad. Did you know that the Chinese use the same word for "crisis" as they do for "opportunity"?*

Homer: *Yes! Cris-atunity.*

THE SIMPSONS, "FEAR OF FLYING" (1994)

parents are still living) may not be able to offer significant emotional or financial help. While adults can and should accept help from others, an increasing number of crises call for independent decisions and actions. For example, many families exist in a state of perpetual crisis, facing multiple challenges relating to work, economic status, family safety and support, and health. Researchers have identified these factors as major causes of stress and have created specific strategies to help families reduce stress (Dacey & Fiore, 2006).

RISK AND RESILIENCE

The stressors that individuals experience are called **risk factors.** Risk factors include poverty, chronic illness, parental mental illness and substance abuse, exposure to violence, and family experiences such as divorce and teenage parenthood. Individuals who deal well with stress are said to have resilience. Researchers have been interested in identifying characteristics of resilient individuals that protect them from stress. Three kinds of **protective factors** have been identified: family environments, support networks, and personality characteristics.

We have explored the value of resilience in several of the other stages of development. In middle adulthood, family environments that protect people from stress include individuals who share responsibilities and workload in the home, and financial stability that supports the well-being of the family in terms of physical and emotional needs. Support networks include informal and formal networks, which can range from work colleagues and close friends or family who share concerns and good humor, to Weight Watchers or Alcoholics Anonymous groups that support people with personal challenges. Individual personality characteristics influence the way people experience life stresses and challenges: A person with an easygoing temperament might not be as concerned if she gets laid off from work, whereas another person might immediately begin worrying about her ability to pay the bills, feed her children, and continue on her career path.

While adults do have more control over their lives than younger people, which can reduce stress, adults tend to experience more stress overload—the tendency to manage many activities and circumstances at the same time. When adults are interviewed, however, interpersonal conflict is the most commonly reported cause of stress in middle adulthood.

Seligman and Csikszentmihalyi (2000) propose that **positive psychology,** as a field of psychology and as a profession, can help people identify their strengths and use them to help them succeed and thrive. Recognizing that most of the time people dwell on what has gone wrong in their lives, positive psychology aims to point out the things that individuals and groups do well that contribute to a more positive life and society. For individuals, positive behaviors and traits include courage, the ability to love and forgive others, and wisdom. For groups, these include responsibility and citizenship, nurturance, and a strong work ethic. In middle adulthood, a positive outlook provides people with strength and inspiration to grapple with the biopsychosocial challenges they encounter and prepares them for the next stage of their lives—late adulthood.

risk factors The stressors that individuals experience, including poverty, chronic illness, and divorce.

protective factors Characteristics of resilient individuals that protect them from stress.

positive psychology A branch of psychology that emphasizes the impact of positive psychological traits on individual and group behaviors.

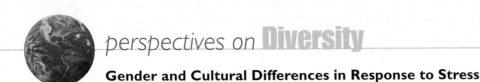
Gender and Cultural Differences in Response to Stress

People often assume that men and women experience stress differently. For example, women are described as responding to stress by nurturing offspring and joining social groups to increase resources, while men have been described in terms of the fight-or-flight response (Taylor et al., 2000).

Other researchers have noted cultural differences related to stress, such as the tendency of Asian and African cultures to be communal, work together, and seek support, compared to the view of American culture as individualistic and aggressive.

Experts on stress note that while gender differences occur *within* a specific ecosystem, cultural differences de-velop *between* ecosystems (Kashima et al., 1995), so how one individual responds to stress is actually more complex than simply gender or cultural design. For example, the feelings of stress that an American woman experiences, though she may be more socially connected than a man (in terms of concern for offspring and social networks), are also entwined with a sense of self and self-orientation that differs, for example, from that of women in traditional Chinese culture. A Chinese woman may experience stress through the cultural lens of emphasis on the good of the larger group. Political, historical, and evolutionary influences must all be considered when making comparisons about gender and cultural differences.

CONCLUSIONS & SUMMARY

What kinds of physical changes affect people in middle adulthood?

- Health concerns in middle adulthood include increasing weight and lower basal metabolism rate.
- In the middle period of adulthood there is a common but often unnecessary decline in muscular ability, due in part to a decrease in exercise.
- Sensory abilities—vision, hearing, smell, and taste—begin to show slight declines in middle adulthood.
- The climacteric, the loss of reproductive ability, occurs at menopause for women but at a much older age for most men.

What are the main factors that affect sexuality among middle-aged people?

- Some minor changes in sexual physiology occur for both sexes, but usually these need not hamper sexual satisfaction.

What are the main factors affecting a person's intellectual development in middle adulthood?

- Horn suggests that, although fluid intelligence deteriorates with age, crystallized intelligence does not.
- Sternberg suggests three types of intelligence: analytical, creative, and practical.
- Creativity, important in a rapidly changing world, manifests itself at different peak periods throughout adulthood.
- Learning in middle adulthood can be enhanced through motivation, new learning experiences, and changes in education systems.

What happens to relationships in middle adulthood?

- Dealing with change is as serious a challenge in midlife as at any other time.
- Learning new ways to get along with one's spouse, parents, siblings, and children is necessary at this time.
- Erikson's theory placed middle adulthood within the stage labeled "generativity versus stagnation." Generativity means the ability to be useful to ourselves and to society without concern for material reward.

What happens to personality during the adult years: Does it typically change or remain continuous?

- Research by trait theorists such as McCrae and Costa generally supports the notion that human beings remain fairly stable throughout life.
- In contrast, theorists such as Levinson and Erikson argue that human beings are best described as constantly changing and developing throughout life.
- Levinson suggested that most men go through a midlife transition in which they must deal with the polarities between young/old, masculinity/femininity, destruction/creation, and attachment/separation.
- Levinson also suggested that females go through a similar experience to that of males, with some notably different influences, such as the conflict women feel regarding work–family.
- McCrae and Costa defined five major personality traits that they believe govern the adult personality: neuroticism, extraversion, openness to experience, agreeableness, and conscientiousness.
- A deepening of friendships begins in middle age and goes on throughout the rest of life.

What are the typical patterns of marriage and family relationships during middle adulthood?

- Middle age offers a time for marriage reappraisal, which proves positive for most couples.
- Middle age is also a time when most people develop improved relationships with their parents, though in some cases the relationship begins to reverse itself when those parents become dependent on their middle-aged children.
- Sibling relationships have the potential to be the most enduring that a person can have.

What are the patterns of work that we most often see in this life stage?

- In recent years, a trend has emerged among employers to recognize some of the concerns of middle-aged employees.
- Considerable attention is now being given to the crisis many people undergo in the middle of their careers.
- One major way of dealing with the midcareer crisis is for the middle-aged worker to help younger employees make significant contributions.

How do adults generally deal with the stress caused by the major events and daily hassles in their lives?

- Calming the nervous system, creating a plan to deal with stress, persistence, and evaluating the plan are strategies that help adults cope.
- People who are exposed to many risk factors but develop few behavioral or psychological problems are called resilient.

KEY TERMS

analytic intelligence *240*

basal metabolism rate (BMR) *234*

climacteric *237*

creative intelligence *240*

crystallized intelligence *239*

downsizing *249*

emotional divorce *247*

empty nest syndrome *247*

five factor model (FFM) of personality *245*

fluid intelligence *239*

generativity *244*

globalization *249*

hormone replacement therapy (HRT) *238*

menopause *237*

midlife transition *243*

positive psychology *250*

practical intelligence *240*

protective factors *250*

risk factors *250*

sandwich generation *247*

stage theorists *245*

stagnation *244*

trait theorists *245*

work–family conflict *249*

For REVIEW

1. When you look at the physical condition of your parents and grandparents, and their attitudes toward health, do you see evidence of stability or change over time?

2. What are some ways that our society might foster the creative abilities of its adult citizens?

3. Describe an ideal strategy for middle-aged people to take care of their ailing, elderly parents, where everyone feels loved, respected, and valued as a member of the family.

Chapter Review Test

1. Basal metabolism rate refers to
   a. the minimum amount of energy an individual tends to use after exercising.
   b. the minimum amount of energy an individual tends to use when in a resting state.
   c. the maximum amount of energy an individual tends to use after exercising.
   d. the maximum amount of energy an individual tends to use when in a resting state.

2. For people over age 50, even one or two drinks a day can be dangerous, but _____ (more than 5 drinks in one sitting) appears to be quite prevalent among this age group, which raises serious concerns about health risks and social supports.
   a. social drinking
   b. drinking to cope
   c. addictive drinking
   d. binge drinking

3. What type of intelligence deteriorates with age, to some extent?
   a. learned
   b. natural
   c. crystallized
   d. fluid

4. What is an example of crystallized intelligence?
   a. arithmetical reasoning
   b. letter grouping
   c. recalled paired associates
   d. dominoes

5. A factor in learning ability during middle adulthood is motivation to learn. It is important for researchers to keep in mind that _____ affects an adult's level of motivation.
   a. level of education
   b. meaningfulness of the task
   c. interest
   d. external distraction

6. If a person is experiencing stress related to a crisis in middle adulthood, the first step in a plan to combat related anxiety is
   a. calming the nervous system.
   b. persisting in the face of obstacles.
   c. evaluating a plan.
   d. denying there is a problem.

7. Dave and Meghan have drifted apart over the years but remain married to each other because of their children. Their relationship illustrates the
   a. functional marriage.
   b. practical marriage.
   c. functional divorce.
   d. emotional divorce.

8. What is the most frequently cited problem of middle-aged adult women?
   a. aging
   b. menopause
   c. caring for their children
   d. caring for their aging parents

9. Research suggests that a typical characteristic of a sibling relationship in middle adulthood is
   a. growing distance.
   b. increased animosity.
   c. mutual caring for aging parents.
   d. rivalry over the inheritance.

10. McCrae and Costa argue that, although habits, life events, opinions, and relationships may change over the lifespan, the basic _____ of an individual does not.
    a. value
    b. orientation
    c. personality
    d. coping mechanisms

Answers: 1b, 2d, 3d, 4a, 5b, 6a, 7d, 8d, 9c, 10c

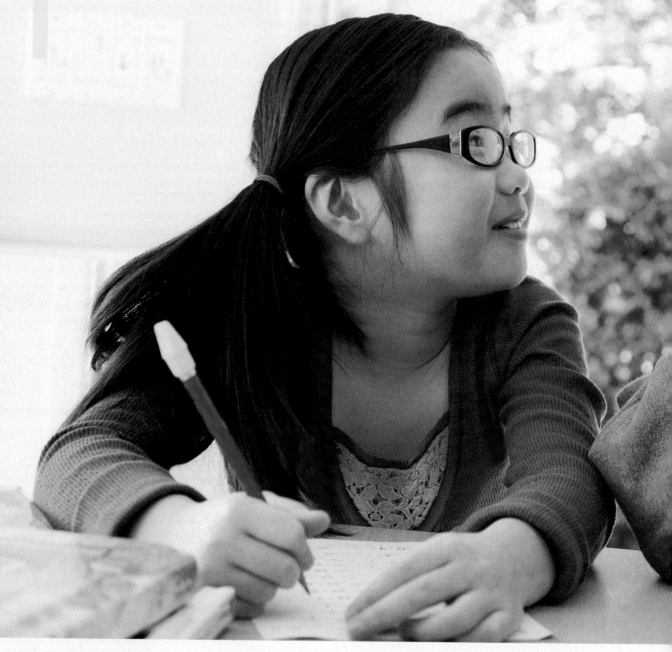

LATE ADULTHOOD

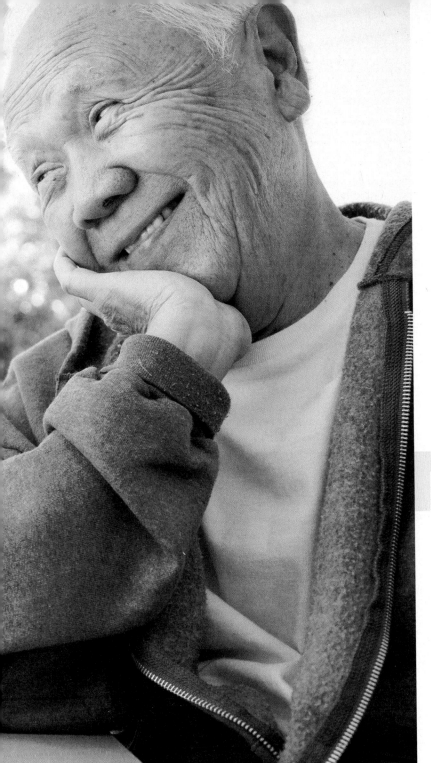

As You READ

After reading this chapter, you should be able to answer the following questions:

- Must we age and die?

- What are the key aspects of physical development among the elderly?

- How is cognitive development affected by old age?

- How do social relationships develop during late adulthood?

- What are major factors affecting the older worker?

- Is personality development any different among older adults?

Must We Age and Die?

Must we all decline as we age, moving inevitably toward death? So far, no person has attained immortality, but not all living things die. Some trees alive today are known to be more than 2,500 years old; they have aged but show no sign of dying. Bacteria apparently are able to live indefinitely, as long as they have the necessary conditions for existence. The fact is, we are not sure why we age, and until we are, we cannot be certain that aging and death are absolutely inevitable. Nor can we overlook those who appear to age well, which is often referred to as "successful aging" (Vaillant & Mukamal, 2001; Westerhof et al., 2001). This uncertainty contributes to fears about adulthood that are felt by even the very young (Cummings, Knopf, & DeWeaver, 2000).

The quote by Vaillant and Mukamal contradicts a stereotypical characteristic of old age, that of declining mental ability. Though sometimes difficult to notice because they can be subtle, such assumptions about older people maintain prejudices that result in **ageism,** a discriminatory attitude against older people based on their age (Levy & Banaji, 2002). Is there some truth to these stereotypes? Does growing old mean doom and gloom for our appearance and abilities, or is there only a relatively slight decline in capacity? Are some negative aspects of aging the result of a self-fulfilling prophecy (people expect to deteriorate, so they stop trying to be fit, and then they do deteriorate)? Could most of us age into capable, happy folks who seem to overcome age and remain vigorous into their nineties and beyond?

Gerontology is the broad term for the field of science that focuses on these questions and assists older adults with issues and problems that they encounter as they age. Gerontology can include facets of the medical profession, social work, and more. A gerontologist, therefore, is a professional who works with older adults in various capacities.

> Old age is not foremost a negative and **problem-ridden** phase of life.
>
> **VAILLANT & MUKAMAL (2001)**

ageism Stereotyping or unfair treatment of individuals or groups because of their age.

gerontology The field of science that deals with issues, problems, and diseases specific to older adults.

life expectancy The number of years that a person born in a specific year is expected to live.

LIFE EXPECTANCY

The concept of successful aging is not only interesting, but also critical to consider as advances in technology and medicine, among other factors, contribute to a greater number of older people living longer and healthier lives. Human **life expectancy** refers to the number of years that a person born in a specific year is expected to live. In the United States, life expectancy has increased 1.4 years over the past decade, reaching nearly 78 years (77.9) in 2009. Women in the U.S. can expect to outlive men by approximately

Successful Seniors

Take a STAND

Even though he is 85, Jimmy Carter's renowned sense of altruism has never left him. The former U.S. president has kept busy volunteering for Habitat for Humanity, serving as a roving U.S. ambassador-at-large, and writing best-selling fiction.

What is there about individuals like Carter that pushes them toward **creation,** as compared to others of the same age who would rather enjoy quiet **recreation?**

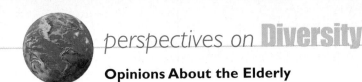

perspectives on Diversity

Opinions About the Elderly

By the time we reach the middle of this century, estimates are that one third of the world's population will be over age 65. Opinions about older adults vary based on cultural values and traditions. For example, some societies demonstrate high levels of respect for older people, as seen in Native American practices involving a circle of elders whose wisdom is sought when important decisions must be made. In contrast, most industrialized societies often describe the elderly using stereotypes and pejoratives.

Because the United States is a diverse nation comprised of many cultural groups, there is variation among as well as within groups, depending on many factors. Communities that welcome elderly citizens as vital members of the social group tend to value personal contributions more than financial ones, and reap physical and psychological benefits associated with this inclusive stance. What are some examples you have seen in your own community that reflect attitudes toward the elderly?

TABLE 11.1

U.S. Population, Over Sixty

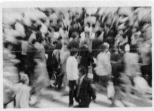

60–64 years	10,805,447
65–69 years	9,533,545
70–74 years	8,857,441
75–79 years	7,415,813
80–84 years	4,945,367
85+ years	4,239,587

Source: U.S. Census Bureau, 2009.

5 years. However, the gap between male life expectancy (75.3 years) and female life expectancy (80.4 years) has narrowed since a peak gap of 7.8 years in 1979. Life expectancy differs among ethnic groups within the U.S. as well as between men and women (Land & Yang, 2006). For example, the average life expectancy for African Americans is 70 years, as compared to non-Latino White Americans at 77 years. Table 11.1 presents population statistics for elderly Americans.

Compared to other countries, the United States has a higher life expectancy rate than some countries (e.g., Mexico and China) and a lower life expectancy than others (e.g., Japan and Israel). Figure 11.1 presents some comparative data. Differences exist because of many interrelated factors, such as quality of and access to medical care, and general health and nutrition.

Because of increases in life expectancy, the United States is experiencing a dramatic increase in the numbers of people who live to old age. Experts note that people are not only living longer, they are also living more active, healthier lives. This includes exercising and participating in other activities that contribute to overall well-being. There is some concern that the impact of recent economic hardships and related stress may have some effects on senior citizens that is yet to be captured in life expectancy data (Parker-Pope, 2009).

FIGURE 11.1

World's "Oldest" Countries Versus the United States, 2006

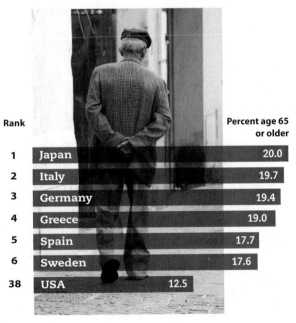

Rank		Percent age 65 or older
1	Japan	20.0
2	Italy	19.7
3	Germany	19.4
4	Greece	19.0
5	Spain	17.7
6	Sweden	17.6
38	USA	12.5

Source: U.S. Census Bureau, 2004 (projected).

Physiological Theories of Aging

It is clear that organisms inherit a tendency to live for a certain length of time. The average human lifespan of approximately 70 years is the longest of any mammal. Elephants, horses, and hippopotamuses are known to live as long as 50 years, but most mammals die much sooner.

Some doctors say, "No one ever dies of old age." This is true. People die of some physiological failure that is more likely to occur as they get older. One likely explanation is that the various life-support systems gradually weaken. Illness and death come about as a cumulative result of these various weaknesses. Several different theories have been suggested to account for aging.

AGING BY PROGRAM

According to the **aging by program** theory, we age because aging is programmed into us. It is hard to understand which evolutionary processes, if any, govern longevity. For example, the vast majority of animals die at or before the end of their reproductive period, but human females average 20 to 30 years beyond the end of their reproductive cycles. This may be related to the capacities of the human brain. For example, in times when food is scarce, older people may remember where it was obtained during the last period of scarcity. However, it may be that we humans have outwitted the evolutionary process and, owing to our medical achievements and improvements in lifestyle, are able to live much longer than our ancestors.

HOMEOSTATIC IMBALANCE

Some researchers have proposed that aging and ultimately death are caused by a failure in the systems that regulate the proper interaction of the organs, rather than wear and tear of the organs themselves. These homeostatic (feedback) systems are responsible, for example, for the regulation of the sugar and adrenaline levels in the blood. Apparently there is not much difference in the systems of the young and the old when they are in a quiet state. It is when stress is put on the systems (death of a spouse, loss of a job, a frightening experience) that we see the effects of the elderly **homeostatic imbalance.** The older body simply isn't as effective reacting to these stresses. Figure 11.2 shows the progress from homeostasis to failure.

CROSS-LINKAGE THEORY

The proteins that make up a large part of cells are composed of peptides. When cross-links are formed between peptides (a natural process of the body), the proteins are altered, often for the worse. This is known as the **cross-linkage theory.** For example, **collagen** is the major connective tissue in the body; it provides the elasticity in our skin and blood vessels. When its proteins are altered, there is an adverse effect on skin (sagging and wrinkles) and vessels (varicose veins).

FIGURE 11.2

Homeostasis and Health

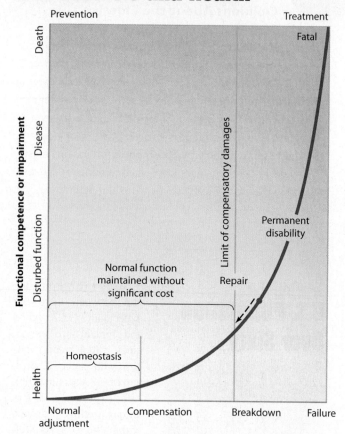

This graph shows the progressive stages of homeostasis from adjustment (health) to failure (death).

Source: Paola S. Timiras, Developmental Physiology and Aging *1972. Macmillan. Fig. 28.1.*

AUTOIMMUNITY

With increasing age, there is increasing **autoimmunity**—the immune system in the body rejects the body's own tissue. Examples of this are rheumatoid arthritis, diabetes, vascular diseases, and hypertension. It may be that the body's tissues become more and more self-rejecting with age. Figure 11.3 shows several influences on adult mental and physical systems.

Autoimmunity could result from the production of new antigens, substances in the blood that produce antibodies, which fight to kill them. An antigen may be a foreign substance such as a bacterium, or it may originate within the body, such as a toxin. These new antigens may come about for one of two reasons:

- Mutations cause the formation of altered RNA or DNA.

- Some cells may be "hidden" in the body during the early part of life. When these cells appear later, the body does not recognize them as its own and forms new antibodies to kill them. This in turn may cause organ malfunction.

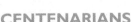

GENETIC THEORIES OF AGING

Little doubt exists that genes affect how long we live. Kallman and Jarvik's (1959) classic research on identical twins still offers strong evidence of this. These researchers found that monozygotic twins (those who developed from the same fertilized egg) have more similar lengths of life than do dizygotic twins (those who developed from two fertilized eggs).

The *telomere shortening theory* proposes that changes in telomeres, tiny pieces of "junk DNA" at the ends of chromosomes that make up the genes of all organisms (including humans), could be a cause of aging. Telomeres protect real DNA during cell division. However, they cannot be copied exactly, so some of the chromosome gets cut off every time a cell divides. As cells continue to divide, the telomeres get shorter until they disappear. At that point, the real DNA copies will be faulty and the cell ages and dies.

CENTENARIANS

There is a distinct group of adults that does not fit neatly into any theory of aging. They are called centenarians—people 100 or older who do not succumb to common causes of death for persons their age. What factors contribute to the survival of these men and women? Smith's (1997) research suggested that these men and women are not necessarily more robust than the peers they've outlived, yet they are more resistant to cancer and other diseases, such as those of the circulatory system.

OTHER MODIFIERS OF AGING

In addition to physiological and genetic factors that affect the individual's rate of aging, other factors can modify a person's level of ability more directly. Many of these modifiers interact with one another in complex ways. Some of the major modifiers are nutritional status, stress level, educational level, occupation, personality type, and socioeconomic status.

For example, although relationships and social networks do not directly affect the survival of elderly people, they are related to their quality of life. Within nursing homes, those who tend to be aggressive and verbally agitated have poor social networks and generally lack intimacy with fellow residents. Because the outcomes of aging are more complex than an analysis of just one factor reveals, the biopsychosocial model is key to a full understanding of the aging process.

FIGURE 11.3

Influences on Adult Mental and Physical Systems

Genetic factors	Physiological factors	Environmental factors
Evolution Telomere theory	Wear and tear Homeostatic imbalance Accumulation of metabolic waste Autoimmunity Cellular aging	Catastrophes Medical advances Economic variables Radiation Viruses

Factors affecting the rate of aging

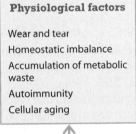

Physical systems (neuromuscular and musculoskeletal systems)	Mental systems (central and autonomic nervous systems)
Muscular ability (speed, strength) Skill Sensory ability Hormonal balance Health Appearance	Intelligence Creative productivity Memory Learning

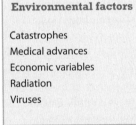

Modifiers of ability

Training	Nutrition	Injury	Occupation
Practice	Organic function	Stress level	Personality type
Motivation	Illness	Education level	Socioeconomic status

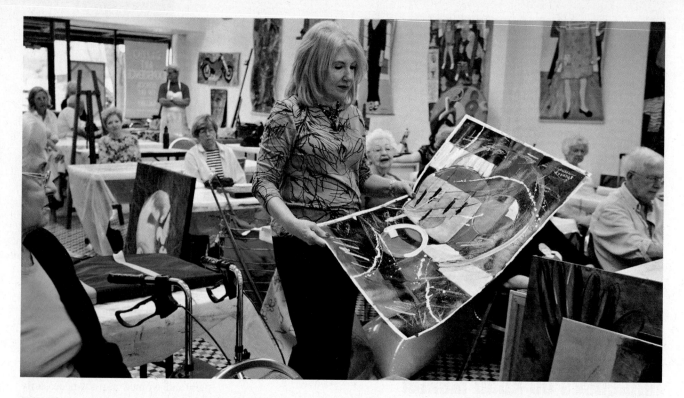

Physical Development

In this section, development is presented from multiple angles—reaction time, sensory abilities, other body systems, and overall health.

REACTION TIME

It is assumed that physical skills decline as people grow older. This appears to be especially true of manual dexterity. Although older people are able to perform short, coordinated manual tasks, a long series of tasks such as playing a stringed instrument becomes increasingly difficult for them. American folk singer and banjo player Pete Seeger and pianist Marian McPartland are notable exceptions.

Do physical skills decline because the human nervous system deteriorates? To answer this question, psychologists have completed numerous studies of **reaction time,** the time between the presence of a stimulus and the actual muscle activity that indicates a reaction to it. Studying reaction time is a scientific way of separating the effects of the central nervous system from the ability of the rest of the body to perform manual tasks. Most studies show that variables other than sheer neural or motor activities influence most change in physical skills over time. Social factors, such as opportunities for activities with peers, or expectations of family and society in general, can also impact physical behaviors.

People's beliefs and feelings about aging also can affect whether or not they age successfully, which can lead to a self-fulfilling prophecy. Persistent messages about declining physical abilities may actually lead to physical decline among older people, as people act the way they feel they should act. Older people may begin to believe that they are less capable than their actual performance reveals.

reaction time The time between the presence of a stimulus and the actual muscle activity that indicates a reaction to it.

SENSORY ABILITIES

In late adulthood, strong patterns of decline occur in the sensory systems—hearing, vision, and balance (Humes & Floyd, 2005; Wong, 2001). Lack of sensory stimulation is one of many factors that emerges during later phases of life and contributes to the aging process. This comes about in part because elderly people are often less active physically and socially, which reduces their exposure to sensory stimulation (such as sports activities) that they may have enjoyed earlier in life.

Although all five senses are affected by the aging process, decline is most obvious in terms of older people's vision and hearing. As people age, their eyes take longer to adjust when moving from a well-lighted room into darkness. This is a major reason why night driving becomes more challenging for the elderly. Older people also lose their acuity when it comes to depth perception. They are less able to distinguish how near or far objects are, such as when trying to park a car, or how high a step is when they are about to climb a flight of stairs.

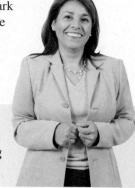

Career Apps

As a music therapist, how could you work with residents of a retirement home to increase their self-esteem using percussion instruments?

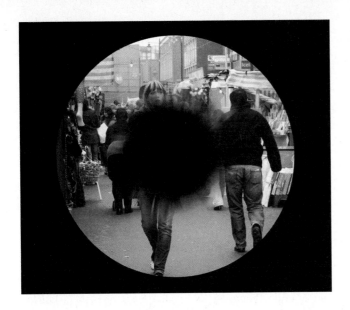

Diseases of the eye further complicate the natural aging effects on eyesight. **Macular degeneration** is caused by declines in the retina of the eye, primarily affecting the center (or focus) of a person's vision. A grandmother may be able to see items with her peripheral vision (around the periphery of the frame of her field of vision), but be unable to see something directly in front of her. The image above demonstrates what a person with macular degeneration experiences every day. **Glaucoma** is damage to the optic nerve caused by pressure that results from a buildup of fluid in the eye. It is detectable with routine eye exams and can be treated with eye-drops but, if left untreated, has the potential to permanently damage a person's vision. **Cataracts,** which are a thickening of the lenses of the eyes, cause blurred, cloudy, or otherwise distorted vision. If needed, a routine surgical procedure can remove cataracts and restore optimal vision.

Hearing decline does not typically impact people in a serious way until they are in their 70s. Many hearing problems can be helped by hearing aids (as discussed in Chapter 10). Sometimes, two different hearing aids are recommended so that each ear can experience the extra support needed for optimal hearing at low and high frequencies.

> **macular degeneration** An eye disease that affects the retina, impacting the center of a person's field of vision.
>
> **glaucoma** Damage to the optic nerve caused by pressure that results from a buildup of fluid in the eye.
>
> **cataracts** Thickening of the eye lenses; cause blurred, cloudy vision.

OTHER BODY SYSTEMS

Included in the category of body systems are the skeletal system, skin, teeth, hair, and locomotion (ability to move about). These systems work in conjunction with specific abilities as part of overall functioning.

While some changes in the body system mostly affect appearance (yellowing of teeth, thickening fingernails, thinning hair), a major concern relates to bone density, which is often mistakenly considered only a woman's problem. Men and women alike experience a loss of bone density in late adulthood, with the result that their bones break more eas-

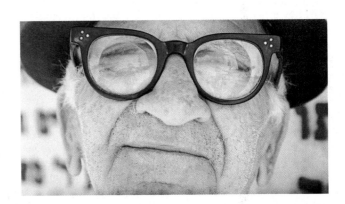

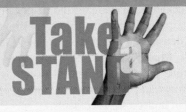

Should the Elderly Lose Their Licenses?

By 2020, up to one in every five Americans will be 65 or older, and the vast majority will possess a driver's license. This is of concern because statistics show that the number of accidents caused by drivers over the age of 75 equals or surpasses the number of those caused by teenagers, who are typically considered the most dangerous group of drivers. Some states are moving to monitor older drivers more aggressively.

However, in those cases where a license is denied or revoked, the drivers may find themselves stranded without crucial transportation.

There is variation among older drivers' abilities just as there is variation among younger drivers' abilities. At what point should generalizations about older drivers' abilities influence public policy?

ily. **Osteoporosis** is a condition in which the bones are thin and brittle due to calcium loss. Routine bone density screening helps doctors identify patients who would benefit from taking calcium or other nutritional supplements. A more visible indicator of osteoporosis is the impact the condition has on a person's height and posture, often seen in a curved spine that resembles a hump, as shown in the accompanying illustration.

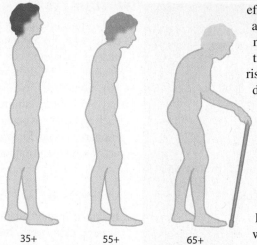

35+   55+   65+

GENERAL HEALTH

As people age, specific health issues come to the fore, such as obesity and arthritis. Our ability to control or influence health decline varies depending on specific biological and environmental factors. A critical factor affecting the health of older American adults is overweight. Although 60% of American adults were found to be overweight in a recent poll (AAHPERD, 2007), only one third were making an attempt to lose weight or exercise. Effective interventions for older Americans include a low-fat diet, multivitamins, and increased exercise to reduce health risks associated with overweight.

Arthritis refers to inflammation that occurs in and around the joints, including fingers as well as knees, elbows, and shoulders, and is characterized by redness, swelling, and possible loss of function in the affected areas. Although arthritis can occur at other stages of life, it is most common in late adulthood.

In late adulthood, concern about general health also includes the incidence of accidents that occur among the elderly population. Clearly, accidents happen randomly throughout the lifespan, but older people face greater consequences as a result of accidents because other body systems are compromised in ways that render them more vulnerable. For instance, misjudging the height of a step on a flight of stairs can cause an elderly person to fall. Decreased bone density results in more frequent fractures and bone breaks, which can contribute to serious injury. Taking some simple precautions, such as installing safety railings on stairways and in bathrooms, can significantly reduce a number of unnecessary accidents.

HEART DISEASE, CANCER, AND STROKE

After the age of 65, the three causes of death with the highest incidence are heart disease, cancer, and stroke. Among men and women, heart disease is the leading cause of death in the United States. Heart disease is linked to hereditary factors, such as race and ethnicity, but also to geographic and educational differences in the general population. Prevention

osteoporosis A condition in which bones are thin and brittle due to calcium loss.

arthritis Tissue inflammation in and around the joints.

efforts by public health agencies aimed at urban, lower socioeconomic communities strive to reduce the disparities among affected groups, as well as risk factors that contribute to the incidence of heart disease.

There are sex differences in the incidence of cancer that are caused by behavior as well as sex hormones. Men have a higher rate of cancers of the stomach and liver. Women have a higher rate of cancers of the gallbladder and thyroid. The incidence of lung cancer is greater in men than in women, but women are catching up.

Prostate cancer is one of the most common forms of cancer in men and one of the leading causes of death among American men (Cohen & Jaskulsky, 2001; Harvard Men's Health Watch, 2004). Recent research shows a promising trend, however, as the incidence of prostate cancer decreased by 4.4 percent each year between 2001 and 2005 (Jemal et al., 2008). Recently, prostate cancer has been linked to lifestyle (Simon, 2007). Lifestyle changes to reduce risk of prostate cancer include

- extremely low-fat vegan diet;
- dietary supplements, such as soy, fish oil, and vitamins E and C;
- exercise regimen of walking 30 minutes 6 days a week;
- stress reduction, including yoga, stretching, breathing, and meditation for an hour daily (Simon, 2007).

Breast cancer is the most common cause of cancer deaths in women over 65 years of age, with more than half of breast cancers occurring in women 65 years of age and older (Silliman, 1998).

Strokes are more frequent in men than women and result from a burst blood vessel or clot in the brain that impedes the flow of blood to some part of the brain. When the affected area of the brain does not receive oxygen for a period of time, then damage results in the form of paralysis, vision problems, and memory loss. Depending on the type of stroke, the specific part of the brain affected, and the brain injury sustained, some effects of stroke are temporary, yet some are permanent. Paralysis or weakness in specific parts of the body are commonly experienced short- or long-term.

Reasons for stroke are not clear, but risk factors include obesity and diabetes, which are somewhat avoidable if healthy lifestyle choices are made with regard to exercise and nutrition.

SUBSTANCE ABUSE

As older adults struggle with daily health challenges, they frequently require medications to combat symptoms that interfere with the quality of their lives. Misuse or abuse of prescription or over-the-counter medication can cause serious health problems, especially complicated by the consump-

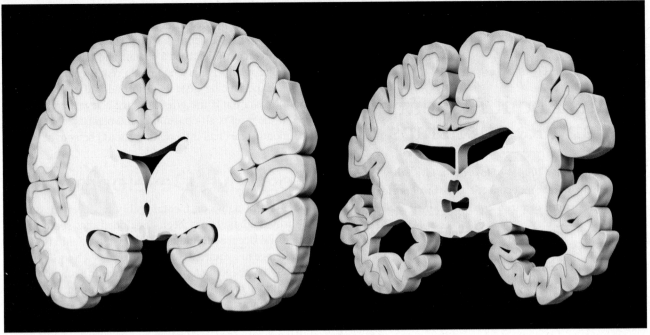

Imaging of a healthy brain (left) compared with a brain affected with Alzheimer's Disease (right).

tion of alcohol or other drugs. Drugs commonly used in late adulthood include medication to treat high blood pressure and high cholesterol, sleeping pills, anti-anxiety pills, and antidepressants. There is serious concern about older adults using medications in combinations that can be dangerous, and even lethal, if taken without proper medical supervision.

The greatest threat to liver health is alcoholism. For adults aged 60 and older, continuous problem drinking and late-onset problem drinking are known to greatly compromise their health. Unfortunately, alcohol abuse is often difficult to recognize in elderly adults, who may exhibit conditions related to aging in general. For those taking medications, alcohol may cause adverse reactions or may interfere in the healthy aging process.

ALZHEIMER'S DISEASE AND DEMENTIA

Much attention has been focused on Alzheimer's disease and the elderly. A disease of the brain, **Alzheimer's disease** involves progressive, irreversible loss of neurons and is manifest as impaired memory, judgment, decision making, orientation to the environment, and language. Alzheimer's disease is a leading cause of **dementia,** the deterioration of cognitive function over time due to brain infection or disease, although other forms of dementia exist and, unlike Alzheimer's disease, are treatable.

Although researchers may have found a gene that is implicated in the cause of Alzheimer's disease, this does not mean they have found a cure. Relatively few of its symptoms respond to any type of treatment, and when they do, it is only in the earliest stages of the disease. Alzheimer's disease usually progresses over many years (Alzheimer's Association, 2009). Although Alzheimer's victims are normal in physical appearance, their brains are undergo-

ing severe changes. Brain autopsies unmask severe damage, abnormalities, and death of neurons.

Until recently the outlook has been bleak for patients and families suffering with Alzheimer's. Breakthroughs appear to be on the horizon on four fronts (Eastman, 2000):

- New ways to combat key enzymes that contribute to Alzheimer's

- New understanding of how to immunize people against a protein that becomes abnormal

- The emergence of human gene therapy capable of vitalizing damaged brain cells

- New educational techniques

An example of educational techniques is reflected in efforts to teach people with early cognitive impairment to recall important information and better perform at daily tasks (Alzheimers.org, 2004). Patients who participate in cognitive rehabilitation therapy experience improved ability to recall faces and names and maintain these and related skills once therapy has concluded. This offers hope for people with early cognitive impairment—they may be able to retain a higher level of functioning despite the disease.

MENTAL HEALTH

The effects of physical decline can affect older adults' mental health. Men and women in late adulthood are at increased risk for suicide and depression, often because they cannot cope with their own medical problems or the death or declining health of a spouse. Depression is both underrecognized and undertreated among the elderly.

Alzheimer's disease Brain disease involving progressive, irreversible loss of neurons and manifesting as impaired memory, judgment, decision making, orientation to the environment, and language.

dementia Deterioration of cognitive function over time caused by brain infection or disease.

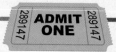
FEATURED MEDIA

Films About Alzheimer's and Relationships

***The Notebook* (2004)** – How can a love story documented in a notebook connect the past and present and sustain the nature of a true love relationship?

***Away From Her* (2006)** – When his wife, institutionalized for Alzheimer's, shows affection for a fellow patient, a man must consider his own ability to ensure her happiness and make a tremendous sacrifice.

***Evening* (2007)** – On her deathbed, a mother relives a critical weekend when she experienced love that forever changed her life, and in sharing her story, her daughters come to terms with their own relationships.

Depressed older adults are at higher risk for poor health and cognitive functioning and physical disability, as well as for suicide than nondepressed older adults. (Huang et al., 2000). Figure 11.4 depicts suicide rates for older adults.

Although comprising only 12% of the U.S. population, people aged 65 and older accounted for 16% percent of suicide deaths in 2004 (NIMH, 2009). Research indicates that Americans at greatest risk for suicide are older White

FIGURE 11.4

Suicide Rates for Ages 65 to 85+

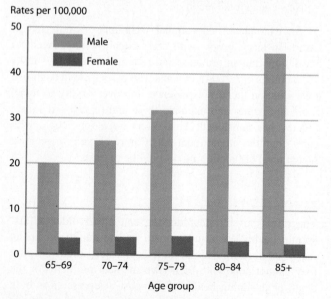

Rates per 100,000

Source: Centers for Disease Control and Prevention, 2006.

men who live by themselves, are socially isolated, use alcohol, and have a history of depression (Lantz, 2001). Older women who have recently become single because of separation, divorce, or death of a spouse and have a number of medical problems are also at greater risk for suicide (Lantz, 2001). Experiencing grief is a normal and expected reaction to loss, even if the grief lasts for a few months. However, if the grief is all-consuming and persists longer than 2 or 3 months, medical intervention should be sought.

Cognitive Development

The effect of aging on mental ability has been the subject of many studies. It has been concluded that some mental deficits do occur with old age. For instance, elderly people take longer to acquire new information, such as learning a different language. Seniors have greater difficulty completing multiple mental tasks at once. In addition, mental illnesses such as dementia or untreated diabetes can greatly limit the mental capacity of older adults.

However, new research suggests that the effects of aging on the human brain are not all negative (Finch, 2003; Pitkin & Savage, 2004; Söderlund et al., 2003; Toussaint, 2003; Tremblay, Piskosz, & Souza, 2003). For example, research by Hess and associates (2003) determined that elders make up for most intellectual limitations with better mental abilities in other areas, such as an increased vocabulary and a greater awareness of political and other world events. These researchers concluded that the extreme differences between the intelligence of younger and older adults as found in previous research was due to biases within the studies. It turns out that some aspects of the testing processes greatly affected the results. For example, it is not surprising that elders performed better when they were tested in the morning and on material that was important in their lives.

Other studies show that the brain will make up for much of the cell loss that happens with age by growing new cells and building new connections among those cells. Dr. Molly Wagster, a researcher at the National Institute on Aging, suggests that there are ways to increase this process of cell growth (Wagster, 2006). According to Wagster, mental exercises, aerobic physical exercise, and good nutrition can lessen the effects of old age on mental competence.

TESTS VERSUS OBSERVATIONS

A major question in the science of elderly cognitive development is which is most reliable: results of tests that rate seniors' intelligence or observations of their actual performance, which are often higher? The answer is not simple. What factors could account for the discrepancy between test scores and actual abilities? Currently there are four hypotheses (Salthouse, 2001):

1. *Differences in type of cognition*. Intelligence tests tend to measure specific aspects of cognitive ability, whereas assessments of real-life activities probably also include

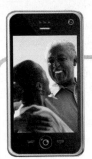
Research Shatters a Long-Standing Belief About Brain Neurons

Scientists have long thought that neurons in the brain are formed only during the fetal period and for a short time after birth. It was assumed that if nerve cells in the brain were damaged or died, the adult human body could not create new ones.

However, that belief has changed dramatically. Researchers have discovered that the human brain does indeed retain the ability to generate neurons throughout life. A study by researchers Peter Eriksson and Fred H. Gage demonstrated that new neurons are generated in the dentate gyrus of the adult human brain (Eriksson et al. 1998), and subsequent research has backed this up. Scientists are hoping that it may soon be possible to stimulate intrinsic brain repair mechanisms to replace neurons lost through age, trauma, and disease. Finding ways to stimulate the formation of new neurons may one day lead to novel therapeutic approaches that influence cognitive performance and treat diseases such as Alzheimer's.

noncognitive capacities, such as personality traits. Thus, some aspects of IQ may decline without causing lowered performance on the job, for example.

2. *Differences in the representativeness of the individuals or observations.* Many examples exist of elderly persons who can perform admirably even into their 90s, but do these individuals really represent the average elderly person? Probably not. It is also likely that only the most competent individuals are able to survive in such demanding situations. Those who are less competent will have dropped out of the competition at an earlier age. Therefore, when we examine the abilities of successful older persons, we may be studying only the "cream of the crop." Finally, it seems likely that observed competence represents only one type of cognitive ability (balancing the company's books, reading music), whereas intelligence testing involves several (verbal, math, reasoning, and other abilities).

3. *Different standards of evaluation.* Most cognitive tests tend to push individuals to their limits of ability. Assessments of real-life tasks, those with which people are quite familiar (such as reading the newspaper), may require a lower standard of testing.

4. *Different amounts of experience.* Doing well on an intelligence test requires one to use traits that are not used every day, such as assembling blocks to re-create

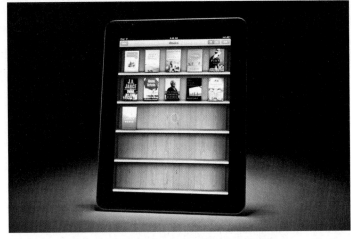

New and engaging tools like the iPad promote learning and creativity.

certain patterns. The skills assessed in real-life situations are more likely to be those the individual has practiced for years. For example, driving ability may remain high if the person continues to drive regularly as he or she ages.

CREATIVITY

The quantity of creative production probably drops in old age, but the quality of production may not. This is based on studies of actual productivity. What about older individuals' potential for creative production? Might it be that the elderly are capable of great creativity but that factors such as motivation and opportunity prevent them from fulfilling this ability? Might later years be a critical period for creative production?

Dacey's theory (1989b) proposes that there are certain critical periods in life during which creative ability can be cultivated most effectively. The basic premise of this theory is that a person's inherent creativity can blossom best during a period of crisis and change. The six periods shown

TABLE 11.2

Peak Periods of Life During Which Creativity May Most Readily Be Cultivated

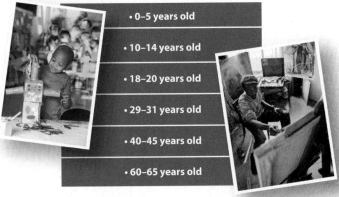

- 0–5 years old
- 10–14 years old
- 18–20 years old
- 29–31 years old
- 40–45 years old
- 60–65 years old

Source: Dacey & Lennon, 1989.

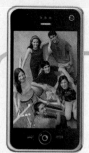
wisdom Superior insight and judgment that can come only from experience.

in Table 11.2 are ages at which most people experience stress owing to life changes.

For most men and women, late adulthood is the period in which they retire. Even if a spouse has not been active in the labor force, both partners have many adjustments to make because of the spouse's retirement. Thus, most adults are faced with a major adjustment of self-concept at this time in their lives.

Whereas some seniors do not cope well with aging and begin withdrawing from society, others take advantage of the change to pursue creative goals that had previously been difficult for them. Obviously a majority of the "young old" (the new term for those who are aged 60 to 70) do not suddenly become creative, but a substantial number do. Of the several thousand highly productive people he studied, Lehman (1953, 1962) found more than 100, or almost 5%, whose major productivity began in the years after 60.

WISDOM

What is the relationship between intelligence and creativity, and how do they relate to the concept of **wisdom**? Robert Sternberg (1990) has compared the concepts of wisdom, intelligence, and creativity, and identified a relationship between the three concepts and the information-processing model of cognition. Higher levels of expertise and automaticity result in deeper wisdom, higher intelligence, and more creative application of ideas, as evident in the processes they engage in (such as problem solving) and products created (such as a negotiated settlement). As people develop differing levels of expertise and performance, and automatic versus effortful ability, they are able to exhibit the qualities (see Table 11.3).

Baltes and Staudinger (2000) offer a somewhat different view of the concept of wisdom, defining wisdom as expert knowledge and judgment about important, difficult, and uncertain questions associated with the meaning and conduct of life. They suggest that wisdom is the result of five factors:

1. intelligence, including both fluid and crystallized types;

2. personality traits, such as openness to experience, generativity (see Erikson's theory later in this chapter), and a continuing willingness to meet life's challenges;

3. the personality-intelligence interface, which includes creativity and social intelligence;

4. life experience; and

5. age (by and large, the older the person, the greater the wisdom).

MEMORY

Not all aspects of memory decline in late adulthood. As a person ages, rather than considering her at a deficit because of abilities lost, the person may be deemed successful by exhibiting strategies to reduce memory loss and adjust to the decline in memory functions. In the field of lifespan development, several kinds of memories have been iden-

TABLE 11.3

Sternberg's Comparison of Wisdom, Intelligence, and Creativity

Aspect	Wisdom	Intelligence	Creativity
Knowledge	Understanding of its presuppositions and meanings as well as its limitations	Recall, analysis, and use	Going beyond what is available
Processes	Understanding of what is automatic and why	Automatization of procedures	Applied to novel tasks
Motivation	To understand what is known and what it means	To know and use what is known	To go beyond what is known

> *You shall more command with your* **years** *than with your* **weapons.**

SHAKESPEARE, *OTHELLO*

tified and examined. First, a distinction has been made between memories relating to the future (**prospective memory**) and memories of things from the past or events that occurred in the past (**retrospective memory**). Examples of prospective memory include remembering to take vitamins or medications each day or water the plants. Older adults can develop simple strategies such as making lists or posting reminders to do the specific task.

Within the category of retrospective memory, there are two kinds of memories. The first, **explicit memory,** refers to facts and experiences that a person can remember and share. Examples of explicit memory include being able to remember the items you were supposed to bring to your grandchildren's house or recalling the plot of a book you've read, or remembering a friend's street address. The second kind, **implicit memory,** refers to an automatic or unconscious process of remembering, that is, memory primarily involved in motor skills. Examples of implicit memory include tying your shoes, driving a car, or even taking a shower. While explicit memory may decline, implicit memory is less affected, partly because our bodies have their own muscle memory that assists us in carrying out the routine tasks.

LANGUAGE

In late adulthood, a decline in memory abilities is often linked to language comprehension—both written and spoken language. Older adults may, for instance, have difficulty comprehending a reading passage or understanding a speaker giving a moderately paced oral presentation or a television commercial featuring information about a specific product. These challenges are related to tasks involved in information processing.

Adults in this age group may also demonstrate difficulties with their own language production, which is linked to memory. They may have trouble recalling specific vocabulary to express a thought or desire, such as the sensation of knowing that they've used a word before but cannot recall it in the moment of need. Research has found that older adults tend to produce fewer words than they did when they were younger (Hough, 2007).

Social Development

Recently, research on the aging process has gotten an encouraging boost from the American Psychological Association (APA). The APA's efforts focus on education and advocacy. For example, its Preparing Psychology for an Aging World Initiative aims to build interest in the field of geropsychology (the psychological study of the elderly) among students, researchers, and practitioners. This will involve understanding that older adults' immediate concerns revolve around their perception of themselves and their lives, as well as relationships with family, friends, and the greater society.

ERIKSON'S THEORY: INTEGRITY VERSUS DESPAIR

The eighth and last stage of Erikson's theory of psychosocial development, covering the age 65 years and older, is termed integrity versus despair. Erikson believed that the resolution of the first seven stages should lead to the achievement of a sense of personal **integrity.** Older adults who have a sense of integrity feel their lives have been well spent and that they have helped create a better life for others. The decisions and actions they have taken seem to them to fit together—their lives are integrated. They are saddened by the sense that time is running out and that they will not get many more chances to make an impact, but they feel reasonably well satisfied with their achievements.

When people look back over their lives and feel that they have made many wrong decisions or, more commonly, that they have frequently not made any decisions at all, they see life as lacking integrity. They feel **despair,** which is the negative resolution of this last stage. Such individuals are angry that there can never be another chance for their lives to make sense. They often hide their fear of death by appearing contemptuous of humanity in general and those of other religions and races in particular.

Erikson (1978) provided a panoramic view of his developmental theory in an analysis of Swedish film director Ingmar Bergman's famous film *Wild Strawberries*. In the movie, an elderly Swedish doctor goes from his hometown to a large city, where he is to be honored for 50 years of service to the medical profession. On the way, he stops by his childhood home and, resting in an old strawberry patch, begins an imaginary journey through his entire life, starting with his earliest memories. In the ruminations of this old man, Erikson saw clear and specific reflections of the eight stages he proposed and in particular that this last stage involved a life crisis. Poignantly, the old doctor struggles to make sense out of the events of his life. He is ultimately successful in achieving a sense of integrity.

prospective memory The process of remembering to do something in the future.

retrospective memory Memory of past event or item.

explicit memory Refers to facts and experiences that a person can remember and share.

implicit memory Refers to an unconscious or automatic process of remembering.

integrity The resolution of each of the first seven crises in Erikson's theory should lead to the achievement of a sense of personal integrity. Older adults who have a sense of integrity feel their lives have been well spent.

despair The negative resolution of Erikson's last stage; individuals look back over their lives and feel that they have made many wrong decisions or no decisions at all and see life as lacking integrity.

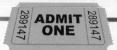
FEATURED MEDIA

Rod Serling's Twist on the Twilight Years

Rod Serling created a tremendously successful television series, the *Twilight Zone,* by combining science fiction, suspense, and horror with sometimes poignant subject matter. Famous actors of the time—some still popular today—portrayed characters whose foibles are hauntingly familiar to viewers. The following episodes feature subject matter relating to topics covered in this chapter:

Season 1, Episode 4: *The 16mm Shrine* **(1959)** – An aging film star lives a life of seclusion in her private screening room.

Season 3, Episode 86: *Kick the Can* **(1962)** – A retirement-home resident thinks that he has found the secret to youth.

Season 3, Episode 96: *The Trade-Ins* **(1962)** – An older couple must decide which one will be made young.

Season 3, Episode 100: *I Sing the Body Electric* **(1962)** – A robotic grandmother helps a widower raise his children.

Season 5, Episode 131: *A Short Drink from a Certain Fountain* **(1963)** – An elderly man who has a young wife takes an experimental youth serum.

GENDER AND SEXUALITY

You might think that by the time people reach the stage of late adulthood their gender roles and attitudes toward sexuality have become pretty well fixed. In fact, researchers generally agree that this is not the case—the major concern for gender roles among the elderly is **role discontinuity,** which refers to an abrupt or disruptive change caused by conflicts among roles in a person's life.

A number of gerontologists have noted that people in late adulthood experience a crossover in gender roles, whereby men behave more like women and women behave more like men. Men may take on a more nurturing role, for example, caring for grandchildren or volunteering. Women may become more assertive and independent, for example, taking trips with friends or arguing/advocating for political issues.

The differences between men and women become less important as we age. With the barriers breaking down, older men and women

role discontinuity Abrupt and disruptive change caused by conflicts among one's various roles in life.

seem to have more in common with each other and thus may be of more comfort to each other as they deal with the disruptive changes of growing old. This is not to say that men and women reverse gender roles. Rather, they move toward androgyny (as discussed in Chapter 9), which means expressing whatever gender role, male or female, is appropriate in a given situation.

Some older individuals often feel that talking about gender or sexual matters is embarrassing, because years ago, people generally thought it was. Many senior citizens still hesitate to discuss their questions or concerns with professionals (Blank, 2000). Another issue is that society sends men and women the message that they are less sexually attractive as they get older. Elderly adults who have a negative physical self-image might not be as likely to initiate sexual activity as when they were younger. Furthermore, fears about sexual performance, such as erectile dysfunction, that often accompany old age create doubts about their sexual desirability.

On the other hand, one study of sexual behavior found that 75% of 65- to 75-year-old men and women reported that they were satisfied with their sex lives (Dunn, Croft, & Hackett, 2000). While more men (30%) tended to report more dissatisfaction with the frequency of sex than women (20%), overall sexual satisfaction did not decline with age. In fact, people over age 65 were generally as satisfied with their sexual activity as people under 65.

One of the biggest fears in aging males is erectile dysfunction—the inability to attain and sustain an erection. Physical changes, nonsupportive partners and peers, and internal fears may be enough to inhibit or terminate sexual activity in males. In many cases a man is capable of having intercourse, but a physical condition such as diabetes impedes it. New types of prosthetic devices can remedy a variety of psychological and physical problems, and drugs such as Viagra have changed the perception of prosthetics as the only solution.

Most sexual issues that women experience are due to hormonal changes. The vaginal walls begin to thin, and intercourse may become painful, with itching and burning sensations. Estrogen pills and hormone creams relieve many of these symptoms. Although women tend to have fewer concerns about sexual performance than men do, they are often worried about losing their attractiveness, which can also have a negative effect on their sex lives.

AGING AND THE FAMILY

Family relationships naturally undergo changes during the aging process. With people living longer, married couples are finding that they have more years together after their children leave home, and they are having longer relationships with generations of their kin (Bengtson, 2001). These relationships remain strong, despite the tremendous diversity of the makeup of families. Most couples go through similar stages in the life cycle. The following are the four basic phases:

1. Child rearing

2. Childlessness before retirement

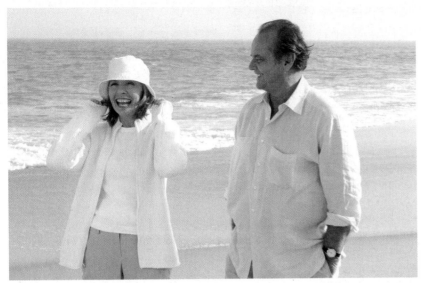
Films like Something's Gotta Give *present the humor and frustration of relationships in late adulthood.*

3. Retirement

4. Widowhood or widowerhood

The duration of each stage in the life cycle and the ages of the family members for each stage vary, of course. Childbearing patterns have a lot to do with life in the later stages of life. Couples who raise children early in their marriage will have a different lifestyle when their last child leaves home than couples who have babies in their 40s or beyond. The latter may have a dependent child at home when they are ready to retire. This can pose serious economic problems for retirees on fixed incomes, trying to meet the considerable costs of education. In addition, with children in the home, saving for retirement is difficult.

As couples spend more years together due to increasing life expectancy, researchers will be interested in seeing whether interactions in a long-term marriage also change or if they remain stable despite individual development. These data will provide evidence for the debate over whether human development is more stable or unstable, which was discussed in Chapter 10.

Conflict is an inevitable part of any relationship, especially those that last a long time. The relationship between elderly parents and their adult children is no exception. Clarke and associates (1999) conducted a study of aging parents and their middle-aged children. They were specifically interested in the emergence of common conflict themes. They found six categories of conflict:

- Communication and style of interaction
- Lifestyle choices and habits
- Parenting practices and values
- Religion, ideology, and politics
- Work habits
- Standards of household maintenance

Interesting generational differences were found. For example, older parents more often reported conflicts over habits and lifestyle choices, such as smoking, while their adult children more often reported conflicts in communication and interaction style, such as whether or not to discuss feelings. Regardless of the source of conflict, relationships between older parents and their adult children also provide a tremendous source of strength, which is greatly needed in times of loss.

WIDOWHOOD

Most married women will become widows because, on the average, they marry men who are somewhat older. The average age of widowhood is 56; in contrast, most men in society will not become widowers until on average around age 85. Widowhood is a tremendously stressful and life-altering event in the lives of older adults. People who experience the sudden death of a spouse have a more difficult time coping than those who have time to anticipate the death of their spouse (Carr et al., 2001). However, there is no significant difference between those who experience the sudden death of a spouse and those who anticipated the spouse's passing, in terms of their *feelings* about the loss—depression, anger, shock, and grief.

The surviving spouse, male or female, faces a number of life changes, from shifting social relationships to the demands of new responsibilities, such as cleaning, cooking, managing household finances, and even needing to find work. Lee and associates (2001) learned that men and women experience similar levels of depression at the loss of a spouse. However, women are more likely to be the surviving spouse because they outlive men by large margins. Only half of women over 65 are living with a partner. Lee and associates (2001) report that women tend to adapt relatively well to widowhood in the long run.

Social networking online creates additional opportunities for women and men to communicate with each other. Technology has had a major impact on relationships and has changed the boundaries of friendship and intimacy. For example, such free socializing websites as Facebook, Twitter, and Second Life offer opportunities to explore relationships of varying degrees of intimacy. Social media make it possible for people to keep in touch regularly, regardless of age or physical distance. This is especially important for older adults, who may have limits on their physical ability and mobility.

Seniors who choose to remarry enjoy much success if the ingredients of love, companionship, financial security, and consent of offspring are present. In one study, partners in long-standing marriages (between 20 and 29 years) showed lower levels of disease and disability, such as hypertension, arthritis, and functional limitations, than did their counterparts in marriages of shorter length (Pienta, Hayward, & Jenkins, 2000). However, widows and divorcees tended to report higher levels of these types of health problems than people of any other marital status. It has been found, however, that those marriages in which one spouse suffers a long-term illness do tend to have more problems (Leinonen et al., 2001).

CARE OF ELDERLY PARENTS

Elderly people identify their adult children, when they have them, as the primary helpers in their lives. When they have both an adult son and an adult daughter, tasks often fall into gender-stereotyped categories, with women attending to housework and personal needs, and men handling yard chores, general home repair, and finances (Mosher & Danoff-Burg, 2004).

In the past, responsibility for any elder care most often fell to unmarried daughters, if there were any. They were expected to do this because it was assumed that the work would be easier for them, as they had no responsibilities for husbands or children. If the elderly person was still employed or had retirement benefits, male and female caregivers would offer less support, regardless of their own employment status.

Support for the caregivers who take care of the elderly is critical. Depression and stress are two of the most common risk factors cited, with the degree of stress and depression experienced associated with specific traits of the caregiver. For example, Meshefedjian and associates (1998) found that the closer the caregiver felt to the elderly person, the higher the caregiver scored on a test of depression. In addition, the less education caregivers have, the more likely they are to be depressed. Having a close relationship with the elderly person often causes the caregiver to feel overwhelmed. Not only is the closeness of the relationship between parent and child a factor in caregiver mental health, but the quality of this association is also important. Poor interactions between caregivers and those in their care even result in verbally and physically aggressive behavior (Cohen-Mansfield & Werner, 1998).

David Guia (2003) has identified a constellation of symptoms that he calls the *caregiver stress syndrome*. This syndrome is the result of stress, either acute or chronic, that results from providing caregiving activities and includes changes in physiological and psychological functioning. Religious and spiritual beliefs, shared caregiving responsibility, and the use of adult day-care facilities have been useful in reducing caregiver stress levels.

Elders who have no kin tend to substitute a close friend whom they persuade to take the place of the absent relative when they need to be cared for. Most family and close friends still feel that they ought to take care of the elderly in their own homes if possible. Racial and ethnic traits play a role in who should be responsible for caring for the older generation. For example, Lee and associates (1998) found that elderly African American parents were more likely to expect to be cared for by their children than were elderly

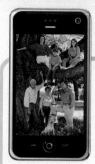

TECH TRENDS

Wii: It's Not Just for Kids!

The Wii, a device that allows playing sports matches on any television set, creates excellent opportunities for exercise and socializing. It has become tremendously popular among older adults (Angela, 2008). Recently, however, doctors are witnessing increases in injuries stemming from marathon Wii sessions. In a recent *New York Times* article on Wii "warriors," one doctor says of an older patient, "I was asking him what happened . . . and he said, 'Well, we bought a Wii system for the grandkids. Next thing I know, my shoulder's killing me'" (Das, 2009). While the benefits of physical activity are significant, anyone starting a new exercise program should always consult a physician. As Dr. Susan Joy says in the same article, "It's good to remember that you're not a kid."

White parents. Burr and Mutchler (1999) found that elderly Latinos were also more likely to agree that the younger generation should care for them.

It is not always the younger generation that provides caretaking for elderly persons. Often, the spouse of the elderly person takes on this role. Much research on wives caring for elderly husbands exists, but less is known about elderly husbands who care for their wives (Cahill, 2000). Older husbands who care for their ailing wives tend to do well when they approach caregiving as a series of tasks or problem-solving activities. They are more likely to seek support services from a variety of sources and are able to place some distance between themselves and their caregiving role (Twigg & Atkin, 1994). Caring for an elderly person with dementia has been found to be extremely stressful (Cahill, 2000). Ory and associates (1999) found that caregivers of dementia patients spend significantly more time each week in their role than other types of caregivers. Further, those who care for dementia patients experience more caregiver strain and report higher levels of physical and mental health problems.

Another option for elderly care is a nursing home. If a family does choose long-term care for an elderly parent, how do they choose the right nursing home for that parent? The U.S. Department of Health and Human Services provides information on over 17,000 nursing homes nationwide at www.medicare.gov. McCarthy (2002) argues that there is a critical need for increased funding for such facilities.

THE CHANGING ROLE OF THE GRANDPARENT

Today, many grandparents play a more integral part in the lives of their grandchildren than grandparents did a generation ago. A survey completed by the American Association of Retired Persons (AARP, 2000) concluded that the state of American grandparenting is for the most part healthy. A 2002 report of the U.S. Census Bureau stated that over 2.4 million grandparents were raising their grandchildren in the United States, and the numbers today are likely higher. Many are raising their grandchildren alone. The parents of these children, the middle generation, are usually absent often due to death, substance abuse, or incarceration. Pruchno (1999) found that among grandmothers, African Americans and Whites differed in two important ways. First, it was more common for African American grandmothers to have peers also raising grandchildren alone. Second, a household containing multiple generations living together was not uncommon among African Americans. These two findings may explain why the Black grandmothers in this study experienced fewer emotional burdens from their caregiving role than did their White counterparts.

Grandparents are also playing a bigger role as day-care providers for their grandchildren. In order for them to have a positive effect on their grandchildren, it is critical that social and financial supports be made available to ease the challenges associated with such care arrangements and contribute to grandparents' well-being (Gerard, Landry-Meyer, & Roe, 2006).

RELATIONSHIPS WITH OTHERS

Contrary to the stereotype, getting old need not, and usually does not, mean being lonely. In fact, the elderly, most of whom have a good deal of free time, use it to develop their social lives. For example, older adults are the fastest-growing group of Internet users and are accessing technology through various venues (Czaja et al., 2006).

What is the optimum pattern of aging in terms of our relationships with other people? For many years, there have been two different positions on this question, known as the activity theory and the disengagement theory.

According to the **activity theory,** human beings flourish through interaction with other people and physical activity. They are unhappy when, as they reach the older years, they have fewer contacts with others as a result of death, illness, and societal limitations, such as lack of access to events due to mobility challenges or financial constraints. Those who are able to keep up the social activity of their middle years are considered the most successful. Retirement simply means choosing other, hopefully more enjoyable, activities.

Disengagement theory (Cummings & Henry, 1961) contradicts this idea. According to this theory, the idea

In three words I can sum up everything I've learned about life: It goes on.

ANONYMOUS

that activity is better than passivity is a bias of the Western world. This was not always so; the Greeks, for example, valued their warriors and athletes but reserved the highest distinction for such contemplative philosophers as Sophocles, Plato, and Aristotle. Many Eastern cultures also value the isolated thinker or the solitary observer. According to disengagement theory, the most mature adults are likely to gradually disengage themselves from their fellow human beings in preparation for death. They become less interested in their interactions with others and more focused on themselves, on such concerns as their health and finances. They accept the decreasing attention of a society that sees them as losing power.

Does this mean that the tendency toward disengagement is more natural than the tendency toward activity? It is now believed that what has appeared to be disengagement is instead a temporary transition from the highly active role of the middle-aged adult to the more sedate, spiritually oriented role of the elderly person. Most humans truly enjoy social contact, so disengagement from one's fellows may be the result of traumatic experience or a physiological disturbance such as clinical depression. However, activity theory, with its emphasis on social involvement, is also now considered too general. For example, many people may reduce social contacts but keep active with solitary hobbies. Activity per se has not been found to correlate with a personal sense of satisfaction with life.

Carstensen (1995, 1996) offered a resolution of the debate with her **socioemotional selectivity theory.** She suggested that humans use social contact to ensure physical survival, to get information they need, to maintain a sense of self, and to acquire pleasure and comfort. These goals exist throughout life, but the importance of each shifts with age. For the elderly, the need for physical support and the need for information from others become less important, while the need for maintaining a sense of themselves grows. They tend to get this support from relatives and close friends (their "social convoy," as they have been called) more and more, whereas the need for support from casual acquaintances such as coworkers declines.

Furthermore, the challenges faced in later life can be quite different. For example, Lang (2001) found that older adults who are able to maintain their close emotional relationships and let other, less important relationships go have a greater sense of well-being. Older African Americans and Whites are likely to have similar small, close social networks made up mainly of kin (Ajrouch, Antonucci, & Janevic, 2001). Thus, the elderly may appear to be disengaging but, in fact, are simply becoming more selective about with whom they wish to spend their social time.

In his keynote address to the APA annual convention in 1997, Nobel

activity theory Humans flourish/thrive through interactions with others and physical activity, and suffer in the absence of such stimulation.

disengagement theory The elderly will remove themselves from many social networks.

socioemotional selectivity theory Humans use social contact for four reasons: to ensure physical survival, to gain information, to maintain a sense of self, and to acquire pleasure and comfort.

Gateball in Japan

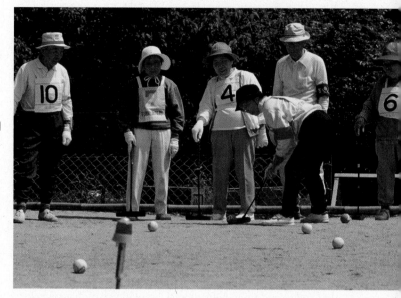

Gateball, developed in post–World War II Japan, is a team sport combining elements of golf and croquet. It employs strategies that exercise both mind and body. Although the object is to score the most points, a great deal of emphasis is placed on the individual's contributions to the team as opposed to individual achievement.

In addition to these benefits, gateball provides a social outlet, building relationships around a common interest. Gateball has become immensely popular among "silver agers," as older people are called by the Japanese. In a modern, crowded, industrial country such as Japan, with early retirement and the highest life expectancy in the world, gateball provides a way for seniors to continue their lifelong pattern of group participation in something worthwhile.

Observations of gateball players in action found people who share information, laughter, and a relaxed sense of belonging. When a player who hadn't been there for some time reappeared, he or she was warmly welcomed back. Exchange of food occurs routinely on the break, and people often encourage others to take some home with them.

In America, this kind of community spirit among seniors is evidenced in some sports (such as golf and bowling), but the stereotype of an elderly person sitting in a rocking chair somehow remains pervasive. Sports provide a means by which older people can remain healthy as well as connected to other people. It is an important lesson we might glean from Japanese culture.

Laureate Elie Wiesel emphasized the need for gratitude to the elderly for their role in helping us remember the lessons of the past, as has been the case with the Holocaust. He defended the rights of the elderly and other often-victimized populations. Focus on elderly issues should help us deal with problems caused by increasing numbers in this age group, particularly in the area of social development.

Patterns of Work

Only a small percentage of all adults aged 65 and older, about 11%, are in the labor force. In the past, many retirements were due to forced retirement.

Career Apps

As an elderly companion, how would you help an elderly person retain a sense of independence and enjoy activities with others?

Today, only airline pilots and public safety workers such as firefighters and police can be forced to retire because of their age. There is a growing trend toward staying in the workforce (Finch & Robinson, 2003). Economists' theories on why people choose to remain in the workforce include: Social Security reforms (the longer a person waits to retire, the larger her Social Security checks will be when she does retire), increased opportunities in the workplace, and freedom from pension constraints (Johnson, 2002). Individuals have their own reasons for seeking personal and professional rewards, such as a desire to feel useful and the pressures of an economic recession.

PERFORMANCE

As a greater number of older people live longer and healthier lives, the baby-boom generation ages, and birthrates decrease, many stereotypes about aging are coming under closer scrutiny. This is because by 2012 over 29% of men and 20% of women aged 65–74 will be in the workforce, and over 8% of men over age 75 will be as well (Phillips, 2004). The stereotype of an older, less effective workforce is bolstered by research on aging that demonstrates a decline in abilities such as dexterity, speed of response, agility, hearing, and vision. If all these abilities decline, then one might conclude that job performance must decline with age. McEvoy and Cascio (1989) conducted an extensive review of 96 studies and found no relationship between age and job performance. It made no difference whether the performance measures were ratings or productivity measures, or whether the type of job was professional or nonprofessional.

What explanation is there for these results? How does the older worker deal with the mild decline of physical abilities that affects most elderly persons? Experience is one answer. There is said to be no substitute for it, and it is certainly valued by employers. Other reasons cited are that older workers have lower absenteeism, turnover, illness, and accident rates. They also tend to have higher job satisfaction and more positive work values than younger workers. These qualifications seem to offset any decreases in physical ability that increasing age causes.

RETIREMENT

The path to retirement for older adults can take many different forms. Although the economic downturn of the early 2010s has forced many older workers to reconsider whether they can afford to retire, for many people, retirement is a welcome relief from work life. For others, it is just as difficult as being unemployed. Retirement requires changing the habits of a lifetime. In 2002, nearly 80% of baby boomers said they planned to work after 65 (www.boston.com). The New Retirement Survey (http://seniorliving.about.com) found that percentage to be almost exactly the same today.

Nevertheless, the great majority of those over 65 have chosen not to work. The decision is a complicated one, but health may be the biggest factor. Morris (2006) sums up the situation wryly:

> *The best is yet to come? That's a falsehood of governmental proportions, absurd on its smiling face and no more plausible after the smile contracts. But it has become one of the lies we live by ... The "senior citizens" who have replaced the former "old" in a powerful national myth are curious and adventurous, well-heeled and free—but for the doctors' appointments and hospital stays around which they have to schedule their adventures. (p. 72)*

Dychtwald (2005) argues that increased life expectancy and potential for high creativity will usher in a new

FIGURE 11.5

Rising Labor Force Participation Rates Among the Elderly

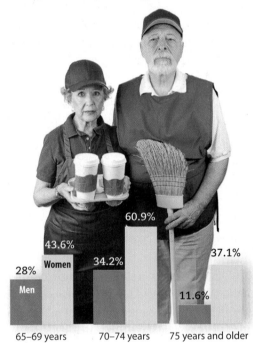

This graph shows the percentage change in labor force participation rates since 1994.

era of retirement, better termed "rehirement" (see Figure 11.5). Many people desire to be useful, and feel youthful and active. Research indicates that the decision to retire is influenced by the retiree's desire to reinvent herself physically or mentally (Lloyd, 2009). Retirement is a time to "do good"—now it can be working at something you really care about rather than just working to pay the bills.

The belief that retired people are an important community resource is growing. Numerous efforts have been made in recent years to tap this powerful resource. A number of national programs now make an effort to involve retired persons in volunteer and paid work as service to society.

CONCLUSIONS & SUMMARY

At the beginning of this chapter we asked, "Must we decline as we age?" The answer is that some decline is inevitable, but the picture is much less gloomy than we have been led to believe. The loss of mental and physical abilities is, on the average, relatively slight; some individuals experience only moderate physical loss and no cognitive loss at all. For many older adults, compensatory skills and abilities may replace lost capacities. The same is true for personal and social development.

What are key aspects of physical development among the elderly?

- A variety of physiological theories regarding aging and death exist. These include aging by program, homeostatic imbalance, and cross-linkage theories.
- Genetic theories of aging suggest that the program for aging exists in certain harmful genes.
- Major modifiers of ability such as training, nutrition, illness, stress level, and personality type also affect one's rate of aging.
- Although reaction time appears to decline with age, some researchers have pointed to several reasons for this decline.
- Variables other than sheer neural or motor activities account for most change in physical skills over time. These include ageism, motivation, depression, anxiety, response strategies, and response style.
- Changes in sensory abilities, the skeletal system, skin, teeth, hair, and locomotion are noticeable in late adulthood.
- For both women and men, hormone production slows down during late adulthood.
- One of the most debilitating conditions of the elderly is Alzheimer's disease.
- A strong relationship exists between physical and mental health.

How is cognitive development affected by old age?

- A number of factors have been suggested as explaining the difference between tested and observed changes in elderly cognition. These include differences in type of cognition, the representativeness of the individuals or observations, standards of evaluation, and amounts of experience.
- Creativity is evidenced in late adulthood and in some cases may be strongest during this time. Although quantity of creative production probably drops in old age, the quality of creative production and potential for creative production probably do not.
- Wisdom refers to going beyond what is known to an understanding of the implication of things. It is the result of intelligence, personality, the intelligence-personality interaction, life experience, and age.
- For Erikson, the resolution of each of the first seven stages in his theory should lead people to achieve a sense of integrity in the last stage. If not, they experience despair.

How do social relationships develop during late adulthood?

- People in late adulthood tend to experience a crossover in gender roles, with older men becoming more like women and older women becoming more like men.
- In late adulthood, males are generally more sexually active than females. Declining sexual activity in the female is usually attributable to her declining interest or to illness in her male partner.
- Elderly people identify their adult children, if they have them, as the primary helpers in their lives. When they have both an adult son and an adult daughter, elderly people most often ask the son to be the primary helper, although the daughter usually does most of the caregiving.
- Research suggests four basic phases through which most middle-aged and aged couples pass: child rearing, childless preretirement, retirement, and widowhood/widowerhood.

What are major factors affecting the older worker?

- Although older people show less interest in working than younger people, discrimination and stereotypes about older workers underestimate their desire to continue to be involved in the workforce.

- Elderly people become more interested in their "inner selves," perceptions of the environment change, psychic energy declines, and gender-role reversals occur.
- For years developmental scientists have held two different positions on what is the optimal pattern of aging: the activity theory of aging (the elderly simply switch activities as they age) and the disengagement theory (most elderly naturally switch from an external to an internal focus). Today, a more accepted explanation of elderly social behavior is Carstensen's socioemotional selectivity theory.

KEY TERMS

activity theory *271*

ageism *256*

aging by program *258*

Alzheimer's disease *263*

arthritis *262*

autoimmunity *258*

cataracts *261*

collagen *258*

cross-linkage theory *258*

dementia *263*

despair *267*

disengagement theory *271*

explicit memory *267*

gerontology *256*

glaucoma *261*

homeostatic imbalance *258*

implicit memory *267*

integrity *267*

life expectancy *256*

macular degeneration *261*

osteoporosis *262*

prospective memory *267*

reaction time *260*

retrospective memory *267*

role discontinuity *268*

socioemotional selectivity theory *271*

wisdom *266*

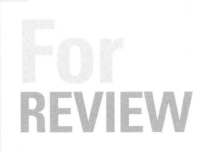
For REVIEW

1. Which of the explanations of why we age and die do you find most persuasive? Support your answer with examples from the text.

2. Programs in which young people meet regularly with elderly adults seem to have rewards for all involved. By what other means might we better tap the knowledge and creativity of the elderly?

3. Some researchers have said that Erikson's first seven stages describe crises in which action should be taken, yet the eighth and last stage, integrity versus despair, is merely reactive. Did Erikson mean to portray the elderly as sitting in rocking chairs and looking back over their lives? How do you interpret the impact of physical, psychological, and social factors on late adulthood?

Chapter Review Test

1. Ageism can be defined as
   a. a type of prejudice toward older adults.
   b. an illness that strikes old people after age 75.
   c. physical changes that occur in late adulthood.
   d. the study of human development.

2. Alzheimer's disease is
   a. caused largely by bacteria.
   b. suffered most by people whose IQ is in the top third of the population.
   c. easily treated and resolved successfully.
   d. one of the two most common forms of dementia that affect the elderly.

3. Dacey (1989b) proposed that there are certain _____ in life during which creative ability can be cultivated most effectively.
   a. critical periods
   b. ages
   c. educational experiences
   d. work-related experiences

4. A failure in the boy's systems to regulate the proper interactions of organs is called
   a. counterpart theory.
   b. homeostatic imbalance.
   c. autoimmunity.
   d. cross-linkage theory.

Answers: 1a, 2d, 3a, 4b, 5a, 6b, 7a, 8c, 9a, 10a

5. Stress level, educational level, motivation, and personality type are examples of
   a. modifiers of ability.
   b. environmental factors.
   c. genetic factors.
   d. physiological factors.

6. The type of memory that allows us to remember something we need to do in the future is called _____ memory.
   a. episodic
   b. prospective
   c. explicit
   d. implicit

7. Older workers make valued employees for all of the reasons listed except
   a. job skills.
   b. absenteeism.
   c. accident rates.
   d. turnover.

8. The first phase of life that most middle-aged couples experience is
   a. widowhood/widowerhood.
   b. the retirement phase.
   c. the child-rearing phase.
   d. the childless preretirement period.

9. A person's decision to retire is largely influenced by the retiree's
   a. spouse.
   b. boss.
   c. teacher.
   d. doctor.

10. When adults distance themselves from others in preparation for death and become less interested in their interactions with others, it is referred to as
    a. disengagement.
    b. separation.
    c. personal well-being.
    d. achievement.

DYING AND SPIRITUALITY

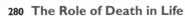
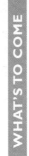
As You READ

After reading this chapter, you should be able to answer the following questions:

- What is the role of death in life?
- What is the purpose of "grief work"?
- What are the factors that cause and determine the nature of suicide?
- What is the meaning of "successful dying"?
- How do psychologists define the nature of spirituality?

The Role of Death in Life

Prior to the 20th century, people were used to seeing death. It was considered a typical part of life. Before the industrial revolution transformed the way people lived in Western societies, one third of all children died within their first year and half died before their 10th birthday. The institution of seemingly simple innovations, such as clean drinking water and organized waste disposal, along with improvements in health care, contributed to a rise in living standards and fall in death rates. Interestingly, over the past 100 years, deaths from some causes (such as tuberculosis, influenza) have declined significantly, while deaths from other causes (for example, cancer) have increased (see Table 12.1).

It remains the case, however, that in modern Western societies, death comes mostly to the elderly. This has been especially true in recent years, as seen in the trend of death rates for men and women over 85 declining by 3.9% for men and 4.1% for women (CDC, 2006c). In the United States, the **mortality rate** has declined from 17 per 1,000 people in 1900 to 8 per 1,000 in 2004 (Minino et al., 2006). The average life expectancy has been reported at

mortality rate The number of deaths in a population for a given year; typically, number of deaths per 1,000 people per year.

an all-time high of nearly 78 years. Overall, a family may expect to live 20 years (on the average) without one of its members dying (see Figure 12.1).

As death rates fell over the past century, and death became less a part of life, ironically, the subject of death seemed to become more and more taboo. Avoidance of death, even discussion of death, has become entrenched in the dominant U.S. culture. As a result, social scientists spent little time studying the role of death in life. Fortunately, in recent decades, this has begun to change, and death has become a more approachable subject of both research and public discourse, including media attention. Research and theory from the social and physical sciences tend to focus on three major concerns: What is death? How do we deal with the death of others? How do we deal with our own death?

WHAT IS DEATH?

Establishing when people are truly and finally dead has been a medical, and therefore social, problem for centuries. Fear of being prematurely buried alive has been one of humankind's oldest fears. The fear was so strong in the 19th century that in 1882 a patent was granted for a life signal called "Fearnaught," a warning flag device that

TABLE 12.1

Death Rates by Cause of Death, 1900–2005 (per 100,000 population)

Year	Tuberculosis, all forms	Malignant neoplasms (cancer)	Major cardiovascular diseaseas	Influenza and pneumonia	Motor vehicle accidents
1900	194.4	64.0	345.2	202.2	N.A.
1920	113.1	83.4	364.9	207.3	10.3
1940	45.9	120.3	485.7	70.3	26.2
1960	6.1	149.2	521.8	37.3	21.3
1980	0.9	183.9	436.4	24.1	23.5
2005	0.2	188.7	288.8	21.3	15.3

Source: 1900–1970, U.S. Public Health Service, Vital Statistics of the United States, annual, Vol. I and Vol. II; 1971–2001, U.S. National Center for Health Statistics, Vital Statistics of the United States, annual; National Vital Statistics Report (NVSR) (formerly Monthly Vital Statistics Report); and unpublished data.

FIGURE 12.1

Average Life Expectancy by Current Age Group

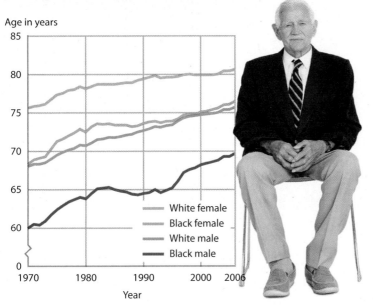

Age in years

White female
Black female
White male
Black male

Year

Source: National Center for Health Statistics, 2005.

FIGURE 12.2

"Fearnaught" Device

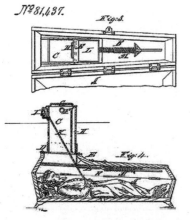

Nº 81,437.

Fig: 3.

Fig: 4.

Patented Aug. 25, 1868.

Fear of being buried alive motivated the invention of this casket device. A rope placed in the hands of the coffin occupant could be pulled to ring the bell above ground.

could be activated if someone was buried alive inside a coffin (see Figure 12.2). It is no coincidence that Edgar Allen Poe, one of the greatest writers of all time, known for his spine-tingling tales of horror and misfortune, wrote a story titled *The Premature Burial* (1850).

Professionals no longer have any serious problem determining whether a person is dead. Of more concern is determining exactly when death occurs. Because all of the body's systems do not cease at once upon death, disagreements sometimes exist over which system is most significant in judging whether a person is dead.

FOUR TYPES OF DEATH

Today, four types of death are recognized: clinical death, brain death, biological or cellular death, and social death.

Clinical Death

In one sense, the individual is dead when his or her breathing and heartbeat have stopped, which is termed **clinical death.** Actually, clinical death is the least useful to the medical profession and to society at large because it can be unreliable and temporary. Owing to the success of **cardiopulmonary resuscitation (CPR),** many individuals, whose lungs and heart would have ceased to function decades ago before the technique was put into practice, have been saved. In other cases, spontaneous restarting of the heart and lungs has occurred after failure. New CPR findings suggest that mouth-to-mouth breathing may not be necessary to sustain a person's life until emergency aid arrives. Pushing on a person's chest approximately 100 times per minute seems to do the trick, according to several recent studies, and pushing to the beat of the Bee Gee's (1977) song "Staying Alive" gives the approximate number of compressions/minute (Harman, 2008).

Brain Death

Death of the brain occurs when it fails to receive a sufficient supply of oxygen for a period of time (usually 8 to 10 minutes) and all electrical activity has stopped. The cessation of brain function occurs in stages,

clinical death The individual is dead when his or her respiration and heartbeat have stopped.

cardiopulmonary resuscitation (CPR) Technique for reviving an individual's lungs and heart that have ceased to function.

According to most studies, people's number one fear *is public speaking. Number two is* death. *Does that sound right? This means to the average person, if you go to a funeral, you're better off in the casket than doing the* eulogy.

JERRY SEINFELD

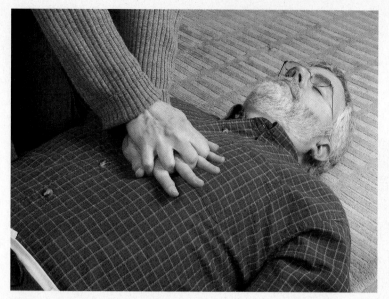

still alive, to save time and complete necessary tasks efficiently.

THE LEGAL DEFINITION OF DEATH

The various definitions pertaining to death can be quite confusing. In the legal profession, where language is of utmost importance and words are examined and interpreted on a case-by-case basis, death is regarded as a status, not a process. Proof of death is required for such status to be acknowledged as fact, meaning that there is no room for competing definitions or ambiguity. In an attempt to narrow the definition of death, the Harvard Ad Hoc Committee to Examine the Criteria of Brain Death suggested the following criteria for **legal death** in 1968: "unreceptivity and unresponsivity, no movements or breathing, no reflexes, and a flat EEG reading that remains flat for 24 hours."

Although people may disagree on the exact nature of death itself, passionate debates have helped inform the field of lifespan development about how people deal, and how they should deal, with the death of their loved ones.

LIFESPAN PERSPECTIVES ON DEATH

Although most people associate dying with late adulthood, we know that death can occur at any point throughout the lifespan—birth through old age. The causes of death can be as varied as the interpretations that people have once death is pending or after it has occurred. A person's age and corresponding level of cognitive development influence that person's perspective of death and dying. For example, infants are certainly attached to their parents and loved ones, but not in the same way as toddlers, for whom attachment is a major focus of their cognitive and social development. If a child is

brain death Occurs when the brain fails to receive a sufficient supply of oxygen for a short period of time (usually 8 to 10 minutes).

Electroencephalogram (EEG) Recording of the electrical activity produced by the firing of neurons in the brain.

biological death Occurs when it is no longer possible to discern an electrical charge in the tissues of the heart and lungs.

social death Point at which a patient is treated essentially as a corpse, although perhaps still "clinically" or "biologically" alive.

legal death A legal pronouncement by a qualified person that a patient should be considered dead under the law.

involving the cortex, the midbrain, and the lower brain stem. When the cortex and midbrain cease functioning, **brain death** has occurred, and the person enters an irreversible coma. However, the body can remain alive in this condition for a long time, because the nervous systems functions such as breathing and heartbeat are governed by the brain stem. When the brain stem ceases functioning, the person is dead. Consciousness and alertness, however, will never be regained (Sullivan, Seem & Chabelewski, 1999). It is the loss of these skills, and associated abilities that we equate with being human, that is commonly linked with the concept of brain death. One indication of death is a flat **electroencephalogram (EEG)** for a specified period of time.

Biological Death

Biological death follows clinical death and brain death, and cells start dying from lack of oxygen. **Biological death** occurs when it is no longer possible to discern an electrical charge in the tissues of the heart and lungs, thus signaling the permanent end of all life functions. If clinical death is responded to quickly enough, it is possible to prevent biological death, although all tissues and organs would sustain injury from lack of blood supply.

Social Death

Researcher David Sudnow (1967) was the first to suggest the concept of **social death,** the point at which an individual is treated as dead although the person is still biologically alive. He cites cases in which body preparation (for instance, closing the eyes) was started while the patient was

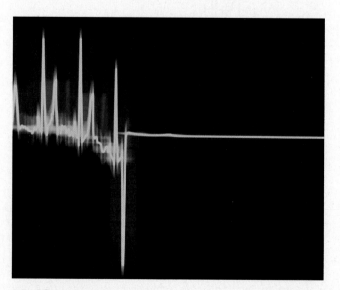

A flat EEG that occurs for a period of time is one indication of brain death.

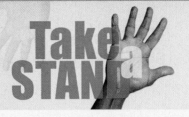

Advances in medical technology have made it possible to prolong a person's time living, but is this desirable? Many people would prefer to die than live in a painful or unconscious state, placing emotional and physical demands on loved ones.

Children, who are dependent on adults to care for them in a safe and consistent manner, are not typically consulted as to their wishes for medical treatment. A recent court case that received national attention focused on Daniel Hauser, a 13-year-old whose family wished to cease chemotherapy treatment for his Hodgkin's lymphoma. The court ruled that Daniel's parents were medically neglectful, even though they had their own preferred methods of treating his lym-phoma—noninvasive treatments that were acceptable based on their religious beliefs. Doctors argued that without chemotherapy and radiation treatment, Daniel's hopes for survival were greatly compromised. The doctors believed that Daniel's health and general well-being outweighed any sort of parental "imperative" in which the parents knew best.

Do you believe there is a specific age that should be reached before someone can make his or her own decisions regarding health and medical treatments? Who should decide the age, and who should enforce or deny a family's wishes?

sick or dying, she might fear that her caregivers will leave her. Hospitalization often requires caregivers to be absent at least some of the time, while children rest or receive treatment, and medical professionals—no matter how kind or well intentioned—are no substitute for close family. If a child's parent or close relative is dying, the child will likely fear abandonment in a similar sense, with very real concerns about "who will take care of me?" Older children often mourn the loss of a pet quite deeply, and their grief is not to be underestimated. Children do not yet have the ability to think abstractly about death, spirituality, or the afterlife, so close contact and reassurance is helpful to their preoperational or concrete operational levels of understanding.

Adolescents, whose thinking is in the formal operational stage of cognitive development and who can think abstractly and reason logically, may still feel confused about death and dying, for they can imagine any number of possibilities to account for their own death or loss of a loved one. Teens, who feel they are invincible to some degree and experience adolescent egocentrism, might not worry about death as younger children do. However, young adults who have served in the military, or have friends or family who have served, have a quite different view of death. They may feel that some kind of cosmic order is not functioning fairly if someone dies before old age.

A rational outlook on death and dying develops during adulthood, as people now care for others—children and/or aging parents—and wish to ensure that their loved ones will receive care as long as possible. Risky behaviors are therefore not as common. Death is something that people

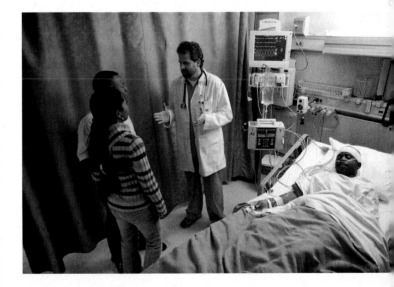

tend to want to avoid as much as possible so that they may see all tasks through to completion with regard to family and career. Adults have a different perspective on death as they begin to see fewer years of living ahead, compared to the number of years behind them.

Once adults reach the stage of late adulthood, they have likely experienced loss of family and friends. Older adults tend to reconcile their feelings about their own mortality, and often loosen previously rigid ideas about individual differences between people of all races, social classes, religions, genders, or sexual orientations. A general sense of acceptance tends to replace resistance to those who are

*No one ever told me that grief felt so like fear. I am not afraid, but the **sensation** is like being afraid. The same fluttering in the stomach, the same restlessness, the yawning. . . . There is a sort of **invisible** blanket between the world and me. I find it hard to take in what anyone says. Or **perhaps,** hard to want to take it in."*

C. S. LEWIS

grief An emotional response to the loss of another; includes feelings of anxiety, despair, sadness, and loneliness.

anticipatory grief Grief that is experienced before the death of a person.

"different," as the imminent journey into the unknown (death) is something that all people will experience together, regardless of race, social class, or other distinctions. Those who are aware of the state of their own health are often compelled to get all of their business in order concerning finances and personal property so that their death does not cause undue stress on loved ones after their passing.

The Role of Grief

Grief is an emotional response to the loss of another person, and includes feelings of anxiety, despair, sadness, and loneliness. Most psychologists who have examined the role of grief have concluded that it is an essential aspect of a healthy encounter with the crisis of death. Grief has a great deal in common with fear, and most grieving people really are afraid, if only unconsciously. They are frightened by the strength of their feelings, and they often fear that they are losing their sanity. Grieving people often feel that they cannot go on, that they are losing control, and that their loss is so great that their own lives are in danger.

Grief not only follows death; when there is advance warning, it frequently precedes it. Known as **anticipatory grief,** it has four phases: depression, a heightened concern for the ill person, a rehearsal of death, and finally an attempt to adjust to what is likely to occur after the death. Indeed, the grieving process can seem to have a yo-yo effect—a person feels less conscious grief one minute and terrible despair the next.

Numerous factors are involved in how one processes grief, including personality, perception, religion, and family dynamics (Dunne, 2004). The fact that people experience grief differently reflects personal, as well as cultural, beliefs and practices (Haas, 2003).

perspectives on Diversity

Victims Left Behind

While the decrease in U.S. deaths from AIDS is significant, it is not the same in other parts of the world, and all too often, children are the ultimate victims who are left behind when a parent (or parents) dies from complications of AIDS. Estimates are that AIDS has orphaned 15 million children around the world, with even more children being

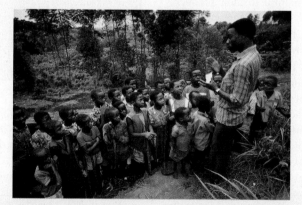

"lost" because their communities are unable to care for them. Statistics show that 11.6 million of these children live in sub-Saharan Africa.

In 2009, in an effort to bring global awareness to the crisis affecting millions of children, an international group (FXB International) proclaimed May 7th to be World AIDS Orphans Day. Founder and president of FXB International, Albina du Boisrouvray, stated, "This day gives a visibility, a voice to a dropped generation, dropped because it does not vote and does not buy and does not count in the global game. Alone we can do nothing, together we can do everything."

perspectives on Diversity

Cultural Variations in the Mourning Process

Grieving is a feeling about the death of a loved one; **mourning** is the action taken as a result. For example, some people mistakenly believe that the Japanese don't grieve because in their society, highly emotional displays of mourning are not shared in public. On the other hand, keening (loud lamentations) is an expected mourning behavior in some Irish cultures, as well as among indigenous peoples in Asia, Africa, and Australia. How do geography and social custom affect the mourning process? There is strong evidence to support biopsychosocial influences on the process of mourning.

In terms of biology, the universal responses to sadness, fear, or despair, such as crying or fainting, occur across cultures. People in all cultures experience other physical symptoms, such as headaches, stomachaches, or sleep disturbances, after a death that is significant to them. In any culture, the deceased person need not be a biological relative to evoke the biological response. For instance, media images showed people around the world crying at the passing of Senator Ted Kennedy in 2009.

Psychological factors, such as love, perception of loss, and sadness, can spark physical and social reactions to the event (such as crying or wearing black). Culture influences the manifestations of how people perceive loss and the mourning practices that follow (such as attending a wake that is boisterous versus one that is somber). Similarly, society as a whole shapes acceptable grieving

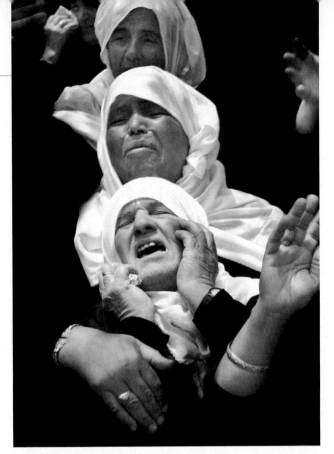

and mourning practices, and sends messages about what is considered normal and what is considered extreme (such as waiting a certain period of time before dating/remarrying or refusing to wash a deceased loved one's clothes). People who experience a death, whether of a family member, celebrity, or a stranger in the obituary column of a newspaper, may experience similar feelings that manifest themselves quite differently because of cognitive and cultural factors.

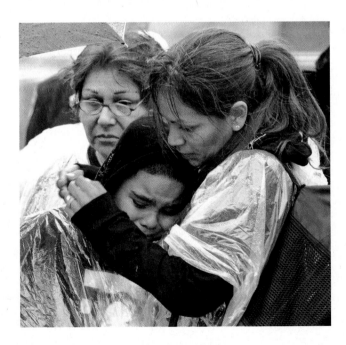

UNRESOLVED GRIEF

The process of grieving, painful as it is, is resolved by most individuals. In some cases, however, morbid grief reactions occur that prevent the successful conclusion of this life crisis. Three types of these grief reactions are delayed reaction, distorted reaction, and complicated grief.

> **mourning** Actions taken as a result of grieving
>
> **delayed grief** Grief that is postponed for an inordinate time.

Delayed Grief

In some cases, the intense reaction of the first stage is delayed for days, months, and in some cases years. In cases of **delayed grief,** a seemingly unrelated incident may bring to the surface an intense grieving that the individual does not even recognize as grief. Take, for example, the case of a 42-year-old man who underwent therapy to deal with a mysterious depression. During conversation he disclosed that when he was 22, his 42-year-old mother committed suicide. Apparently, the occurrence of his own 42nd birthday

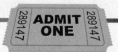
distorted grief Normal grief carried to an extreme degree; adoption of deceased person's ailments.

psychosomatic Physical illness or symptom brought about by mental factors.

complicated grief Prolonged and intensified grief; may take weeks or months to pass.

brought to the surface many feelings that he had managed to repress.

Distorted Grief

In most cases, **distorted grief** reactions are normal grief symptoms carried to an extreme degree. They include adopting the behavior traits of the deceased, such as aspects of the deceased's fatal illness or other **psychosomatic** ailments—physical illness or symptoms caused by mental factors such as stress. One example is a young man whose mother died of lung cancer. At the end of her life, she often had painful coughing fits and sometimes coughed up blood. Some weeks after she died, her son began experiencing pain in his chest and started coughing. Upon examination, he was found to be in perfect health, and his chest X-ray appeared normal. His doctor decided that the only explanation of the symptoms was the young man's grief over the loss of his mother. The ultimate distorted reaction is depression so deep that it causes the physical deterioration—even death—of the surviving loved one. This is especially likely to happen to widowers (Asch-Goodkin & Kaplan, 2006).

Complicated Grief

With **complicated grief,** the grieving process is prolonged and intensified. Complicated grief can last a long time,

whereas distorted grief is not characterized by length of time. Frequently, people suffer from impaired physical and/or mental health caused by complicated grief. The difference between complicated grief and distorted grief is that while people who experience distorted grief reactions may adopt the symptoms of the deceased, people who experience complicated grief can bring about an illness that may be quite different than what the deceased experienced. Extensive therapy helps people experience normal and healthy grief and move on with their lives.

Experts on the grieving process believe that open confrontation with the loss of a loved one is essential to accepting the reality of a world in which the deceased is no longer present. Attempts to repress or avoid thoughts about the loss are only going to push them into the subconscious, where they will continue to cause problems until they are dragged out and fully accepted. Dealing with grief is difficult and can exact a cost. For example, the mortality rate among grieving persons is seven times higher than it is for a matched sample of nongrieving persons.

THE ROLE OF THE FUNERAL

One of the most difficult aspects of dealing with the death of a loved one is deciding how the funeral (if there is to be one) is to be conducted. Funerals have historically been an important part of American life, whether the elaborate burial rituals practiced by Native Americans, the simple funerals of the colonial settlers, or the diverse practices of the numerous ethnic groups that have immigrated to the United States.

Once the intimate responsibility of each family, care for the dead in the United States has been transferred to a paid service industry. The need for this new service was brought about by changes in society during the first part of the 20th century. The more mobile, urbanized workforce had less family support and less time to devote to the task of caring for the dead. In a relatively short time, funeral homes and funeral directors became the accepted form of care for one's dead relatives.

This commercialization of care for the dead has had mixed results. Although the services that external agents provide take some of the burden away from grieving families, they also potentially prevent the family from confronting the realities that death entails. This emotional buffer is reinforced by some funeral businesses. For example, during the 1950s and 1960s, funeral homes came under stinging criticism for their high costs and their low levels of sensitivity to the needs of the surviving family members. In recent years, coffins have become available for pur-

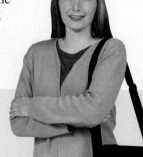

Career Apps

As a grief counselor, how would you assist an adult son deal with the sudden loss of his parents due to an accident?

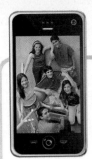
Many people suffering from grief and the anger that often accompanies it believe that their only option is to "wait it out" and "just get through it." In fact, grief sufferers have a number of options available online that afford people as much or as little communication with others as they want. Options range from websites with information about grief and anger, such as facts and frequently asked questions, to discussion groups and chat rooms where people can meet and exchange thoughts and feelings. Here are a representative sample of online resources:

Website – Grief Recovery Online (http://www.groww.com/index.htm) is a comprehensive site providing answers to common questions and opportunities to communicate with others, news, and other information.

Discussion/Support Group – Webhealing.com (http://www.webhealing.com), established by Tom Golden in 1995, was the first interactive website on the Internet. It offers discussion forums as well as general information.

Podcast – "Healing the Grieving Heart" is a free podcast subscription available through iTunes. Created by a marriage and family therapist and adjunct faculty member at Columbia University, the content is geared toward parents of children who have died and their grieving siblings.

Application – "Stress Relief–Blowaway" is an application available on iTunes that incorporates breathing and visualization. Users can view the peaceful scene of a windmill and tulips, and the interactive feature allows users to blow the windmill into action or blow flower petals away. The use of breath encourages breathing practices, which are fundamental to relief from anxiety, anger, and stress.

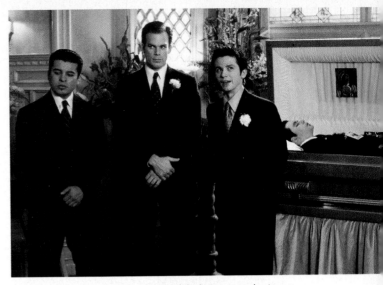

The HBO series Six Feet Under *presented the humorous and poignant sides of life and the commercial aspects associated with death.*

> *If you know not how to die, never trouble yourself.* Nature *will in a moment fully and sufficiently* instruct *you; she will exactly do that business for you; take you no care for it.*

MICHEL DE MONTAIGNE, ESSAY XIX, *OF PHYSIOGNOMY* (1580)

chase in warehouse stores, such as Costco, and the juxtaposition of such items with everyday staples such as eggs and light bulbs takes the concept of one-stop shopping to a whole new level.

Dealing Successfully With One's Own Death

Many people find facing death a much harder experience than Michel de Montaigne, an essayist of the French Renaissance, would have us believe. The acceptance of death is quite painful to many people, who often choose to deny it, and yet concern over death can occur in every stage of human development. At the root of most anxiety is a person's belief that she will die if the thing that she most fears comes to pass. For example, a woman who fears flying may truly believe at the deepest level that she will die if she rides in an airplane.

Psychiatrist Elisabeth Kübler-Ross is the most famous student of the process of death and dying. Kübler-Ross discovered that, far from wanting to avoid the topic of death, many dying patients have a strong urge to discuss it. She interviewed hundreds of terminally ill people in the 1960s and, on the basis of these interviews, developed a five-stage theory describing the emotions underlying the process of dying (see Figure 12.3). The stages in her theory are flexible, in that people can move through them quickly, slowly, or not at all. Some fluctuation occurs between the stages, but by and large people tend to move through them in this order:

FIGURE 12.3
Kübler-Ross's Stages of Grief

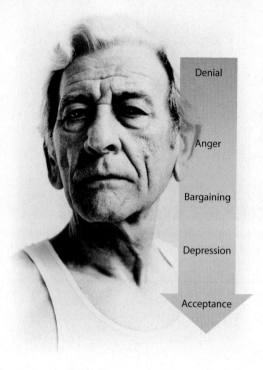

Denial

Anger

Bargaining

Depression

Acceptance

1. *Denial.* In the first stage, a person denies that death is going to happen. This often happens when a terminal diagnosis is first given, but eventually the person must interact with others to consider the practical and logistical matters that need to be addressed.

2. *Anger.* Once a person can no longer deny the fact that death is a reality, she often experiences anger and resentment. A dying person may feel robbed of time on earth, goals unattained, or bitterness that it is her and not another person who will meet this end. A loved one may feel angry at the dying person for abandoning her, at God or another higher power for taking this person away, or the medical professionals for being unable to save the dying person.

3. *Bargaining.* In the third stage of dying, a person comes to hope that the death can be avoided or delayed in exchange for other thoughts or behaviors. Promises are sometimes made to oneself, others, or God in hopes of making a narrow escape a reality.

4. *Depression.* In the fourth stage of dying, the dying person or loved one begins to accept the inevitable conclusion. The dying person may attempt to isolate herself from others, to disconnect from relationships in preparation for death and to help loved ones disconnect. Kübler-Ross deemed this behavior appropriate, as the person needs to confront the reality of dying.

5. *Acceptance.* In the final stage of dying, a person comes to a state of peace and resolution, and no longer attempts to resist the end of her life. Any pain or suffering is no longer viewed as a burden but, rather, part of the natural cycle of life. A feeling of greater connectedness to a higher power is common.

One criticism of Kübler-Ross's stage theory is that no scientific evidence confirms that her sequence of stages is typical or universal. Another criticism is that her theory overlooks the effects of personality, ethnic, or religious factors. For example, people in cultures such as some Native American and Asian ethnic groups view death as just another stage of existence and do not dread it. Whether or not you choose to accept Kübler-Ross's model, the biological, psychological, and social aspects of the process of dying are obviously very complex. Knowledge gained through careful research can help answer questions that emerge as a result of examining the model, but her theory, like all good theories, continues to provide us with constructs that help guide research.

Another theory, also based on observation and describing five stages, is that of psychologist and bereavement researcher Catherine Sanders (1989), who identified five states of the grief process: shock, awareness of loss, withdrawal, healing, and renewal. The similarities with Kübler-Ross's stages are noteworthy. Many researchers agree with the themes presented by Kübler-Ross and Sanders, but suggest that they do not occur in set stages for all people. Rather, these studies find that the themes are intermingled, with some people ending on a positive note and others ending with feelings of anger or depression.

Death and dying are complicated and important topics that have an important place in the study of life. Over the course of the lifespan, humans have options to cope with death in various ways that are influenced by biological, psychological, and social factors.

DEATH WITH DIGNITY

No doubt most people would rather not suffer serious physical pain when they die, and many would prefer to avoid the emotional pain that often attends death. Until recently, however, it was the rare occasion when a person would have any choice. Today, debates have formed around two alternatives, both of them forms of **euthanasia** ("good death" in Greek), the act of ending a life in a painless manner to relieve or prevent suffering.

Passive euthanasia refers to refraining from continuing efforts to sustain someone's life, such as turning off life-

euthanasia The ending of a life, usually in a person with a terminal illness, to prevent a prolonged and painful death.

passive euthanasia Refraining from continuing efforts to sustain someone's life.

living will Legal document that describes specific life-prolonging medical treatments.

health-care power of attorney Legal document giving someone authority to make health-care decisions if one is incapacitated.

active euthanasia Intentionally ending a person's life.

physician-assisted suicide (PAS) Active euthanasia whereby doctors give patients death-inducing drugs.

The Funeral in Other Times and Countries

Looking at the funeral practices of former cultures shows us not only how they buried the dead, but also something about their values.

Ancient Egypt. Egyptians believed in life eternal, and thus the body of the dead person was embalmed, or treated with preservatives, in order to prevent decomposition. The body was placed in a tomb, the elegance of which was determined by family wealth and prestige.

Ancient Greece. Within a day after death the body was washed, anointed, dressed in white, and laid out for 1 to 7 days, depending on the social prestige of the deceased. The ancient Greeks prepared their tombs and arranged for subsequent care while they were still alive. About 1000 B.C.E. the Greeks began to cremate their dead. Although earth burial was never superseded, they came to believe in the power of the flame to free the soul.

The Roman Empire. For reasons of sanitation, burial within the walls of Rome was prohibited; consequently, great roads outside the city were lined with elaborate tombs erected for the well-to-do. For the poor, there was no such magnificence; for slaves and aliens, there was a common burial pit outside the city walls.

Anglo-Saxon England. The body of the deceased was placed in a hearse for the funeral procession, which included

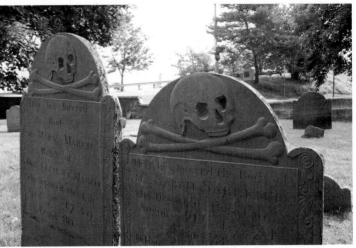

priests, friends, relatives, and strangers who deemed it their duty to join the party. Mass was sung for the dead, the body was laid in the grave (generally without a coffin), the mortuary fee was paid from the estate of the deceased, and alms in the form of money, food, or clothing were given to the poor.

Colonial New England. Neighbors or a nurse washed and laid out the body. The local woodworker built the coffin, and in special cases, metal decorations imported from England were used on the coffin. Funeral services consisted of prayers and sermons said over the cloth-covered coffin. Sermons often were printed (with skull and crossbones prominently displayed) and distributed to mourners.

---

support systems or withdrawing medicine or food. These methods can be covered by a **living will** (legal document that describes a person's wishes for specific life-prolonging treatments) or determined by the patient's **health-care power of attorney** (legal document giving someone authority to make health care decisions for one who is incapacitated).

Active euthanasia means intentionally ending a life, either through directly killing the person or by **physician-assisted suicide (PAS),** which occurs when a doctor gives a patient death-inducing drugs. It is against the law almost everywhere for the physician to give the patient a death-inducing drug, and Dr. Jack Kevorkian is a Michigan-based doctor who gained notoriety for doing precisely that. He served 8 years of a 10- to 25-year prison sentence for second-degree murder before being paroled in 2007 due to good behavior and his own failing health.

In the Netherlands, doctors administer lethal drugs to patients who request them, but with strict legal guidelines. Closer to home, a law was passed in Oregon in 1997 (upheld in 2006 by the U.S. Supreme Court) called the Death With Dignity Act. This law allows doctors to prescribe lethal medications to patients who

Career Apps

As a licensed practical nurse (LPN), what would you do if a close colleague asked you for help ending her pain and suffering by administering potentially lethal drugs to her?

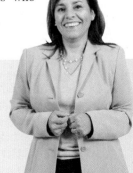

Legal attention has been brought to the subject of whether a person has the right to enlist the help of a physician to end his or her life.

> The right of a competent, terminally ill person to avoid excruciating pain and embrace a timely and dignified death bears the sanction of history and is implicit in the concept of ordered liberty. A state's categorical ban on physician assistance to suicide—as applied to competent, terminally ill patients who wish to avoid unendurable pain and hasten inevitable death—substantially interferes with this protected liberty interest and cannot be sustained.

American Civil Liberties Union, Amicus Brief, *Vacco v. Quil* (1996)

The history of the law's treatment of assisted suicide in this country has been and continues to be one of the rejection of nearly all efforts to permit it. That being the case, our decisions lead us to conclude that the asserted "right" to assistance in committing suicide is not a fundamental liberty interest protected by the Due Process Clause.

U.S. Supreme Court Majority Opinion, *Washington, et al., v. Harold Glucksberg et al.* (1997)

Which of these court decisions do you agree with? Why?

request them, but the patients must administer the medications themselves (Oregon.gov, 2007).

There is debate over the appropriateness of physician-assisted suicide (Bernat, 2001). Those who support it claim a number of advantages for the option: the time of death is up to the patient; it can be used by those for whom the hospice or hospital is inappropriate; and death is painless if the patient is given a high enough dose of morphine.

Almost 80% of Americans die in hospitals, and 70% of those deaths involve some aspect of medical technology such as breathing, feeding, and waste-elimination equipment. Therefore, it is essential that those who do not want to be maintained on life-support systems if they become terminal put their wishes in writing according to their state's laws. Open communication with one's doctor is also essential (von Gunten, Ferris, & Emanuel, 2000). This type of decision making before the end of one's life seems to be increasing and is practiced in many European countries (van der Heide et al., 2003). In England and Wales, living wills are called *advance decisions,* while in nearby Ireland they are known as *advance health-care directives.*

An increasing number of cases illustrate the ethical problems involved with maintaining the life of individuals, with the support of technical equipment, in the absence of such legal documents. Terri Schiavo collapsed in her home in 1990, due to heart failure that may have been associated with bulimia. Her husband Michael, as her legal guardian, battled against her blood relatives to allow her to be taken off the life-support mechanisms and die peacefully,

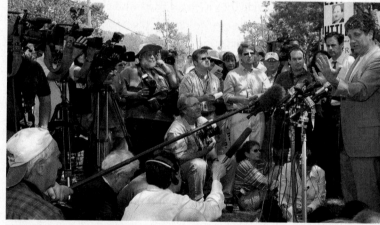
Media coverage closely followed the Terri Schiavo case.

as he claimed she would have wanted. In 2005, the courts determined that Terri Schiavo was in a vegetative state from which she could never return, and therefore her feeding tube was removed. She died 15 days later. A number of medical professionals, philosophers, and theorists have debated the issue of life support, arguing whether maintaining life under these conditions is wrong.

THE HOSPICE: "A BETTER WAY OF DYING"

In 1978, *Time* magazine brought attention to the **hospice,** a program providing comfort and supportive services to those near the end of life and to their families, stating that it provides patients "a better way of dying." At that time, hospices were still considered a new form of care, although the concept of hospice care dates back many centuries. The first U.S. hospice opened in New Haven, Connecticut, in 1974. Hospices became a more mainstream part of the American medical establishment when the hospice Medicare benefit was enacted in 1982. Since then, the National Hospice Organization has been formed to help promulgate this movement, and hundreds of groups have organized hospice programs that focus on often-neglected areas of care, such as pain management, psychological counseling for patients and their families, and recognition of terminal illness. Figure 12.4 illustrates the number of hospices per county in the United States. Currently, hospice programs in the United States are primarily home-based care, with the sponsorship of such programs evenly divided between hospitals and community agencies. Approximately 1.45 million patients were treated in U.S. hospice settings in 2008, and many insurance programs now cover hospice care.

The hospice is a relatively new philosophy of patient care in the United States. Hospice care is different from other types of care because it provides

- a team approach to caring for the individual,
- attention to the spiritual and psychological needs of patients and their families,
- pain and symptom control,
- services in the home or hospice setting, and
- family conferences and bereavement care.

The collaborative nature of hospice care is one of the major factors that distinguishes such care from hospital treatments. Hospice teams include doctors, nurses, social workers, and spiritual supports. Families are consulted to ensure that decisions are made with as much input as possible from all concerned parties.

> **hospice** A program providing comfort and supportive services to those near the end of life and to their families.

Because there is an emphasis on quality of life for the patient and family, as opposed to impending death, control of pain and symptoms are goals of hospice care. A patient is typically treated for pain with over-the-counter pain medications such as ibuprofen, aspirin, or acetaminophen. For terminally ill patients, pain levels often increase to the point where these medications no longer help. At that point, the physician will prescribe narcotic medications alone or in combination with other medications. The main objective of medication is to relieve symptoms that interfere with one's quality of life. A major goal of the hospice is to keep the person's mind as clear as possible at all times. A person whose mind is clear can think more cogently about the dying process and to explore the feelings associated with death and the meaning of dying (Dobratz, 2003).

Suicide: The Rejection of Life

There are times that people feel that their personal pain outweighs their ability to cope with the pain. Such thinking occurs in different people for different reasons, at different

FIGURE 12.4
Hospice Statistics

This map shows the number of hospices per county per capita in 2007.

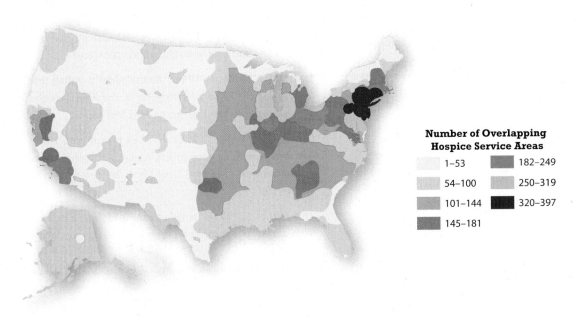

Number of Overlapping Hospice Service Areas

1–53		182–249	
54–100		250–319	
101–144		320–397	
145–181			

TABLE 12.2

Fact Sheet on Suicide: Adolescents and Young Adults

- The rate of suicide increases tenfold between early adolescence (ages 10–14) and young adulthood (ages 20–24). Suicide rates continue to increase in adulthood until age 49, decrease between ages 50-74, then increase again at age 75.

- Adolescent and young adult males aged 10–24 have a consistently higher suicide rate (84%) than their female peers.

- American Indian/Alaskan Native non-Hispanics have the highest suicide rate, 2 to 4 times that of same-age males in other racial/ethnic groups and 11 times that of same-age females. Suicide is the second leading cause of death for American Indian/Alaskan Native non-Hispanic males age 10–24. Black/non-Hispanic and Hispanic females are least likely to commit suicide (National Adolescent Health Information Center, 2006).

times of life, regardless of socioeconomic class, religion, race, or gender (see Table 12.2).

Although suicide ranks as the second leading cause of death among people 13 to 19 years of age, the rate for those 65 and older is higher—17.4 per 100,000, for non-Hispanic males (CDC, 2006b). For the elderly, poor health is often a cause of suicide because it is linked to depression.

THE INFLUENCE OF GENDER

At all ages, there are major gender differences in suicide. Males are about four times more likely to die of suicide attempts than are females, owing to the methods used, the lethality of the attempt, and a person's present state of mental health (CDC, 2006b). Attempt rates show even more dramatic gender differences. Failed attempts at suicide among females are much higher than those for males (Curran, 2006). A major reason for the high survival rate among females is the method used. Whereas males often resort to such violent and effective means as firearms and hanging, females tend to choose less violent and less deadly means, such as drug overdose. Suicide attempts for men and women may be influenced by factors such as alcohol and drug use, unemployment, divorce, and death of a spouse or other close friend or relative.

No single factor is in itself a clear cause of suicide, and no one warning sign can be a clear indicator of intent. Several factors or warning signs, however, are cause for concern (see Figure 12.5). Anyone talking about committing suicide should be taken seriously and a mental health professional should be consulted, even when you feel sure the person is only seeking attention or sympathy.

Health-care professionals can play an important role in suicide prevention, providing support and information that highlight alternatives to choosing to end one's life. Examining the practical role of community support in relation to

death sheds light on the way we handle the reality of death, which is a fundamental part of the lifespan.

Spirituality

Spirituality refers to issues affecting the spirit or soul. It may involve the attempt to better understand the reasons for living through striving to know the intentions of a higher power. While spirituality is not the same as religion, there is a clear spiritual element to organized religion, which often involves reflective practice, gathering in a specific place, and considering the self in relation to other people and places, and it specifies an accepted body of teachings that defines answers to spiritual questions.

A basic spiritual goal is trying to discern life's purpose. People engage in spiritual practices by, for example, examining historical trends and biological changes (such as the study of written texts or scientific advances) to debate the forces underlying human existence. In any case, spirituality includes all of our efforts to gain insight into the forces of life. For many, it is the only justification for moral and ethical behavior.

Spirituality does appear to develop with age. A number of theories have been offered as to how and why this is so, including those of Viennese psychoanalysts Viktor Frankl and Carl Jung and American sociobiologist E. O. Wilson.

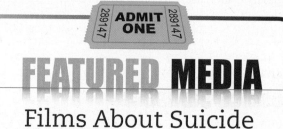

FEATURED MEDIA

Films About Suicide

Harold and Maude (1971) – After a chance meeting at a funeral, how does a life-changing relationship between a teenage boy and a 79-year-old woman blossom?

Scent of a Woman (1992) – How does a young man handle the challenge of caring for a cranky ex-colonel who has his own agenda—to end his life?

Leaving Las Vegas (1995) – When a man who thinks he's lost everything goes to Las Vegas to drink himself to death, can new love save him? Or is he determined to end his life?

The Hours (2002) – How are three different women, from three different generations, affected by the same novel?

FRANKL'S THEORY OF SPIRITUALITY

Frankl (1967) described human life as developing in three interdependent stages, according to the primary dimension of each stage:

1. *The somatic (physical) dimension.* According to the somatic dimension, all people are motivated by the struggle to keep themselves alive and to help the species survive. This intention is motivated entirely by instincts. It exists at birth and continues throughout life.

2. *The psychological dimension.* Personality begins to form at birth and develops as a result of instincts, drives, capacities, and interactions with the environment. The psychological dimension and the somatic dimension are highly developed by the time a person reaches early adulthood.

3. *The noetic dimension.* The noetic dimension has roots in childhood but primarily develops in late adolescence and beyond. It is spiritual in the totality of the search for the meaningfulness of life.

Frankl believed that development in the physical and personality dimensions results from the total sum of the influences bearing upon an individual. The developmental nature of the theory is recognizable here, as individuals acquire more skills and understanding throughout their lives, based on interactions with others and the environment. The noetic, however, is greater than the sum of its parts. This means that we as adults are responsible for inventing (or reinventing) ourselves! Whatever weaknesses or challenges we may have been given through biology or our environment, they need not govern our lives; we can and should try to overcome them.

JUNG'S THEORY OF SPIRITUALITY

Carl Jung, a student of Freud's, agreed to a large extent with Freud's description of development in the first half of human life. But he felt that Freud's ideas were inadequate to describe development during the second half of life, middle adulthood and beyond.

The First Half of Life

In Jung's view, the personality develops toward individuation, or the process of coming to know, giving expression to, and harmonizing the various components of the psyche. Most people are well individuated by the middle of life, at approximately age 35; that is, we have become distinct individuals and are most different from one another at this age (see Figure 12.6).

The Second Half of Life

The goal of human development in the second half of life is just the opposite. Somewhere around midlife, people begin turning inward, turning attention to the development of their inner self, which marks the beginning of true adult spirituality. The goals of this introspection are to discover a meaning and purpose in life, determine which values and activities one is willing to invest energy and creativity in, and prepare for the final state of life—death.

By nourishing qualities of oneself that are less developed (such as typically gender-stereotyped characteristics like sensitivity or assertiveness), one comes to recognize the spiritual and supernatural aspects of existence. The Dalai Lama has been a source of inspiration for millions of people who wish to learn how mindfulness and meditation lead to greater awareness of life's ordinary moments—pleasant as well as challenging.

WILSON'S THEORY OF SPIRITUALITY

In contrast to the self-determination of spirituality seen in Frankl's and Jung's psychological points of view, sociobiology sees spirituality as determined almost entirely by instinct—that is, as a function of genes and heredity. Harvard sociobiologist Edward O. Wilson, the leading spokesperson for the sociobiological point of view, argued that religion and spirituality are inseparable and that together they grant essential benefits to believers.

In Wilson's view, religion is one of the few uniquely human behaviors. He argues that all societies, from hunter-gatherer bands to socialist republics, have religious practices with roots that go back at least as far as the Neanderthal period. Wilson argued that humans have a need to develop simple rules for handling complex problems. Furthermore, religious learning is almost entirely unconscious—most religious tenets are taught and deeply internalized early in life.

> I find hope in the **darkest** of days, and focus in the **brightest.** I do not judge the universe.

DALAI LAMA

FIGURE 12.6

Jung's Theory, Differentiation by Age

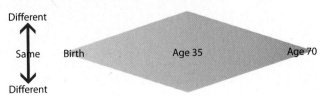

The predisposition to religious *belief is the most complex and powerful force in the human mind and in all probability an* **ineradicable** *part of human nature.*

E. O. WILSON

The sociobiological explanation of spirituality, then, is that through religious practice, the survival of practitioners is enhanced. Those who practice religion are more likely to stay alive (or at least they were in the past) than those who do not practice religion. The potential for self-sacrifice can be strengthened in this manner because the willingness of individuals to relinquish rewards or even surrender their own lives will favor group survival. The first responders who died trying to save lives in the 9/11 attacks are an excellent example.

Wilson saw science as taking the place of theology today, because science has explained natural forces more effectively than theology. In fact, he asserted that science has explained theology itself. Although he saw theology as being phased out, he argued that the demise of religion is not at all likely. As long as religions make people more likely to survive and propagate themselves, Wilson suggested, they will continue to enjoy popularity.

If I Had My Life to Live Over

The following question was asked of 122 retired people:

> If you could live your life over again, what would you do differently?

Most people responded that the pursuit of education would be the area they would most like to choose if given

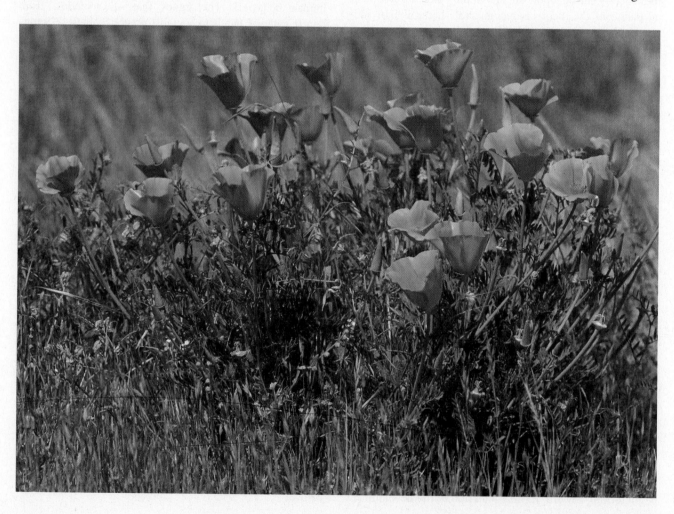

another chance. This emphasis among retirees may be because they feel their lack of education led to missed or limited opportunities. Although people indicated they would have spent more time doing a variety of things, they said that they would have spent less time worrying about work.

These feelings are summed up in this poem, attributed to Nadine Stair, an 85-year-old poet:

If I had my life to live over,
I'd dare to make more mistakes next time.
I'd relax. I would limber up.
I would be sillier than I have on this trip.
I would be crazier. I would be less hygienic.
I would take more chances, I would take more trips.
I would climb more mountains, swim more rivers, and
watch more sunsets.
I would burn more gasoline. I would eat more ice cream
and less beans.
I would have more actual troubles and fewer imaginary
ones.
You see, I am one of those people who lives
Prophylactically and sensibly and sanely,
Hour after hour, day after day.
Oh, I have had my moments
And if I had it to do over again, I'd have more of them.
In fact, I'd try to have nothing else.
Just moments, one after another.

Instead of living so many years ahead each day.
I have been one of those people who never go anywhere
Without a thermometer, a hot water bottle, a gargle, a
raincoat, and a parachute.
If I had to do it over again, I would go places and do
things.
I'd travel lighter than I have.
If I had my life to live over, I would start barefooted
Earlier in the spring and stay that way later in the fall.
I would play hooky more. I wouldn't make such good
grades except by accident.
I would ride on merry-go-rounds.
I'd pick more daisies!

As you have reached the end of this book, think back to the case study of Amshula Khare presented in Chapter 2. Knowing what you now know about lifespan development, about the biopsychosocial forces that influence us across the lifespan, what do you predict for Amshula? How might she experience adolescence, middle adulthood, or old age, based on what you know about her early childhood situation and family dynamics?

The study of the lifespan allows us to make some educated guesses about the "why" beneath all of human development. Hopefully your curiosity has been piqued and you found ideas that challenged as well as validated your opinions. Best wishes as you continue your own life's journey!

CONCLUSIONS & SUMMARY

The goal of living a good life has many meanings and takes different forms. The same may be said for achieving a successful death. The stages of death and grief reflect the values of a society and culture, and our interpretation and responses to death and spirituality, in turn, contribute in some small way to achieving a good life.

What is the role of death in life?

- Today, four types of death are recognized: clinical death, brain death, biological death, and social death.
- In modern Western societies, death comes mostly to the old. Unfortunately, this is not true in many other areas of the world.

What is the purpose of grief?

- Grief both follows and can precede the death of a loved one.
- In some cases, morbid grief reactions occur that prevent the successful conclusion of the life crisis. These are known as delayed reactions, distorted reactions, and complicated grief.
- Most experts who have examined the role of grief have concluded that it is a healthy aspect of the crisis of death.
- Funerals have always been an important part of American life. Research has indicated that the rituals surrounding funerals have therapeutic benefits that facilitate the grieving process.
- Kübler-Ross has offered five stages of dying: denial, anger, bargaining, depression, and acceptance.

What is the meaning of "successful dying"?

- The hospice movement and death with dignity legislation have provided people with more control over their own death, making it easier to accept.

What are the factors that cause and determine the nature of suicide?

- There are major gender differences in suicide, with men being more likely to die from suicide attempts than women.

How do psychologists define the nature of spirituality?

- In recent decades, participation in religious activities has been changing in a number of ways.
- Theories of spirituality have been presented by Frankl, Jung, and Wilson.

KEY TERMS

active euthanasia *288*

anticipatory grief *284*

biological death *282*

brain death *282*

cardiopulmonary resuscitation (CPR) *281*

clinical death *281*

complicated grief *286*

delayed grief *285*

distorted grief *286*

Electroencephalogram (EEG) *282*

euthanasia *288*

grief *284*

health care power of attorney *289*

hospice *291*

legal death *282*

living will *289*

mortality rate *280*

mourning *285*

passive euthanasia *289*

physician-assisted suicide *289*

psychosomatic *286*

social death *282*

[For REVIEW

1. It has been suggested that people in Western society typically avoid, or are generally uncomfortable, talking and thinking about death. If so, what factors contribute to this attitude?

2. Are there some old people—those who have lost their spouse and friends or those who are terminally ill—who should be allowed to take their own lives? If so, how should these people be supported?

3. What are some ways that you find a spiritual connection in the world, to a higher power or within yourself?

Chapter Review Test

1. The three steps involved in brain death include the cortex stopping, the midbrain failing, and function ceasing in the
   a. pituitary glands.
   b. stomach.
   c. brain stem.
   d. optic nerve.

2. The phases of anticipatory grief are
   a. depression, a heightened concern for the ill person, a rehearsal of death, and an attempt to adjust to the consequences that are likely to occur after the death.
   b. depression and rehearsal of death.
   c. a heightened concern for the ill person, a rehearsal of death, and an attempt to adjust to the consequences that are likely to occur after the death.
   d. depression, a heightened concern for the ill person, and a rehearsal of death.

Answers: 1c, 2a, 3b, 4b, 5c, 6b, 7a, 8a, 9c, 10a

3. According to Kübler-Ross's theory, dying need not be a(n) _____ experience.
   a. religious
   b. unexpected
   c. unhappy
   d. expensive

4. A young man, whose father died from lung cancer, is displaying grief known as distorted reaction. He has
   a. experienced grieving stages that are prolonged and intensified to an abnormal degree.
   b. developed some of the same symptoms his father had, which his doctor determined were entirely psychosomatic.
   c. created a shrine in memory of his father.
   d. experienced anticipatory grief.

5. Legislation that grants adults the right to instruct physicians to withhold or withdraw life-sustaining procedures in the event of a terminal condition refer to
   a. "right to life."
   b. "living with integrity."
   c. "death with dignity."
   d. None of the answers is correct.

6. Care for terminally ill people is known as
   a. visiting nurses.
   b. hospice care.
   c. behavioral medicine.
   d. home health care.

7. Whether life is worth living and why it is worth living are the major premises of
   a. spirituality.
   b. religion.
   c. separation anxiety.
   d. None of the answers is correct.

8. In what stage of Frankl's theory of spirituality are people motivated by the struggle to keep themselves alive and to help the species survive?
   a. somatic dimension
   b. psychological dimension
   c. noetic dimension
   d. None of the answers is correct.

9. According to Jung, by the age of 35, most people are well
   a. established.
   b. prepared for life's work.
   c. individuated.
   d. on their way to developing a wholeness of personality.

10. The sociobiological point of view states that we develop religion through what steps?
    a. objectification, commitment, mythification
    b. commitment and mythification
    c. objectification and mythification
    d. objection and commitment

13

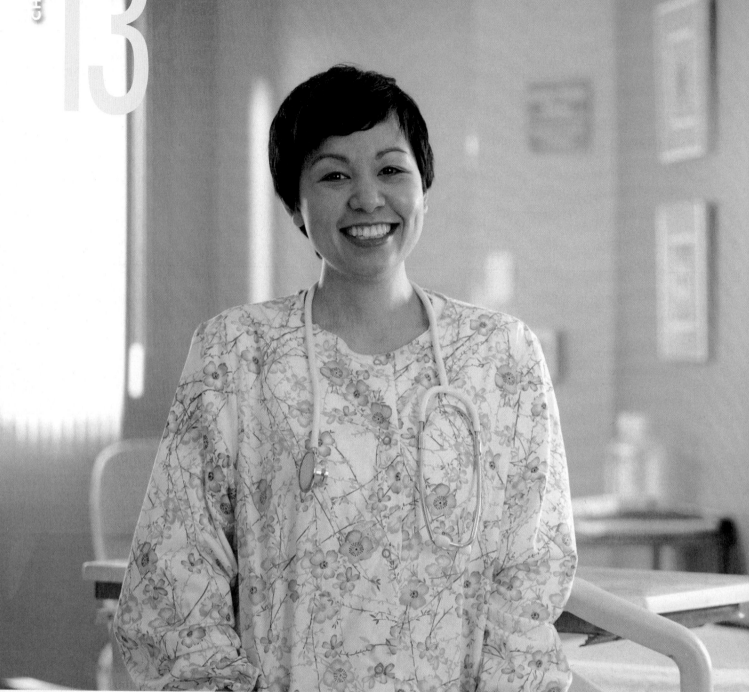

PUTTING IT ALL TOGETHER:

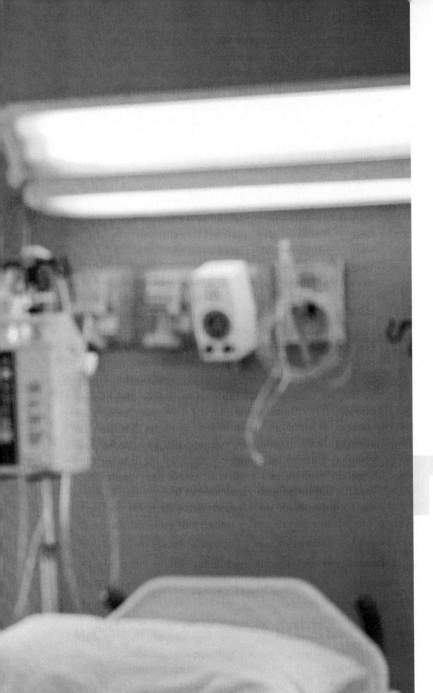

LIFESPAN DEVELOPMENT IN ACTION

As You READ

After reading this chapter, you should be able to answer the following questions:

- How are human development theories actualized in daily life?
- Who are the stakeholders in the interest of successful lifespan development?
- What are some current concerns in the field of lifespan development?
- How does history inform current practices?
- What are some careers for people interested in lifespan development?
- How can people successfully advocate for others?
- Where is the intersection between legislation and lifespan development?

Lifespan Development: It's All About You

This book began by asking you to think about one of the most compelling questions in lifespan development: "Why?" You've had an opportunity to learn about the stages of lifespan development, as well as theories that attempt to explain the way biology, psychology, and social forces influence you throughout your life. And now that you've come to the final chapter of this book, a new question is likely on your mind: "Now what?"

This chapter is focused precisely on the "Now what?" of lifespan development; *Now* that you've read the material and engaged in related classroom discussions and activities, *what* can you do to interpret and apply classic theories and facts in our current context, to consider technology as both tools and learning resources, and ultimately to consider your future? You have the power to choose to live your life in ways that reflect a set of values and expectations and that carry consequences for yourself and for the communities you live in. This chapter marks not the end but, rather, a beginning—to help you recognize the intersection between multiple forces that exist all around you and how to participate as an individual as well as a member of a group of human beings.

PUTTING THEORY INTO PRACTICE

In Chapter 2, we explored how theories present one way of interpreting a particular aspect of human development. You have learned about theories that apply to physical, cognitive, and social phenomena, and have likely felt drawn to some theories and have criticized others. Recognizing that no one theory can explain every aspect of development from all angles, across all cultures, throughout history, it is interesting to consider theories as sets of ideas that invite consideration of lifespan development from different perspectives.

Theories are essential for constructing meaning out of facts. They suggest explanations for things you witness everyday, such as why toddlers sometimes cry when they are separated from their parents or why a middle-aged man might lease a red Corvette when he turns 50. While you may be a bit more tuned in to human behavior as a result of your study of lifespan development, you many also want more than rudimentary understanding—you might seek further information or crave action. You might want to validate what you observe daily and what is important to you in your current life or work. What does it mean to actually apply a theory of lifespan development?

inquiry Investigating, questioning, following a hunch to see what happens.

action research Formal methodology that involves collaborative investigation and co-learning to solve immediate problems and contribute to greater society.

The concepts of informal inquiry, and the more formal action research, are two ways people may choose to explore and apply lifespan theories. **Inquiry** entails investigating a hunch—asking questions about something you have noticed and seeing what happens if _____.

For example, you may notice certain behaviors that people exhibit when they walk past a homeless man holding a sign on a street corner. Some people may avert their eyes; others may cross to the other side of the street to avoid contact with him, whereas other people may engage him in conversation or share money and other items with him. You may recall Maslow's hierarchy of needs and remember how challenging it is to feel self-actualized when one's basic physiological (food, shelter) and safety needs aren't met. You may wonder what would happen if people were able to view homelessness through a different lens.

Action research is a more formal methodology that includes the characteristics of an informal inquiry, but addresses the short-term problem or question identified by an individual or group, while also addressing the long-term benefit to society. Collaboration is an important aspect of action research, and participants learn together while they ask questions and attempt to solve inherent problems.

The way you put a theory into practice may be more or less direct, depending on the theory. For example, Piaget's theory of cognitive development is described in terms of specific stages, and therefore specific measures can assess which stage of development an individual is in, based on responses to specially designed questions or observational guidelines. Gardner's theory of multiple intelligences, on the other hand, does not have a specific set of benchmarks or levels that an individual is expected to reach by a certain age. Rather, individuals can use Gardner's ideas to guide how they create curriculum for children or how they assess a person's level of expertise in a specific domain, such as music. The theories can inform choices that all of us make, but they do not need to be the sole basis on which decisions are made. The lifespan is a complex experience for any one individual. Because people do not exist in isolation, lifespan development defines individual experiences that combine to impact human interactions and existence.

THE FIELD OF LIFESPAN DEVELOPMENT

The field of lifespan development has experienced tremendous growth over the past century. Lifespan development began as a field dedicated to the study of developmental psychology. Developmental psychology emerged because people recognized that the mental functions and behaviors that are the focus of traditional psychology exist in different forms at different times of life. No one had named those specific times as stages or defined them while also taking into account major areas discussed in this book, such as intelligence and personality. The influence of social factors (such as culture/ethnicity and socioeconomic status) became more important to include, and therefore it is now widely acknowledged that although a person may possess a certain intellect or personality, she cannot be examined without considering her context.

Careers that utilize the knowledge of lifespan development will continue to expand and evolve in the future. As mentioned in the previous chapter, people are living longer and more active lives, which affords more opportunities for new jobs and research on individual and interpersonal levels. Some jobs are more obviously anchored in psychology and connected to lifespan development, such as a nurse, art therapist, or director of a retirement home, than others are. Examples of jobs that have found a new and welcome home in the field, even though they are not immediately associated with lifespan development, are advertising executive (targeting different populations to sell them a given product), business manager (ensuring a business is most effective and efficient), and human resources administrator (coordinating employees and benefits for organizations). As you think about careers that interest you, what might be some future directions for the field of lifespan development?

A newer and cutting-edge area in lifespan development relates to how technology impacts human resources. A recent article featured on the National Public Radio website (http://www.npr.org) noted that the growth of social networking sites, such as Facebook, is creating a tremendous stir in the online scene. With approximately 400 million members, Facebook is the dominant social site in the United States, but it is aggressively marketing itself to users in other countries (Weeks, 2010). The connections to human resources vary. For example, someone who lives in Colorado can apply for a job in Florida, and the hiring manager can go on Facebook to see if the candidate from Colorado has a profile on Facebook or another site, simply by putting the individual's name into a web browser such as Google. This underscores the importance of recognizing that online content is public domain. In light of cyberbullying mentioned earlier in this text, that cannot be emphasized enough, and it is prompting people to rethink what types of information they put online.

From a cultural perspective, it is interesting to note that some countries, such as China, block access to social networking sites like Facebook. While this allows alternative sites, such as Qzone and RenRen, to flourish in China, it raises questions about relative values and belief systems, and politics. Other restrictions are related not to culture, but to age. The site Faceparty, based in England, was once open only to members under 36 years of age. Most sites, regardless of region, require members to be at least 13 years old to join, which links the notions of rites of passage and transitions to adulthood to these technological tools that are becoming such an important part of many societies.

Some people consider social networking sites to be a waste of time, or frivolous, but more organizations and individuals are using the sites as opportunities to bring attention to causes (such as parenting education or environmental groups) and connect with people from their past. In terms of lifespan development, there are also opportunities for technology to help alleviate human suffering. For example, work is being done to develop new sources of energy that can do everything from purifying water to generating electricity. Technology is helping some people diagnosed with cancer to live longer than once predicted. Whereas 100 years ago people were somewhat isolated, technology

is helping people connect as part of a **global community,** and this has important implications. People can no longer act and assume that they are the only ones who will experience the consequences of their actions.

> I believe that to meet the **challenge** of our times, human beings will have to develop a greater sense of universal **responsibility.** Each of us must learn to work not just for his or her own self, family or nation, but for the benefit of all **mankind.**

HIS HOLINESS, THE 14TH DALAI LAMA OF TIBET

MEET THE STAKEHOLDERS

Who are the stakeholders in the global community? The term **stakeholder** is used to refer to individuals who are affected by the actions of a larger group or organization. In a business context, the stakeholders could be the employees, administrators, or investors who are affected by the overall actions of the company. Regardless of geographic location, culture, age, or gender, people have a vested interest in their own development and basic freedoms—physical, social, emotional, economic, and political. Throughout the lifespan, people attempt to secure these freedoms in ways appropriate to their developmental stage. For example, a 3-year-old might struggle to wear a yellow sundress in winter, an adolescent might argue to stay out past parents' curfew, and a 72-year-old might strategize as to how she can best extend her pension benefits before retirement.

While we are all individuals interested in our own small pursuits, public figures such as the Dalai Lama have suggested that we need to open our eyes to the ways in which we must act for the benefit of others. The field of lifespan development recognizes the impact that psychology has on all aspects of our lives and that we are all stakeholders in the outcomes. Figure 13.1 illustrates how other countries view the U.S.

It is important to acknowledge the complex relationship between stakeholders and the environment in the global context. For example, politicians and military figures interact in the interest of multinational goals

global community Consideration of all humans in the world as being closer because of advances in technology and communication; people are united in common interests relating to health and basic freedoms.

stakeholder Individual who is affected by the actions of a larger group or organization.

humanitarian Efforts dedicated to improving the lives of human beings.

Ten lowest ratings		Ten highest ratings	
Germany	30%	Ivory Coast	88%
Indonesia	29%	Kenya	87%
Malaysia	27%	Ghana	80%
Egypt	21%	United States	80%
Jordan	20%	Mali	79%
Argentina	16%	Israel	78%
Morocco	15%	Ethiopia	77%
Pakistan	15%	Nigeria	70%
Palestinian Territories	13%	Senegal	69%
Turkey	9%	Uganda	64%

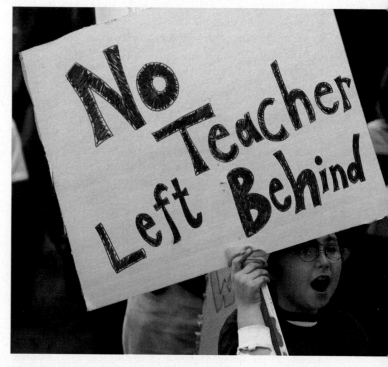

FIGURE 13.1

International U.S. Favorability Ratings

Because we exist in an interdependent global network, the consequences of our actions, both large and small, reverberate throughout the world.

Source: Kohut, 2007.

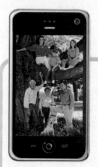

TECH TRENDS

Global Participation via Online Action

The following websites provide information and invitations to action in various **humanitarian** efforts impacting human beings on a global scale. Human, natural, and other resources are considered in different ways by different organizations, and there are volunteer opportunities for stakeholders of all ages and backgrounds.

Action Against Hunger *www.actionagainsthunger.org* – This organization is dedicated to ending world hunger, through such efforts as providing safe access to water and food, and advocating for higher levels of nutrition and sanitation.

Doctors Without Borders *www.doctorswithoutborders.org* – This international organization originated in France and provides medical aid and attention to countries whose people are threatened by crises (war, malnutrition, natural disaster).

UNICEF *www.unicef.org* –This humanitarian organization strives to improve the lives of children around the world through multiple efforts and media channels.

World Resources Institute *www.wri.org* – This organization works with businesses, governments, and the broader society to confront environmental issues that impact everyday life.

(such as nuclear arms reduction), and advances in technology make communication possible between industry leaders despite physical boundaries or language barriers. For example, an increase in migration around the world, as people move to increase their opportunities for improved quality of life, is an example of how communication facilitates human development (Human Development Report, 2009) in terms of jobs and resources. As we encounter similar issues relating to health, resources, and education, we become closer to others in those common interests that ultimately inform the chances of our survival. For this reason, even the youngest citizens are equal stakeholders, as they too share the benefits and burdens of future development.

New Horizons

The current growth potential for the field of lifespan development is distinguished by a convergence of interests (political, social, economic) that makes this a unique time in history—one rich with opportunity, but also fraught with controversy.

CURRENT CONCERNS AND CONTROVERSIES

Due to numerous advances in what we know about human development across the lifespan, and previously mentioned gains in technology and communication, different stakeholders can combine their resources and interests in new or existing programs that fall under the lifespan development umbrella. This has the potential to expand the existing range and depth of benefits to a broader scope of recipients, but it also creates conflicts.

An example of a major concern in the U.S. for the past few decades is in the education of children, primarily in public schools. The overlap with lifespan development (and the basis of conflict with educators and policymakers) exists in terms of expectations for children and what is developmentally appropriate for them in classrooms. This controversy is often summed up in debates over standardized testing. Teachers are expected to cover specific curriculum content to meet state and national standards, and schools and school districts are held accountable for student outcomes. In efforts to ensure that children indeed meet

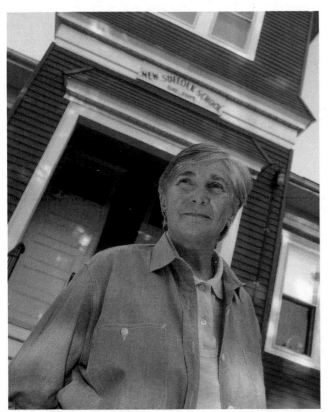

Education historian, Diane Ravitch

the standards, practices have been put in place that have resulted in teachers often "teaching to the tests," rather than to children's interests. In her latest book, *The Death and Life of the Great American School System* (2010), Diane Ravitch—an education historian who served in the offices of Presidents George H. Bush and Bill Clinton—discusses how legislation designed to advance children's learning (the No Child Left Behind Act of 2001) resulted in punitive practices such as firing teachers and withholding funds from underperforming schools. She argues that the critical variable in academic performance is not poor teaching, but poverty.

Attempts to address poverty on a grand scale require much greater effort and collaboration among government officials (national, state, and local) and all citizens. This is an example akin to what the Dalai Lama calls "universal responsibility"—doing what is right for humankind rather than focusing on narrower self-interests—and has been difficult to achieve.

HOW HISTORY INFORMS CHANGE

In recent decades, a focus on government funds and monies available to support initiatives that impact humans across the lifespan (such as health care and education) has shifted conversations from a focus on what different programs *do* to the visible *outcomes* of these programs. Figure 13.2 illustrates the decisions that federal government has made in funding state and local programs. Rather than examine how Head Start programs (begun in 1965 during Lyndon B. Johnson's presidency) support family engagement, for example, there is much research aimed at comparing math and literacy test scores of children who attended Head Start programs with children who did not attend Head Start programs. Rather than examine how Social Security (begun in 1935 during Franklin D. Roosevelt's presidency) benefits the elderly population, there is a focus on the amount of tax dollars being allocated to Social Security funds and new possibilities for spending or reallocating funds. The outcomes of research studies (such as many featured in this book) determine the success or lack of success as perceived through a particular lens. Definitions of success and subsequent funding decisions often lead to action on the part of concerned stakeholders.

You now know about physical, cognitive, and social aspects of development for people of all ages. To use the terminology of Piaget's theory, you are in the formal operational stage, which means that you can hypothesize about what is in the best interest of U.S. citizens and our global community. What this further means for you is that as debates continue to evolve as to how best support efforts aimed at improving life and livelihood in the United States and around the world, you can make educated decisions that impact the future. You can choose a career or volunteer opportunity that engages you as an agent of change.

A **change agent** is someone who helps bring about change to better

> **change agent** Someone who helps bring about change to better human lives or conditions.

Federal Grants to States and Localities, 2008

Source: Office of Management and Budget, "Aid to State and Local Governments," Budget of the United States, Fiscal Year 2008. Accessed online at www.whitehouse.gov on August 24, 2007.

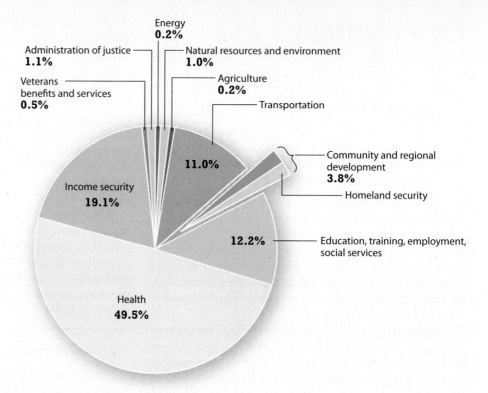

Energy
0.2%

Administration of justice
1.1%

Veterans benefits and services
0.5%

Natural resources and environment
1.0%

Agriculture
0.2%

Transportation

11.0%

Income security
19.1%

Community and regional development
3.8%

Homeland security

12.2% Education, training, employment, social services

Health
49.5%

human lives or conditions. In relation to lifespan development, change agents are people who

- *Live firmly planted in the present but are aware of future possibilities and needs.* It is one thing to be "future minded," but without a keen understanding of the impact that change will have on present-day living, future planning will remain unrealistic and often unrealized. An example of this is in the work of educator and advocate Geoffrey Canada and the many people who live and work in the Harlem Children's Zone (see Chapter 6). Canada directs the efforts of a vast network of employees, volunteers, and participants, and remains fully cognizant of the work required to get from day-to-day experiences to future success.

- *Find inspiration in their work and, in turn, motivate others to join the effort.* People often feel disappointed if their efforts don't bring about immediate results, and they miss the impact that small change can have on a broad group of people. An example of an individual who was inspired to make a difference in people's lives and spread inspiration to others is Blake Mycoskie, originator and Chief Shoe Giver at TOMS—a socially conscious company based in Santa Monica, Calif., that sells shoes on the "One for One" premise. For every pair of TOMS shoes that is purchased, TOMS donates one pair of new shoes to a child in need. Estimates are that 300,000 pairs of shoes will have been delivered to children living in developing countries by the end of 2010, and the movement is gaining momentum on college campuses and among celebrities.

- *Understand people and acknowledge them as the most important resource.* It is important to motivate people to

enact change, but it is critical to recognize that without human effort behind the change, the change will likely not have any powerful, long-term impact. An example of a person who embodies this aspect of change is Michelle Bachelet, who recently ended her term as first female president of Chile. Bachelet grew up the daughter of a military general who was charged with treason during the 1973 coup of General Augusto Pinochet and died during imprisonment. Bachelet studied medicine so that she could have a career that would directly impact human lives. In 2000, she was appointed minister of health in Chile, and in 2006, she was elected president. Her 4-year term as president received extremely high and low approval ratings, but she ended her tenure as president with an approval rating of 84%. During her term, she made social protection and equal opportunities her priorities, which included the building of thousands of day-care facilities and free health-care benefits to her fellow citizens. Chile does not allow successive terms for presidents, but Bachelet has not ruled out running in 2014. She was featured in the top 25 lists of *Forbes* magazine and *Time* magazine for power and influence.

LEADERSHIP OPPORTUNITIES

Leadership relating to lifespan development exists in many arenas, ranging from psychology to teaching to public health to politics. Opportunities for leadership are constantly changing. Leadership in the field of lifespan development involves coordinating existing networks of individuals and organizations, and reaching local, state, and national levels to advance specific interests. Today's leaders in the field will help define the field for tomorrow, and therefore it is important to iden-

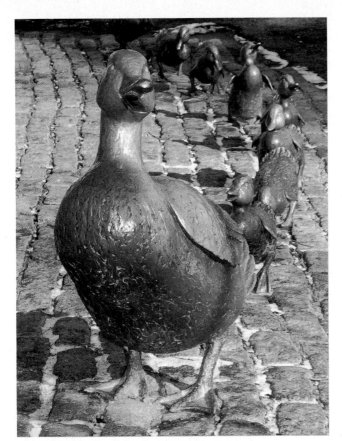

The Make Way for Ducklings statue in Boston's public garden represents determination and caring.

tify some traditional leadership roles, while acknowledging the prospect of new leadership territory.

An example of a leader in the field of lifespan development is Marion Wright Edelman, the founder and president of the Children's Defense Fund. In her leadership role for the organization, Edelman crosses boundaries that often separate distinct fields (political, business, health) as she advocates for children and families who are disadvantaged due to poverty or other life circumstances. She is as active promoting the development of Freedom Schools (designed to provide summer and after-school experiences aimed at improving children's academic skills and love of learning) as she is lobbying Congress to pass legislation that will impact health care for American citizens. The Children's Defense Fund Freedom Schools model is growing to include elementary schools across the country. Edelman embodies the passion and knowledge of human development needed to inspire action in others that will impact not only the present lives of many individuals, but future generations as well.

Other leadership opportunities exist on a more humble scale but have tremendous impact. Parents of a child diagnosed with cancer started an organization named Cookies for Kids' Cancer, based on the simple "bake sale to raise money" concept. Committed to help fight pediatric cancers and raise awareness while providing other people with a vehicle to help, this organization has grown and is helping to support research for new treatments and therapies. Inspiring others to hold bake sales, the leaders of this orga-

nization have watched the mission continue to reach greater numbers of people who want to make a difference, and it doesn't require a professional degree, just passion.

Professionalism in the Field of Lifespan Development

Because the field of lifespan development is strongly rooted in psychology, the bulk of careers in the field tend to be linked to psychology and to a general area referred to as the **helping professions.** Helping professions are professions that relate to people's physical, cognitive (including psychological and intellectual), and social-emotional (including spiritual) well-being.

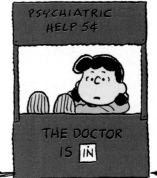

PEANUTS © United Features Syndicate, Inc.

CAREER CHOICES AND CONSIDERATIONS

Knowledge of lifespan development is beneficial, if not required, in many fields. People who possess an understanding of the physical, cognitive, and social interactions throughout the lifespan will have greater insight into what is developmentally appropriate in a variety of areas. It may seem obvious that teachers and nurses need to possess knowledge about what constitutes typical development (physical, cognitive, and social) at different ages. But other fields, such as business and technology, also benefit from knowledge of lifespan development. For example, the manager of a company who recognizes that his employees need support in their role as parents, due to dual demands of family and career, will seek to provide an environment that reflects care and consideration for families. Similarly, an employee who recognizes the importance of social networking, and the opportunities afforded by technology, will be able to anticipate new opportunities for increasing social interactions between age groups and perhaps carve out a new niche in this rapidly expanding area.

Specific coursework relating to psychology has been shown to make a difference in the career choices students make. Macera and Cohen (2006) conducted a study with 168 undergraduate students enrolled in a course titled "Psychology as a Profession." The researchers found that the course affected the career plans of nearly all the students—62% of students reported changing their career plans as a result of the course, and 20% of the students claimed to feel

helping professions
Professions that relate to people's physical, cognitive, and social-emotional well-being.

TABLE 13.1

Careers in Lifespan Development/Helping Professions

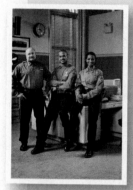

Business
Personnel Department Specialist, Human Resources Administrator, Employee Mental Health Coordinator, Department Manager

Communications
Editor, Librarian, Museum Curator, Journalist

Criminal Justice
Correctional Officer, Lawyer, Probation Officer, Police Detective

Education
PreK-12 Classroom Teacher, Early Childhood Teacher, College Professor, Educational Tutor, School Administrator

Elderly Services
Senior Living Manager, Nursing Home Manager, Recreation Advisor

Medicine
Physician, Physician Assistant, Nutritionist/Dietician, Nurse, Certified Nursing Assistant, Developmental Disabilities, Program Manager, Health Violations Inspector, Communicable Disease Prevention Coordinator, Muscular Therapist, Acupuncturist, Epidemiologist (epidemics specialist)

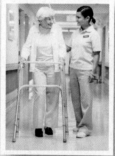

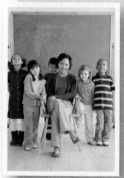

Mental Health
Clinical psychologist, Psychotherapist, Art/Expressive Therapist, Holistic Health Specialist, School Counselor, Life Coach, Substance Abuse Counselor

Public Service
Social Worker, Homeless Assistance Program Coordinator, Agricultural Agent, Public Health Agent, At-Risk Youth Program Coordinator, Parenting Educator, Veterans Service Manager

idea. A human development specialist would be able to assist in the development of programs in public schools, for instance, as the specialist would know about expectations for today's children and aspirations for tomorrow's adults. There are currently jobs and licensure requirements, such as for social workers and child life specialists, with enough overlap in the knowledge and expertise required in those roles, that demand for a human development specialist is not great enough to warrant immediate action by the APA. The absence of a license can, however, cause some confusion about just what human development experts are qualified to do. There are, however, a wide range of jobs for those with a background and interest in lifespan development, as Table 13.1 shows.

Some jobs in the field of lifespan development require a graduate degree, such as a master's degree in clinical psychology or social work, which leads to very specific jobs. This preparation has the advantage of assuring recipients that they will be prepared to pass licensing tests and qualify for a specific job. This works well when jobs are plentiful, but in times of economic crisis, job choices may become limited as more qualified people vie for fewer positions.

Most services provided by people in the helping professions are rendered by individuals who possess a master's degree, whereas supervisory and administrative positions in the field are often held by people who possess a doctoral degree. Depending on the specific job, there are considerations to be made about graduate schools and the programs they offer, such as whether or not an institution is accredited. For example, those in the field who hire new professionals in the field of psychology are aware of the difference between a master's-level licensed mental health provider and a clinical psychologist with a PhD. The main distinction is that a doctorate involves more research and applied theory and assessment than a master's degree.

There are two categories of doctoral work that a person interested in a psychology career should investigate—doctor of philosophy (PhD) and doctor of psychology (PsyD). Both doctorates lead to a license in psychology that entails postdoctoral supervised experience hours, but PsyD programs tend to be less research-oriented and more practice-oriented than PhD programs. When considering careers, it is important to explore all possibilities before making a commitment in terms of time and expenses.

EFFORT REWARDED: FINANCIAL VERSUS EMOTIONAL COMPENSATION

In a recent report, *Money* magazine listed the top 10 jobs in America (Table 13.2) based on responses to survey data that asked more than 35,000 workers questions about job flexibility, stress, satisfaction, and quality of life. The list was first compiled using criteria that included jobs predicted to grow 10% or more over the next 10 years (as determined by the U.S. Bureau of Labor Statistics); require at least a bachelor's degree; demonstrate a median pay of at least $65,000 a year for experienced workers; and have

more confident about their career plans as a result of the course. The results suggest that an undergraduate psychology course that includes academic advising and career planning is quite helpful in guiding students along their career paths.

The options for graduates with a background in lifespan development coursework are plentiful. Although there is not yet a specific job called "licensed human development specialist," there has been some discussion within the American Psychological Association (APA) about this

TABLE 13.2

Best Jobs in America (2009)

Rank	Job Title	Job Growth (10 yr. forecast)
1	Systems Engineer	45%
2	Physician Assistant	27%
3	College Professor	23%
4	Nurse-Practitioner	23%
5	Information Technology Project Manager	16%
6	Certified Public Accountant	18%
7	Physical Therapist	27%
8	Computer/Network Security Consultant	27%
9	Intelligence Analyst	15%
10	Sales Director	10%

Source: Adapted from CNNMoney.com, 2009.

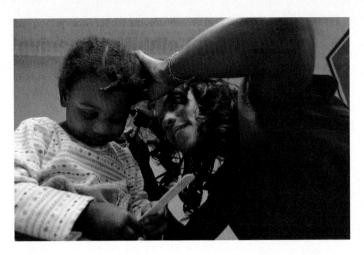

more than 10,000 positions of record nationwide. The list was whittled down further by eliminating jobs that fared poorly during the recession.

It is interesting to see several jobs listed in the top 10 that fall directly under the category of helping professions: physician assistant, college professor, nurse-practitioner, and physical therapist. Other jobs, such as intelligence analyst or sales director, have an indirect relationship to lifespan development in terms of work with people and information that will impact people's lives. Jobs that are heavily linked to technology offer a new perspective on "helping" in that they too can have a more or less direct impact on the lifespan, depending on the specific tasks involved in the work.

Among the jobs listed in the helping professions, there is a clear difference in salary. For example, a physician assistant earned an average of $64,094 in 2009, while a college professor earned $47,559. Compare these salaries with the 2009 salary of New York Yankees shortstop Derek Jeter ($21,000,000) or Miley Cyrus's 2009 earnings estimated at $29,000,000. There is often a moment of soul-searching that people who choose careers in the helping professions experience: They notice the salaries that top athletes and performers receive and question the respect for helping professions in society when compensation and direct impact on human lives seems so unbalanced.

It is provocative to consider the impact of jobs in sports and entertainment on human lives and livelihood compared to that of careers in medicine and education, but it is not realistic to draw a clean comparison between those dramatically different fields. It is important to remember that the small number of elite athletes and performers rests at the tip of a mountain of aspiring athletes and performers who do not receive millions of dollars for their work.

Recent research indicates that the impact of strong teachers does indeed last a lifetime (Leonhardt, 2010). Convinced that quality early education is essential, Tennessee researchers involved in Project Star gathered data to propose an estimated kindergarten teacher salary of $320,000. While the likelihood of such a teacher's salary seems small in our culture and economy, it is important to consider the value of investments—both personal and financial.

perspectives on Diversity

Teacher Salaries Around the World

An investigation into the salaries of teachers around the world reveals some interesting differences in amount of compensation. Further investigation is required to fully understand the values and practices that are intricately woven into the decisions about how much an elementary school teacher earns yearly in the following countries:

Japan — 156,500 yen a month (new teacher)– 292, 500 yen a month (head teacher) Equivalent to $1,704.51–$3,185.74 U.S. dollars a month

New Zealand — 56,467–70,583 New Zealand dollars a year Equivalent to $40,000–$50,000 U.S. dollars a year

South Africa — 115,276–146,088 South African rand Equivalent to $15,511.88–$19,658.97 U.S. dollars

United States — $51,000 new teacher salary

Data adapted from http://www.educationworld.net and http://www.teacherportal.com.

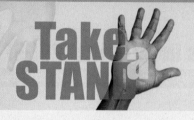

Estimates for the jobless rate in the United States are 9.9–10.1% for 2010, 8.2–8.6% for 2011, and 6.8–7.5% for 2012 (Lanman, 2009). While the slight decline in potential unemployment is encouraging, the percentages still translate into thousands of people who will be out of work. Yet a person walking down the main streets of most cities will no doubt see plenty of people drinking cups of coffee purchased from a local coffee chain or wearing clothes featuring designer labels.

What factors into a person's decision to spend money? Is there a distinction between "extras" versus necessities, and what role does each play in people's perceptions of their own success or happiness?

Individual passions and personality traits motivate people toward the careers they ultimately pursue. Researchers have found that people who are drawn to careers in psychology tend to have higher levels of empathy than those who pursue other careers (Harton & Lyons, 2003). Empathy or compassion may indeed impact a person's decision to choose a career that is not as potentially lucrative as other careers, but is satisfying for its positive impact on other people. Other characteristics and life circumstances can influence decisions as well, such as discipline and desire to interact with people on a daily basis.

RESPONSIBILITY TO SELF AND OTHERS

As you contemplate career paths and professionalism in the field of lifespan development, consider too the levels of responsibility associated with different choices. Different jobs require different levels of accountability to oneself and to the public. Those working in the field of lifespan development or helping professions often are held accountable to public opinion. This accountability is critical, because funding and support for programming relies on public confidence. For example, if the public perceives that impoverished students who attended Head Start programs receive higher scores on math tests than impoverished students who did not, then chances are great that Head Start programs will receive funds to continue their work. If the public sees that a decision to increase the minimum wage increases employment, then services that are utilized to financially support unemployed citizens will be less burdened and those funds can be reallocated into other programs.

In the United States, the democratic underpinnings of society place fundamental emphasis on the power of an

FIGURE 13.3

Voter Turnout in Presidential Elections, 1948–2008

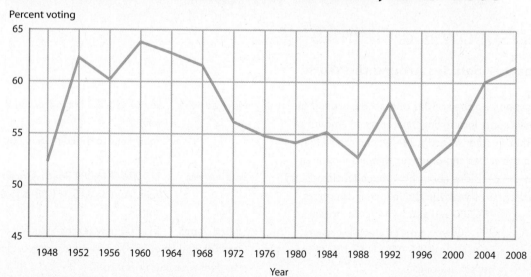

Source: U.S. Census Bureau, Voting Age Citizen Population.

individual to make decisions that represent the interests and needs of a larger group. Every time an election takes place, individuals exercise their rights to make decisions. Figure 13.3 illustrates the levels of voter participation in U.S. elections between 1972 and 2004. The political system relies on individuals to realize these interests and advocate for causes that benefit individuals across the lifespan. If certain groups of people are not voting in public elections, it is important to consider the impact that the absence of representation has on their daily lives and future development. Efforts to represent people who cannot or choose not to represent their own interests are prominently represented in the field of lifespan development.

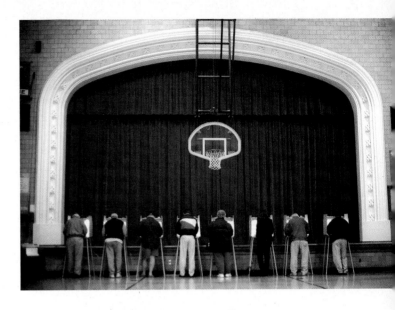

Advocacy in the Field of Lifespan Development

To **advocate** is to actively work on behalf of a person, cause, or idea. You have every opportunity to actively work with or for others in the interest of a topic that relates to lifespan development.

SURVEYING THE LANDSCAPE

The landscape is consistently changing in the field of lifespan development. Every new scientific study seems to give rise to a new recommendation that has the potential to influence people's lives. As you have seen throughout this book, one theory or set of ideas inspires other people to question or validate the tenets of the theory. Sometimes the only visible changes stem from discussions about a given topic, much as you have experienced discussions in your classes. The impact of small changes, however, can be quite large.

> **advocate** To actively work on behalf of a person, cause, or idea.
>
> **policy** A course of action to guide and determine decisions.

Throughout history, individuals have taken steps to advocate for people who are unable to pursue their own best interests, often at personal cost. For example, Nelson Mandela served 27 years in a South African prison because of his anti-apartheid activism. As a result, his political notoriety brought attention to the racial segregation activities of countless African groups. In 1994, Mandela was elected president of South Africa in the country's first fully democratic election.

IMPLICATIONS FOR POLICY AND PRACTICE

When the efforts of a person or group change others' everyday experiences, the results are sometimes large enough to result in new thinking and behavior in the field. Leadership can frame the future, but policy ensures that change is enforced in a uniform way. A **policy** may be defined as a course of action to guide and determine decisions, and typically emerges as a response to a specific problem that has been identified through advocacy efforts.

Policies exist on federal, state, and local levels, and are often (but not always) linked to legislation. For example, there are national policies related to employment, such as the Family Medical Leave Act (FMLA), which ensures that family members have the right to leave work for an extended period of time (12 weeks within a calendar year) to care for newborn children or for family members with a serious health condition. If an employer fails to abide by the guidelines spelled out in FMLA, the company can face

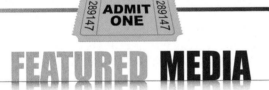

Films About Advocates and Advocacy

The Blind Side (2009) – What inspires a woman to adopt a homeless boy and support him and his dreams of playing football?

The Client (1994) – How can a young boy bring down a mob family and escape from harm under the support of a determined lawyer?

Gandhi (1982) – How does a lawyer lead the Indian revolution against British rule, inspiring others through peaceful protest?

Up (2009) – How do a 78-year-old man and an 8-year-old boy reconcile their dreams and engage in the adventure of a lifetime?

Individuals with Disabilities Education Act (IDEA) Law that details rights and guidelines for students with disabilities in the United States.

serious consequences, such as high fines.

Universities often maintain attendance policies that are detailed in student handbooks or academic websites. If students fail to adhere to the details of an attendance policy, they face penalties that can negatively impact their grades. Preschool teachers may create a policy about how much time children can spend on tricycles before it is another classmate's turn. If a child fails to share the tricycle, a teacher may need to enforce the consequences. Although policies can be linked to legislation, it is clear that legal strings need not be attached to influence behavior. There is a developmental quality to policy—regardless of a person's age, there is a requisite willingness of individuals to follow the policy and the need for appropriate consequences to enforce it.

Legislation and Lifespan Development

In lifespan development, policy decisions that are legally enforced often stem from tragic events and personal experiences, in attempts to protect the greater good. For example, Upton Sinclair's novel *The Jungle,* published serially in 1905, was an exposé about unsafe practices in the meatpacking industry in Chicago that helped lead to the Pure Food and Drug Act of 1906.

Some examples of legislation that has been developed in the past century to protect individuals' rights throughout the lifespan include laws related to disabilities, sexual orientation, and gender.

- *IDEA.* The **Individuals with Disabilities Education Act (IDEA)** is the law that specifies rights and guidelines for students in the United States who require special education services. The law describes the services that

schools must provide and how parents can advocate so that their children receive the benefits of these services. Two key features of the law are that students with disabilities are entitled to a free appropriate public education and that it occurs in the least-restrictive environment.

- *Matthew Shepard Act.* This law (officially the *Matthew Shepard and James Byrd, Jr. Hate Crimes Prevention Act*) was signed in October 2009 and expands federal hate crimes law enacted over 30 years ago. The law now includes crimes directed against a person due to the individual's real or perceived gender, sexual orientation, or disability. It is the first federal law to extend protection to transgender individuals. The law removes previous requirements that the victim be in the process of a federally protected activity at the time of the crime, such as voting or attending public school. It also grants federal authorities more rights to investigate crimes, despite efforts (or lack of) on the part of local law enforcement.

- *Title IX.* Renamed in 2002 the *Patsy T. Mink Equal Opportunity in Education Act,* but commonly referred to as Title IX, this law specifies that no U.S. citizen can, on the basis of sex, be denied the right to participate in or receive benefits from, or be subjected to discrimination under, an education program or activity that receives financial assistance from the U.S. government. This law is typically associated with high school and collegiate athletics even though the original focus of the law was on all aspects of academic life.

These examples illustrate how people in the United States have responded to the social and political forces around them in the interest of basic freedoms. As you continue to explore the nuances of lifespan development, primarily by living it, you may be inspired to bring positive change to the lives of others in the capacity that best fits your needs and interests. You are the protagonist in your own lifespan—so let the curtain rise as a new chapter begins.

CONCLUSIONS & SUMMARY

What are the implications of the study of lifespan development on multiple facets of a person's life?

- Lifespan development theory can be applied to everyday life in many ways.
- The field of lifespan development involves stakeholders of all ages and all levels of power within our societal framework.

How do some ideas change with the times to remain current, while some enduring ideas exist and reemerge throughout history?

- Recognizing one's role as an individual and as a member of a larger group reflects U.S. political history (democracy) and contemporary priorities in lifespan development. Opportunities to advocate for others and as change agents position individuals in roles that can benefit a larger group.

Why do career choices in lifespan development tend to center on the helping professions?

- Different expectations and qualifications exist for specific jobs and career paths.
- There is a distinction between jobs that bring financial reward and fame and jobs that provide emotional fulfillment, although they are not mutually exclusive.
- Leadership opportunities exist for people engaged in specific efforts across the lifespan.

How can individuals and groups use advocacy efforts to affect societal change?

- The current landscape affords opportunities for development of policy in the interest of the greater good.
- Some examples of legislation that has been developed in the past century to protect individuals' rights throughout the lifespan include laws related to disabilities, sexual orientation, and gender.

KEY TERMS

action research *300*

advocate *309*

change agent *303*

global community *301*

helping professions *305*

humanitarian *302*

Individuals with Disabilities Education Act (IDEA) *310*

inquiry *300*

policy *309*

stakeholder *301*

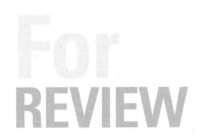

1. What theories (or aspects of theories) of lifespan development most inspire you? How might you incorporate some of those theories into activities that are important to you?

2. What actions can you take to influence policy around a practice or idea that you have observed in the media or in your own life?

3. Describe your dream job. What steps will you need to take to achieve your goals?

Chapter Review Test

1. Theories are essential for constructing meaning out of
   a. facts.
   b. documentaries.
   c. development.
   d. distractions.

2. Developmental psychology emerged because people realized that the mind and related _____ exist in different forms at different times of life.
   a. body
   b. career choices
   c. behaviors
   d. characters

3. An example of a job *not* typically associated with lifespan development is
   a. nurse.
   b. psychologist.
   c. college professor.
   d. advertising executive.

4. A cutting-edge area of lifespan development relates to technology and how it can be used to alleviate
   a. back pain.
   b. human suffering.
   c. teacher salaries.
   d. discrimination.

Answers: 1a, 2c, 3d, 4b, 5c, 6b, 7a, 8a, 9d, 10c

5. The notion that all humans in the world are closer because of advances in technology and communication defines
   a. advocacy.
   b. change agent.
   c. global community.
   d. helping profession.

6. Politicians, military figures, investors, industrial leaders, and young children are all equal _____ in lifespan development.
   a. advocates
   b. stakeholders
   c. physicians
   d. activists

7. Someone who acts in the interest of making people's lives better is known as a
   a. change agent.
   b. supervisor.
   c. mentor.
   d. probate officer.

8. Individuals who choose jobs in the helping professions have been shown to have high levels of
   a. empathy.
   b. serotonin.
   c. intelligence.
   d. fairness.

9. There is a distinction between jobs that garner financial reward and those that provide _____ compensation.
   a. physical
   b. lucrative
   c. autonomous
   d. emotional

10. A person who actively works on behalf of a person, cause, or idea is called a(n)
    a. mentor.
    b. guru.
    c. advocate.
    d. equalizer.

Glossary

accommodation   Piaget's term to describe the manner by which cognitive structures change.   *35*

achieved identity   A sense of one's self based on personal effort and commitment.   *210*

action research   Formal methodology that involves collaborative investigation and co-learning to solve immediate problems and contribute to greater society.   *300*

active euthanasia   Intentionally ending a person's life.   *289*

activity theory   Humans flourish/thrive through interactions with others and physical activity, and suffer in the absence of such stimulation.   *271*

adaptation   One of the two functional invariants in Piaget's theory.   *35*

adolescent egocentrism   Self-centered thinking patterns of childhood that sometimes occur in the teen years.   *192*

adoption   The process of voluntarily taking a child of other parents as one's own.   *64*

advocate   To actively work on behalf of a person, cause, or idea.   *309*

afterbirth   Stage 3 of the birth process in which the placenta and other membranes are discharged.   *82*

ageism   Stereotyping or unfair treatment of individuals or groups because of their age.   *256*

aging by program   Theory that we age because aging is programmed into us.   *258*

AIDS (acquired immune deficiency syndrome)   Disease caused by the HIV virus, which can invade a newborn baby's immune system, thus making it vulnerable to infections and life-threatening illnesses.   *72*

Alzheimer's disease   Brain disease involving progressive, irreversible loss of neurons and manifesting as impaired memory, judgment, decision making, orientation to the environment, and language.   *263*

amniocentesis   Fetal testing procedure that involves inserting a needle through the woman's abdomen, piercing the amniotic sac, and withdrawing a sample of amniotic fluid.   *68*

amniotic sac   Fluid-filled uterine sac that surrounds the embryo/fetus.   *65*

analgesics   Mild medications used to alleviate pain; may be used before and during labor.   *84*

analytic intelligence   Sternberg's term to describe a person's ability to break down a problem or situation into the smaller parts of the whole.   *240*

androgyny   Gender-role identification that allows expression of both male and female gender roles.   *217*

anesthetics   Stronger medications used during labor to control pain; can numb mother to pain in the various stages of labor.   *84*

animism   Children's preoperational activity in which they consider inanimate objects to possess human thought, feelings, and actions.   *133*

anorexia nervosa   An eating disorder characterized by low body weight and distorted body image.   *190*

anoxia   Insufficient oxygen supply during labor and delivery, which can cause fetal brain damage or death.   *87*

anticipatory grief   Grief that is experienced before the death of a person.   *285*

Apgar scale   A test to evaluate a newborn's basic life signs administered at 1 minute and 5 minutes after birth.   *94*

apnea   Brief periods when breathing is suspended.   *92*

arthritis   Tissue inflammation in and around the joints.   *262*

artificial intelligence   Human intelligence simulated by machines; a specific field of computer science.   *107*

ascribed identity   A sense of one's self based on determination of others, not the individual.   *210*

assimilation   Piaget's term to describe the manner in which we incorporate data into our cognitive structures.   *35*

assisted reproduction technologies   External fertilization procedures; fertilization occurs with help outside the woman's body.   *64*

asthma   Lung disorder resulting in bronchial tubes filling with mucus and tightening.   *157*

attachment   Behavior intended to keep a child (or adult) in close proximity to a significant other.   *121*

attention deficit disorder   A disability related to inattention and lack of focus.   *159*

attention deficit hyperactivity disorder (ADHD)   A disability related to inattention, hyperactivity, and impulsivity.   *159*

authoritarian parenting   Baumrind's term for parents who are demanding and want immediate obedience as the most desirable trait in a child.   *143*

authoritative parenting   Baumrind's term for parents who respond to their child's needs and wishes; they believe in parental control and attempt to explain the reasons for it to their child.   *143*

autoimmunity   Process by which the immune system in the body rejects the body's own tissue.   *258*

autonomous morality   Piaget's term for moral development in children after age 11; actions must be thought of in terms of intentions and consequences.   *168*

axons   Branchlike ends of neurons that send electrochemical signals between cells.   *106*

B

babbling Infants' production of sounds approximating speech between 5 and 7 months. *117*

Babinski reflex Automatic response in which an infant's toes spread out in response to stroking the sole of the foot from heel to toes. *93*

basal metabolism rate (BMR) The minimum amount of energy a person uses when in a resting state. *234*

battered child syndrome A combination of physical and other signs that indicate a child's injuries result from physical abuse. *179*

bioecological model The continuity and change in the biopsychosocial characteristics of human beings, both as individuals and as groups. *42*

biological death Occurs when it is no longer possible to discern an electrical charge in the tissues of the heart and lungs. *282*

biopsychosocial interactions Biological, psychological, and social/environmental forces that combine to impact human development across the lifespan. *5*

blastocyst The fertilized egg when it reaches the uterus (about 7 days after conception). *65*

body mass index (BMI) Measurement used to compare a person's height and weight to determine a healthy body weight. *158*

bonding The formation of a close connection between newborn and caregiver, typically parents. *96*

brain death Occurs when the brain fails to receive a sufficient supply of oxygen for a short period of time (usually 8 to 10 minutes). *282*

Braxton-Hicks contractions Relatively mild muscle contractions that occur before real contractions begin. *80*

Brazelton Neonatal Behavioral Assessment Scale Device to assess an infant's behavior; examines both neurological and psychological responses. *94*

breech birth Birth in which the baby is born feet first, buttocks first, or in a crosswise position (transverse presentation). *85*

bulimia nervosa An eating disorder featuring binge eating and purging. *191*

bullying The act of using verbal or physical means to intimidate or embarrass someone else. *175*

C

cardiopulmonary resuscitation (CPR) Technique for reviving an individual's lungs and heart that have ceased to function. *282*

cataracts Thickening of the eye lenses; cause blurred, cloudy vision. *261*

centration Feature of preoperational thought; the centering of attention on one aspect of an object and the neglecting of any other features. *134*

cerebral palsy A condition resulting from an inability of the brain to control the body; result of brain damage before, during, or after delivery. *88*

cesarean section Surgery performed to deliver the baby through the abdomen if the baby cannot come through the birth canal. *85*

change agent Someone who helps bring about change to better human lives or conditions. *303*

child abuse Infliction of injury to a child; commonly includes physical, sexual, and emotional abuse, or neglect. *179*

cholesterol Substance in the blood that can adhere to the walls of the blood vessels, restricting blood flow and causing strokes and heart attacks. *211*

chorionic villi sampling (CVS) A prenatal test that examines a small section of the embryo's outer layer. *68*

chromosomes Threadlike structures in the cell that come in 23 pairs (46 total) and contain the genetic material DNA. Each parent contributes half of each chromosome pair. *54*

circular reactions Piaget's term for infants' motor activity that is repeated in developing stages. *112*

classical conditioning The learning process in which a neutral stimulus produces an involuntary response that is usually elicited by another stimulus. *39*

classification Ability to group objects with some similarities within a larger category. *134*

climacteric The midlife change in hormone levels that affects fertility. *237*

clinical death The individual is dead when his or her respiration and heartbeat have stopped. *281*

clique Group of friends who share similar interests and activities. *196*

closed adoption Adoption procedures in which the biological parents know nothing about the adopting parents. *64*

code of ethics A guiding set of principles for members of a particular group. *22*

cognitive structures Piaget's term to describe the basic tools of cognitive development. *34*

cohabitation A living arrangement in which unmarried partners share a residence and personal assets and sometimes have a child. *221*

collagen Major connective tissue in the body; provides the elasticity in human skin and blood vessels. *258*

competence The ability to do something well. *173*

complicated grief Prolonged and intensified grief; may take weeks or months to pass. *286*

concrete operational stage Piaget's third stage of cognitive development, between the ages of 7 and 11 years, in which children's thinking is much more flexible than in early childhood. *160*

conservation The understanding that an object retains certain properties even though surface features change. *135*

constructivism The belief that children create, organize, and transform knowledge through active engagement in their environment. *136*

constructivist approach Learning approach in which children are encouraged to be active participants in constructing knowledge and learn by interacting with their environment. *138*

continuity The lasting quality of experiences; development proceeds steadily and sequentially. *16*

convergent thinking Thinking used when a problem to be solved has one correct answer. *193*

cooing Early language sounds that resemble vowels. *117*

coordination of secondary schemes Piaget's term for when infants combine secondary schemes to obtain a goal. *113*

crawling Movement on hands and knees; the trunk does not touch the ground. *108*

creative intelligence Sternberg's term to describe a person's ability to solve problems in unique ways and to feel comfortable with new or different situations and ideas. *240*

creeping Movement whereby the infant's abdomen touches the floor and the weight of the head and shoulders rests on the elbows. *107*

cross-linkage theory The theory that, when cross-links are formed between peptides, the proteins are altered, often for the worse. *258*

cross-sectional studies Studies that compare groups of individuals of various ages at the same time. *20*

crowd Reputation-based group whose members may or may not spend time with one another. *196*

crystallized intelligence Accumulated information and verbal skills over time, reflecting the effect of culture and learning; allows a person to make connections between information and/or objects. *239*

culture The customs, values, and traditions inherent in one's environment. *14*

cystic fibrosis (CF) Chromosomal disorder producing a malfunction of the exocrine glands. *60*

cytomegalovirus (CMV) A widespread infection, often unrecognized in pregnant women, that can cause severe fetal damage. *72*

D

date rape Coercive sexual activity between a victim and an offender who is known or an acquaintance. *214*

day care Services and care for children provided outside the children's home. *145*

decentration The ability to focus on several features of an object or task. *161*

decode To pronounce words correctly using knowledge of letters and sounds. *159*

defense mechanisms Psychological strategies to cope with anxiety or perceived threats. *30*

deferred imitation Children's preoperational behavior that continues after they witnessed the original action or event. *134*

delayed grief Grief that is postponed for an inordinate time. *286*

dementia Deterioration of cognitive function over time caused by brain infection or disease. *263*

dendrites Branchlike ends of neurons that receive and conduct the electrochemical signals between the cells. *106*

descriptive studies Studies that gather information on subjects without manipulating them in any way. *17*

DES (diethylstilbestrol) A synthetic hormone that was administered to pregnant women in the late 1940s and 1950s supposedly to prevent miscarriage. It was later found that the daughters of the women who had received this treatment were more susceptible to vaginal and cervical cancer. *73*

despair The negative resolution of Erikson's last stage; individuals look back over their lives and feel that they have made many wrong decisions or no decisions at all and see life as lacking integrity. *267*

developing readers Readers who use letter sounds, words, illustrations, and their own knowledge to predict meaning. *170*

developmental risk Risk to children's well-being involving a range of damaging biopsychosocial conditions. *70*

developmental systems theory Set of beliefs leading to the conclusion that we construct our own views of the world. *44*

development The process of changing and the changes that occur through the lifespan. *7*

dilation The first stage of the birth process, during which the cervix dilates to about 4 inches in diameter. *81*

discontinuity Behaviors that are apparently unrelated to earlier aspects of development. *16*

disengagement theory The elderly will remove themselves from many social networks. *271*

distorted grief Normal grief carried to an extreme degree; adoption of deceased person's ailments. *286*

divergent thinking Thinking used when a problem to be solved has many possible answers. *193*

DNA (deoxyribonucleic acid) A molecule with the shape of a double helix that contains genetic information. *54*

doula A woman trained as a caregiver to provide ongoing support to pregnant women before, during, and after delivery. *84*

downsizing A reduction in a company's workforce to improve its total revenue. *249*

Down syndrome Chromosomal disorder caused by an extra copy of chromosome 21. *57*

dual-career family Family in which both partners work, usually full time. *225*

E

early-onset trajectory Criminal behavior that begins before puberty. *201*

egocentric speech The form of speech in which children carry on lively conversations with themselves or others. *117*

egocentrism Piaget's term for the child's focus on self in early phases of cognitive development. *112*

ego Freud's notion of the central part of our personality; keeps id in check. *30*

elaboration An association between two or more pieces of information that are not necessarily related. *167*

Electroencephalogram (EEG) Recording of the electrical activity produced by the firing of neurons in the brain. *282*

embryonic period 3rd through the 8th week following fertilization. *65*

emergent readers Children who possess skills, knowledge, and attitudes that are developmental precursors to formal reading. *170*

emerging adulthood Transition from adolescence to adulthood (approximately ages 18 to 25 years) that includes exploration and experimentation. *208*

emotional divorce Sometimes partners learn to "withstand" each other. The only activities and interests they shared are ones that revolve around the children. *247*

empty nest syndrome The feelings parents may have as a result of their last child leaving home. *247*

epigenetic view View of lifespan development that stresses the ongoing interaction between heredity and the environment. *13*

episiotomy A surgical cut made to widen the vaginal opening. *81*

equilibration Piaget's term to describe the balance between assimilation and accommodation. *36*

ethics of care Gilligan's perspective on moral thinking in which people view moral decisions in terms of relationships and responsibilities to others. *169*

ethology Scientific field that stresses behavior is strongly influenced by biology and is linked to evolution. *121*

euthanasia The ending of a life, usually in a person with a terminal illness, to prevent a prolonged and painful death. *289*

evolutionary developmental psychology Explanation of development that rests on the assumption that our physiological and psychological systems resulted from evolution by selection. *45*

executive functioning Cognitive efforts involving attention and critical thinking. *193*

exosystem Environment in which the developing person is not present but that nevertheless affects development. *43*

explicit memory Refers to facts and experiences that a person can remember and share. *267*

expressive language The language children use to express their ideas and needs. *141*

expulsion Stage 2 of the birth process; the baby passes through the birth canal. *81*

extinction The systematic process in which behaviors are de-conditioned or eliminated. *40*

F

failure to thrive (FTT) Medical term for infants whose weight gain and physical growth fall far below average during the first years of life. *109*

fallopian tube Either of a pair of tubes that join the ovary to the uterus. *62*

fast mapping Children's use of surrounding context to understand words' meaning. *115*

feminist movement A social and political movement that seeks to establish equality for women in all aspects of life. *216*

fetal alcohol syndrome The condition of babies whose mothers drank alcohol during pregnancy that is characterized by growth deficiencies, physical abnormalities, and CNS dysfunction. *74*

fetal monitor Electronic device used to monitor the baby's heartbeat throughout labor. *86*

fetal period Period that extends from beginning of the 3rd month to birth. *67*

fine motor skills Small muscle skills involving hands and fingers that result from physical development. *132*

five factor model (FFM) of personality McCrae and Costa's theory that there are five major personality traits, which they believe govern the adult personality. *245*

fluid intelligence The ability to think and act quickly and solve problems, as well as the ability to use abstract thinking. *239*

forceps Metal clamps placed around the baby's head to pull the baby through the birth canal. *86*

formal operational stage Piaget's fourth stage of cognitive development, featuring abstract thought and scientific thinking. *191*

fragile X syndrome Chromosomal disorder caused by an impaired X chromosome. *58*

fraternal twins Twins who develop from two eggs fertilized by separate sperm; individuals do not share identical genetic makeup. *62*

G

gamete intrafallopian transfer (GIFT) An ART technique in which sperm and egg are surgically placed in a fallopian tube with the intent of achieving fertilization. *64*

gender identity The conviction that one is either male or female. *146*

gender role Culturally defined expectations about how females and males should act. *146*

gender Social/psychological aspects of being male or female. *146*

gender stereotypes   Rigid beliefs about characteristics of males and females.   *146*

gene   A segment of DNA that is a unit of hereditary information.   *54*

generativity   Erikson's term for the ability to be useful to self and to society.   *244*

genital herpes   Infection that can be contracted by a fetus during delivery; the infant can develop symptoms during the first week following the birth.   *72*

genome   All of the hereditary information needed to maintain a living organism.   *55*

genotype   A person's genetic makeup that is invisible to the naked eye.   *55*

germinal period   First two weeks following fertilization.   *65*

gerontology   The field of science that deals with issues, problems, and diseases specific to older adults.   *256*

glaucoma   Damage to the optic nerve caused by pressure that results from a buildup of fluid in the eye.   *261*

global community   Consideration of all humans in the world as being closer because of advances in technology and communication; people are united in common interests relating to health and basic freedoms.   *301*

globalization   The outsourcing of much work to a less expensive labor supply in foreign countries.   *249*

goodness of fit   Concept coined by Chess and Thomas (1977) that describes the match between a child's temperament and his/her environment.   *123*

grasping reflex   Automatic response in which an infant's fingers curl toward palm of hand when object or finger is placed in palm.   *93*

grief   An emotional response to the loss of another; includes feelings of anxiety, despair, sadness, and loneliness.   *285*

gross motor skills   Large muscle skills resulting from physical development enabling children to perform smooth and coordinated physical acts.   *132*

H

habituation   A decrease in an infant's attention.   *110*

hazing   The practice of initiating individuals into group membership through arduous and demeaning tasks.   *208*

Head Start   Government-supported early childhood program that provides education, health, and parenting education services to low-income families.   *139*

health-care power of attorney   Legal document giving someone authority to make health-care decisions if one is incapacitated.   *289*

helping professions   Professions that relate to people's physical, cognitive, and social-emotional well-being.   *305*

heteronomous morality   Piaget's term for moral development in children aged 4 to 7; they conceive of rules as unchangeable.   *168*

heterosexual   Sexual attraction to members of the opposite sex.   *196*

HIV (Human Immunodeficiency Virus)   Virus that attacks T cells of the human immune system.   *72*

holophrases   One word that can communicate many meanings and ideas.   *117*

homeostatic imbalance   Theory that aging is due to a failure in the systems that regulate the proper interaction of the organs.   *258*

homosexual   Sexual attraction to members of the same sex.   *196*

hormonal balance   Change in hormone levels, one of the triggers of puberty.   *187*

hormone replacement therapy (HRT)   Menopause treatment whereby women receive hormone supplements.   *238*

hospice   A program providing comfort and supportive services to those near the end of life and to their families.   *290*

humanitarian   Efforts dedicated to improving the lives of human beings.   *301*

hypothesis   A prediction that can be tested through research and subsequently supported or rejected.   *17*

I

identical twins   Twins who develop from a single fertilized egg that divides after conception; individuals share identical genetic makeup.   *62*

identity crisis   Erikson's term for those situations, usually in adolescence, that cause us to make major decisions about our identity.   *33*

identity statuses   Marcia's categories that depict levels of crisis and commitment that contribute to a sense of identity.   *194*

id   Freud's structure of mind relating to our basic instincts; strives to secure pleasure.   *30*

imaginary audience   Adolescents' perception that others are constantly scrutinizing their behavior and appearance.   *192*

immanent justice   Piaget's term for a child's belief that broken rules will be punished immediately.   *168*

implantation   Attachment of the fertilized egg to the uterine wall.   *62*

implicit memory   Refers to an unconscious or automatic process of remembering.   *267*

inclusion   A child with special needs is educated in the regular classroom.   *162*

independent readers   Competent, confident readers who use skills to derive meaning and enjoyment from reading.   *171*

individualized education plan (IEP)   A written document (similar to a contract) that details an educational plan for a child to succeed under the supervision and guidance from the family, teachers and professionals, and administrators.   *162*

Individuals with Disabilities Education Act (IDEA) Law that details rights and guidelines for students with disabilities in the United States. *310*

individuation Refers to our developing a separate and special personality, derived less and less from our parents and teachers and more from our own behavior. *218*

induced labor Labor initiated by doctors through use of medication and by breaking the amniotic sac. *86*

infantile amnesia The inability to remember events from early in life. *105*

infertility Inability to achieve pregnancy after 1 year of unprotected intercourse. *63*

information-processing theory Cognitive theory that uses a computer metaphor to understand how the human mind processes information. *37*

inner speech Internal speech that often accompanies physical movements, guiding behavior. *117*

inquiry Investigating, questioning, following a hunch to see what happens. *300*

integrity The resolution of each of the first seven crises in Erikson's theory should lead to the achievement of a sense of personal integrity. Older adults who have a sense of integrity feel their lives have been well spent. *267*

intelligence A person's problem-solving skills and use of everyday experiences to inform learning. *163*

intelligence quotient (IQ) Stern's concept of a child's intelligence, calculated by dividing mental age by chronological age, and multiplying by 100. *165*

internalization of schemes Children's use of symbols to think about real events without actually experiencing them. *113*

intimacy Erikson's stage that represents the ability to relate one's deepest hopes and fears to another person and to accept another's need for intimacy in turn. *219*

intrauterine insemination (IUI) An ART technique in which sperm are injected directly into the uterus as part of the fertilization procedure. *64*

in vitro fertilization (IVF) An ART technique in which fertilization occurs in a petri dish and the resulting embryos are transferred to the woman's uterus. *64*

isolette Specially designed bed for premature infants that is temperature-controlled and enclosed in clear plastic; often referred to as an incubator. *89*

K

kangaroo care Practice of skin-to-skin contact, positioning baby against caregiver's bare chest. *90*

Klinefelter syndrome Chromosomal disorder in males caused by an XXY chromosomal pattern. *58*

knowledge-acquisition components Sternberg's term for intelligence components that help us learn how to solve problems in the first place. *164*

L

Lamaze method Natural childbirth method that stresses breathing and relaxation with the support of a partner. *83*

late-onset trajectory Criminal behavior that begins after puberty. *201*

learning disability A neurological disorder that impacts the brain's functioning. *159*

least restrictive environment: A child with a disability must be educated in a setting that is similar to that of children who do not have disability. *162*

legal death A legal pronouncement by a qualified person that a patient should be considered dead under the law. *283*

LGBT An acronym referring to lesbian (female), gay (male), bisexual, and transgender individuals; it can include a Q for queer or questioning (LGBTQ). *196*

life course theory Theory referring to a sequence of socially defined, age-graded events and roles that individuals enact over time. *44*

life crisis Erikson's term to describe the main tension that individuals experience and seek to resolve during each of eight life stages. *32*

life expectancy The number of years that a person born in a specific year is expected to live. *256*

lifespan development An examination of the biological, cognitive/psychological, and social changes that occur over the course of a human life. This is one perspective in the broader psychology discipline. *5*

lifespan psychology Study of human development from conception to death. *7*

living will Legal document that describes specific life-prolonging medical treatments. *289*

longitudinal studies Studies in which the researcher makes several observations of the same individuals at two or more times in their lives. Examples are determining the long-term effects of learning on behavior; the stability of habits and intelligence; and the factors involved in memory. *19*

M

macrosystem The blueprint of any society. *43*

macular degeneration An eye disease that affects the retina, impacting the center of a person's field of vision. *261*

manipulative experiments Experiments in which the researcher attempts to keep all variables (all the factors that can affect a particular outcome) constant except one, which is carefully manipulated. *18*

meiosis Cell division in which the number of chromosomes is halved to 23. *57*

menarche A girl's first menstruation. *187*

menopause Cessation of women's menstruation, typically occurring in the late 40s or early 50s. *237*

mental age Binet's measure of an individual's mental development compared to that of others. *165*

mentoring The act of assisting another, usually younger, person with his or her work or life tasks. *224*

mesosystem The relationship among microsystems. *43*

metacomponents Sternberg's term for intelligence components that help us plan, monitor, and evaluate our problem-solving strategies. *164*

microsystem The home or school. *43*

midlife transition Levinson's term to describe the period of life that bridges early and middle adulthood approximately ages 40 to 45. *243*

midwife A woman trained in delivering babies; typically a nurse. *84*

mitosis Cell division in which the number of chromosomes remains the same (46). *57*

modeling Bandura's term for observational learning. *40*

moral development Thinking, feeling, and behaving based on rules and customs about how people interact with others. *167*

Moro reflex Infant's automatic response to sudden change in position or unexpected movement; arms and legs flail out in back in toward chest and back arches. *92*

mortality rate The number of deaths in a population for a given year; typically, number of deaths per 1,000 people per year. *280*

mourning Actions taken as a result of grieving. *285*

mutation A change in DNA, affecting the genes, that occurs during mitosis by accident or because of environmental factors. *57*

myelination Process by which speed of information traveling through nervous system increases, due to a fatty layer of cells on nerve cells in the brain. *131*

myelin Sheath of insulation around axons that facilitates communication between neurons. *106*

N

naive psychology Vygotsky's stage in which children explore objects and label objects as they acquire the grammar of their speech. *117*

natural childbirth (or prepared childbirth) Term to describe techniques women use prior to and during the birth process to create the most natural experience possible during delivery. *83*

naturalistic experiments Experiments in which the researcher acts solely as an observer and does as little as possible to disturb the environment. "Nature" performs the experiment, and the researcher acts as a recorder of the results. *19*

negative reinforcement An event that, when it ceases to occur, makes that response more likely to happen in the future. *39*

neonate An infant in the first days and weeks after birth. *90*

neurons Nerve cells that transmit information with electrochemical signals. *106*

New York Longitudinal Study Long-term study by Chess and Thomas of the personality characteristics of children. *124*

No Child Left Behind Act Federal legislation based on the notion that high standards and measurable goals improve individual educational outcomes; requires assessments in basic skills to be given to all students in certain grades. *170*

non-stage theorists Reading theorists who argue that reading develops naturally, as does language. *170*

novice phase Levinson's phase of human development that captures the early adult transition, entering the adult world, and the age 30 transition. *219*

O

obesity Based on BMI, greater than 85th percentile for sex and age. *158*

object permanence Refers to children gradually realizing that there are permanent objects around them, even when these objects are out of sight. *113*

object permanence The realization that objects continue to exist even when they cannot be seen, heard, or touched. *34*

observational learning Bandura's term to explain the information we obtain from observing other people, things, and events. *40*

one-time, one-group studies Studies carried out only once with one group of participants. *19*

open adoption Adoption procedure in which biological parents have considerable input into the adoption process. *65*

operant conditioning The use of consequences (reinforcement, punishment) to modify or shape voluntary behavior or actions. *39*

organization Memory strategy that entails discovering and imposing an easy-to-remember structure on items to be memorized. *136*

organogenesis Process by which organs are formed; occurs around 6 to 7 weeks of pregnancy. *66*

organ reserve The part of the total capacity of our body's organs that we do not normally need to use. *210*

osteoporosis A condition in which bones are thin and brittle due to calcium loss. *262*

overextensions A language irregularity in which children apply a word in a broad manner to objects that do not fit. *141*

overregularization Children's strict application of language rules they have learned. *141*

ovulation The process in which the egg bursts from the surface of the ovary. *61*

oxytocin Hormone secreted by the pituitary gland that stimulates uterine contractions; has been linked to bonding between caregivers and infants. *80*

P

passive euthanasia Refraining from continuing efforts to sustain someone's life. *289*

perception The process of obtaining and interpreting information from stimuli. *110*

performance components Sternberg's term for intelligence components that help us execute the instructions of the metacomponents. *164*

permissive parenting Baumrind's term for parents who take a tolerant, accepting view of their child's behavior and rarely make demands or use punishment. *143*

personal fable Adolescents' tendency to think of themselves in heroic or mythical terms. *192*

phenotype A person's observable characteristics or traits. *55*

phenylketonuria (PKU) Inherited disease caused by a gene mutation. *60*

phonology Sounds of a language. *117*

physician-assisted suicide (PAS) Active euthanasia whereby doctors give patients death-inducing drugs. *289*

placenta Supplies the embryo with all its needs, carries off all its wastes, and protects it from harm. *65*

plantar reflex Automatic response in which an infant's toes curl inward when pressure is placed on balls of feet. *93*

play Activity people engage in because they enjoy it for its own sake. *148*

policy A course of action to guide and determine decisions. *309*

positive psychology A branch of psychology that emphasizes the impact of positive psychological traits on individual and group behaviors. *250*

positive reinforcement An event that increases the likelihood of a desired response in the future. *39*

postformal thought A proposed cognitive development stage after Piaget's formal operations in which people acknowledge the relativistic nature of problems and answers. *215*

postpartum depression Feelings of sadness and emotional withdrawal that continue for many weeks or months after delivery. *95*

postpartum period Period lasting approximately 6 weeks after birth as mother adjusts physically and psychologically. *95*

practical intelligence Sternberg's term to describe "common sense"—a simple, logical understanding of a situation and how to work through a problem. *240*

pragmatics Ability to communicate with others. *117*

preintellectual speech Vygotsky's category for cooing, crying, babbling, and bodily movements that develop into more sophisticated forms of speech. *117*

premature birth Early birth; occurs at or before 37 weeks after conception and is defined by low birth weight and immaturity. *88*

preoperational period Piaget's second stage of cognitive development, extending from about 2 to 7 years. *133*

primary circular reactions Infants' actions that are focused on their own bodies and reflexes. *113*

prospective memory The process of remembering to do something in the future. *267*

protective factors Characteristics of resilient individuals that protect them from stress. *250*

psychoanalytic theory Freud's theory of the development of personality; emphasis on the role of the unconscious. *29*

psychosocial theory Erikson's stage theory that emphasizes the impact of social experiences throughout human development. *31*

psychosomatic Physical illness or symptom brought about by mental factors. *286*

puberty The process of physical changes by which a child's body becomes an adult body capable of reproduction. *187*

punishment Process by which an unpleasant response is paired with an undesired behavior to decrease the likelihood of that behavior occurring in the future. *40*

R

rape Forced sexual intercourse when a person does not consent. *214*

reaction time The time between the presence of a stimulus and the actual muscle activity that indicates a reaction to it. *260*

receptive language The ability of the child to understand written and spoken language. *141*

reciprocal interactions Interactions that shape relationships with others. *119*

reflex An inborn, automatic response to certain stimuli. *92*

rehearsal Mnemonic strategy that describes a person repeating target information. *136*

reinforcement Anything that increases the likelihood a response will occur in the future. *39*

REM (rapid eye-movement) sleep A period of deep sleep marked by eye movements; when vivid dreams occur. *109*

representation A child's application of abstract thinking during the preoperational period. *133*

resilient children Children who sustained some type of physiological or psychological trauma yet return to a normal developmental path. *179*

respiratory distress syndrome (RDS) Problem common with premature babies; caused by lack of a substance that keeps air sacs in the lungs open. *110*

reticular activation system (RAS) Complex subcortical system that protects the brain from being overwhelmed. *192*

retrieval Memory strategy that enables obtaining information from memory; includes recognition and recall. *137*

retrospective memory Memory of past event or item. *267*

reversibility A cognitive act in which a child recognizes that she can use stages of reasoning to solve a problem and then trace the steps back to the original question or premise. *135*

Rh factor Involves possible incompatibility between the blood types of mother and child. If the mother is Rh-negative and the child Rh-positive, miscarriage or even infant death can result. *88*

risk factors The stressors that individuals experience, including poverty, chronic illness, and divorce. *250*

role discontinuity Abrupt and disruptive change caused by conflicts among one's various roles in life. *268*

rooting reflex Automatic response in which an infant turns toward a finger or nipple placed gently on her cheek, attempting to get it into her mouth. *92*

rubella (also known as German measles) An infectious disease that can cause serious birth defects. If a woman contracts the disease during pregnancy, extremely dangerous to a fetus during the first trimester. *71*

S

sandwich generation Term used to describe adults who are simultaneously caring for their children and their aging parents. *247*

scaffolding The systematic use of support to assist a child in his or her performance on a given task. *136*

schemes Piaget's term for organized patterns of thought and action. *36*

scientific method An approach to investigation that includes empirical research, data collection, and testing. *17*

secondary circular reactions Piaget's term for infants' activities that are directed toward objects and events outside themselves. *113*

secular trend The decreasing age of the onset of puberty. *189*

self-concept A person's evaluation of himself or herself. *173*

self-efficacy A person's belief that she can behave in a certain way to achieve a desired goal. *42*

self-esteem One's personal sense of worth and value. *173*

self-regulation An individual's ability to initiate, terminate, delay, or modify thought, emotion, behavior, or action. *174*

semantics Meaning of words and sentences. *117*

sensitive periods Montessori's term for periods of children's development marked by sensitivity/readiness to learn. *139*

sensitive responsiveness The ability to recognize the meaning of a child's behavior. *124*

sensorimotor period The first 2 years of life. *112*

sequential (longitudinal/cross-sectional) studies Cross-sectional studies done at several times with the same groups of individuals. *20*

seriation The ability to order items along a quantitative dimension such as length or weight. *162*

sex Biological maleness or femaleness. *146*

sex cleavage Youngsters of the same sex tend to play and do things together. *147*

sexual harassment Unwelcome sexual advances, such as repeated requests for sexual favors, or other comments or physical contact that lead to a very difficult work or other environment for the victim. *214*

sexual identity How one thinks of oneself in terms of sexual and romantic attraction, linked to genetic traits/physical characteristics of male and female. *216*

sexually transmitted diseases (STDs) Diseases that may cause infertility. *64*

sibling underworld Familial subsystem, or coalition, of brothers and/or sisters. *144*

sickle-cell disease Blood disorder resulting in abnormal hemoglobin. *60*

small for date Term used for babies born or assessed as underweight for the length of the pregnancy. *89*

social (cognitive) learning Bandura's theory that refers to the process whereby the information we glean from observing others influences our behavior. *40*

social constructivism The belief that children construct knowledge through social interactions. *136*

social death Point at which a patient is treated essentially as a corpse, although perhaps still "clinically" or "biologically" alive. *282*

socioemotional selectivity theory Humans use social contact for four reasons: to ensure physical survival, to gain information, to maintain a sense of self, and to acquire pleasure and comfort. *271*

spina bifida Genetic disorder resulting in the failure of the spinal column to close completely. *60*

spindle cells Neurons that play a large role in emotion. *192*

stage theorists Reading theorists who argue that reading occurs in distinct developmental stages. *169*

stage theorists Theorists who consider stages of change across the lifespan and how one's personality interacts with the world. *245*

stagnation Erikson's term for boredom, self-absorption, and the inability to contribute to society. *244*

stakeholder Individual who is affected by the actions of a larger group or organization *301*

stepping reflex Automatic response in which the neonate, held under the arms with feet touching a flat surface, makes stepping movements similar to actual walking. *93*

STORCH diseases Syphilis, toxoplasmosis, other infections, rubella, cytomegalovirus, herpes. *71*

strange situation Measure designed to assess the quality of attachment. *122*

stress Anything that upsets a person's equilibrium—psychologically and physiologically. *178*

sudden infant death syndrome (SIDS) Unexpected death of an apparently healthy infant, usually between 2 and 4 months of age. *109*

superego Freud's concept of our conscience; internal determinant of right and wrong. *30*

surrogate mother A woman who carries another woman's fetus. *64*

symbolic play Children's mental representation of an object or event and reenactment of it in their play; one object may represent a different object in the play scenario. *134*

synapse A small gap between neurons. *106*

syntax The way in which words are put together to construct sentences. *117*

syphilis Sexually transmitted disease that, if untreated, may adversely affect the fetus. *71*

T

Tay-Sachs Genetic disorder caused by the lack of an enzyme that breaks down fatty material in the CNS. *60*

telegraphic speech Initial multiple-word utterances, usually two or three words. *117*

temperament Individual differences; unique and stable styles of behaving. *123*

teratogens Any environmental agents that harm the embryo or fetus. *70*

tertiary circular reaction Piaget's term for repetition with variation; the infant is exploring the world's possibilities. *113*

thalidomide Popular drug prescribed during the early 1960s that was later found to cause a variety of birth defects when taken by women early in their pregnancies. *73*

theory A belief or idea that develops based on information or evidence; a proposed explanation for observed phenomena. *28*

theory of mind Children's understanding of their own thoughts and mental processes. *137*

theory of multiple intelligences Gardner's theory that attributes eight types of intelligence to humans. *163*

time-variable designs A specific amount of time (duration) is allowed for a given study, or there is a specific number of times a measure is used in a given study. *19*

tonic-neck reflex Automatic response in which an infant extends arm and leg on same side as the direction in which she is looking, while flexing other arm and leg. *93*

toxoplasmosis Infection caused by a parasite; may cause damage to a fetus. *71*

trait theorists Researchers who look at pieces of the personality (personality traits), as measured by detailed questionnaires. *245*

transitivity The ability to understand relationships and combine them mentally to draw new conclusions. *162*

triarchic theory of intelligence Sternberg's theory that intelligence consists of componential, experiential, and contextual parts. *164*

Turner syndrome Chromosomal disorder in females caused by an XO chromosomal pattern. *58*

U

ultrasound Use of sound waves and special equipment to produce an image that enables a physician to detect internal structural abnormalities. *68*

umbilical cord Contains blood vessels that go to and from the mother through the arteries and veins supplying the placenta. *65*

uninvolved/neglectful parenting Term for parents who are undemanding and emotionally unsupportive of their child. *143*

V

vacuum extractor Plastic cup attached to a suction device that pulls the baby through the birth canal. *86*

validation Fromm's term for the reciprocal sharing of deep secrets and feelings that allows people to feel loved and accepted. *221*

W

wisdom Superior insight and judgment that can come only from experience. *266*

word spurt Rapid increase of vocabulary from 18 months to 3 years. *117*

work–family conflict Phenomenon that occurs when a person's roles as caregiver and worker conflict or overlap. *249*

X

XYY syndrome Chromosomal disorder in males caused by an extra Y chromosome. *58*

Z

zone of proximal development Vygotsky's term for a range of ability in a given task, where the higher limit is achieved through interaction with others. *37*

zone of proximal development (ZPD) The range of ability a child possesses on a given task, from working independently to working with assistance from adults or older children. *136*

zygote The cell that results when an egg is fertilized by a sperm. *54*

A

AARP (2000, February). Grandparents and kids: Getting along fine. *AARP Bulletin,* 21.

Ackerman, S., Zuroff, D., & Moskowitz, D. (2000). Generativity in midlife and young adults: Links to agency, communion, and subjective well-being. *International Journal of Aging & Human Development, 50,* 17–41.

Ahrons, C. (2004). *We're still family.* New York: HarperCollins.

Ainsworth, M. (1973). The development of infant–mother attachment. In B. Caldwell & H. Riccuti (Eds.), *Review of child development research.* Chicago: University of Chicago Press.

———. (1979). Infant-mother attachment. *American Psychologist, 34,* 932–937.

Ainsworth, M., & Bowlby, J. (1991). An ethological approach to personality. *American Psychologist, 46,* 333–341.

Ajrouch, K., Antonucci, T., & Janevic, M. (2001). Social networks among blacks and whites: The interaction between race and age. *Journal of Gerontology, 56B,* S112–S118.

Alland, A. (1983). *Playing with form: Children draw in six cultures:* New York: Columbia University Press.

Alzheimer's Association. (2009). Alzheimer's disease facts and figures. *Alzheimer's and Dementia, 5*(3).

Alzheimers.org. (2004). Studies suggest people with early AD can still learn. Retrieved from http://www.alzheimers.org/nianews/nianews67.html.

American Alliance for Health, Physical Education, Recreation, and Dance. (2007). Accepting overweight. *Journal of Physical Education, Recreation, and Dance, 78*(1), 3.

American Cancer Society. (2008). *At a glance—Nutrition and physical activity.* Retrieved from http://www.cancer.org/docroot/PED/content/PED_3_2X_Recommendations.asp?sitearea=PED

American Psychiatric Association. (2000). *Diagnostic and statistical manual of mental disorders* (4th ed., text rev.). Washington, DC: Author.

American SIDS Institute. (2009). Retrieved from http://www.sids.org.

Anderson, S. E., Dallal, G. E., & Must, A. (2003). Relative weight and race influence average age at menarche: Results from two nationally representative surveys of US girls studied 25 years apart. *Pediatrics, 111*(4), 844–850.

Angela. (2008). *Wii for the elderly—A report.* Retrieved from http://www.wiicentre.com/wii-for-the-elderly—-a-report-441/

Arenson, J., & Drake, P. (2007). *Maternal and newborn health.* Sudbury, MA: Jones and Bartlett.

Asch-Goodkin, J., & Kaplan, D. (2006). When a spouse is hospitalized (bereavement effect in spouse death). *Patient Care for the Nurse Practitioner.*

B

Bakalar, N. (2005, November 22). Premature births increase along with C-sections. *The New York Times.* Retrieved from http://www.nytimes.com/2005/11/22/health/22birth.html?_r=1

Balcazar, H., & Mattson, S. (2000). Nutrition. In S. Mattson & J. Smith (Eds.), *Core curriculum for maternal-newborn nursing.* Philadelphia: W. B. Saunders.

Ball, J., & Bindler, R. (2006). *Child health nursing: Partnering with children and families.* Upper Saddle River, NJ: Prentice Hall.

Balsam, R. H., & Fischer, R. S. (2006). Mothers and daughters II. *Psychoanalytic Inquiry, 26*(1). New York: Routledge.

Baltes, P., Lindenberger, U., & Staudinger, U. (1998). Lifespan theory in developmental psychology. In R. M. Lerner (Ed.), *Handbook of child psychology: Vol. 1. Theoretical models of human development.* New York: Wiley.

———. (2006). Lifespan theory in developmental psychology. In W. Damon & R. Lerner (Series Eds.) & R. Lerner (Vol. Ed.), *Handbook of child psychology: Vol. 1.Theoretical models of human development.* New York: Wiley.

Baltes, P. B., & Staudinger, U. M. (2000). Wisdom: A metaheuristic (pragmatic) to orchestrate mind and virtue toward excellence. *American Psychologist, 55*(1), 122–136.

Bandura, A. (1997). *Self-efficacy: The exercise of control.* New York: Freeman.

Bandura, A., Barbaranelli, C., Caprara, G., & Pastorelli, C. (2001). Self-efficacy beliefs as shapers of children's aspirations and career trajectories. *Child Development, 72*(1), 187–206.

Bandura, A., Ross, D., & Ross, S. (1963). Imitation of film-mediated aggressive models. *Journal of Abnormal and Social Psychology, 66,* 3–11.

Bandura, A., & Walters, R. (1963). *Social learning and personality development.* New York: Holt, Rinehart & Winston.

Baumrind, D. (1967). Child-care practices anteceding three patterns of preschool behavior. *Genetic Psychology Monographs, 75,* 43–88.

———. (1971). Current patterns of parental authority. *Developmental Psychology Monographs, 4,* 1–103.

———. (1986). *Familial antecedents of social competence in middle childhood.* Unpublished manuscript.

———. (1991a). The influence of parenting style on adolescent competence and substance use. Special Issue: The work of John P. Hill: I. Theoretical, instructional, and policy contributions. *Journal of Early Adolescence, 11*(1), 56–95.

———. (1991b). To nurture nature. *Behavioral and Brain Sciences,* XIV, 386.

———. (1991c). Parenting styles and adolescent development. In R. Lerner, A. Peterson, & J. Brooks-Gunn (Eds.), *The encyclopedia of adolescence.* New York: Garland.

Beausang, C. C., & Razor, A. G. (2000). Young Western women's experiences of menarche and menstruation. *Health Care for Women International, 21,* 517–528.

Beeson, R., Horton-Deutsch, S., Farran, C., & Neundorfer, M. (2000). Loneliness and depression in caregivers of persons with Alzheimer's disease or related disorders. *Issues in Mental Health Nursing, 21,* 779–806.

Bem, S. (1999). *An unconventional family.* New Haven, CT: Yale University Press.

———. (2001). Exotic becomes erotic: Integrating biological and experiential antecedents of sexual orientation. In A. D'Augelli & C. Patterson (Eds.), *Lesbian, gay, and bisexual identities and youth: Psychological perspectives.* (pp. 52–68) London: Oxford University Press.

Bengtson, V. (2001). Beyond the nuclear family: The increasing importance of multigenerational bonds. *Journal of Marriage and the Family, 63,* 1–16.

Berg, S. J., & Wynne-Edwards, K. (2001). Changes in testosterone, cortisol, and estradiol levels in men becoming fathers. *Mayo Clinic Proceedings, 76,* 582–592.

Bergh, S., & Erling, A. (2005). Adolescent identity formation: A Swedish study of identity status using the EOM-EIS-II. *Adolescence, 40*(158), 377–397.

Bernas, K. H., & Major, D. A. (2000). Contributors to stress resistance: Testing a model of women's work–family conflict. *Psychology of Women Quarterly, 24,* 170–178.

Bernat, J. (2001). Ethical and legal issues in palliative care. *Neurologic Clinics, 19,* 969–987.

Berzonsky, M., & Kuk, L. (2000). Identity status, identity processing style and transition to university. *Journal of Adolescent Research, 15*(1), 81–98.

Beutel, M. E., Weidner, W., & Brahler, E. (2006). Epidemiology of sexual dysfunction in the male population. *Andrologia, 38*(4), 115–121.

Bianchi, S., Robinson, J., & Milkie, M. (2006). *Changing rhythms of American family life* (Rose Series in Sociology). New York: Sage.

Birren, J., & Fisher, L. (1992). Aging and slowing of behavior. In Berman & Sonderegger (Eds.), *Psychology and aging: Nebraska Symposium on Motivation 1991.* Lincoln: University of Nebraska.

Bjorklund, D. (2000). *Children's thinking: Developmental function and individual differences.* Belmont, CA: Wadsworth.

———. (2005). *Children's thinking.* Belmont, CA: Wadsworth.

Bjorklund, D. F., & Pellegrini, A. D. (2000). *The origins of human nature.* New York: Oxford University Press.

Black, M., Dubowitz, H., Krishnakumar, A., & Starr, R. (2007). Early intervention and recovery among children with failure to thrive: Follow-up at age 8. *Pediatrics, 120*(1), 59–69.

Blackman, J. (1997). *Medical aspects of developmental disabilities in children birth to three.* Gaithersburg, MD: Aspen.

Blakeslee, S. (2003, December 9). Humanity? Maybe it's in the wiring. *The New York Times,* p. D1.

Blank, J. (2000). *Still doing it: Women and men over sixty write about their sexuality.* New York: Down There Press.

Blazer, D. G., & Wu, L. (2009). The epidemiology of at-risk and binge drinking among middle-aged and elderly community adults: National Survey on Drug Use and Health. *American Journal of Psychiatry.* Retrieved from http://ajp.psychiatryonline.org/cgi/reprint/appi.ajp.2009.09010016v1

Block, R., Krebs, N., the Committee on Child Abuse and Neglect, & the Committee on Nutrition. (2005). Failure to thrive as a manifestation of child neglect. *Pediatrics, 116*(5), 1234–1237.

Bornstein, M. (2002). Parenting Infants. In M. Bornstein (Ed.) *Handbook of parenting: Vol. 1.* Mahwah, NJ: Erlbaum.

Bornstein, M. (Ed.). (2002). *Handbook of parenting* (2nd ed.). Mahwah, NJ: Erlbaum.

Brazelton, T., & Nugent, K. (1995). *Neonatal behavioral assessment scale.* London: MacKeith Press.

Briken, P., Habermann, N., Berner, W., & Hill, A. (2006). XYY chromosome abnormality in sexual homicide perpetrators. *American Journal of Medical Genetics B: Neuropsychiatry and Genetics, 141,* 198–200.

Brim, O., & J. Kagan (1980). *Constancy and change in human development.* Cambridge, MA: Harvard University Press.

Broadbent, D. E. (1954). The role of auditory localization in attention and memory span. *Journal of Experimental Psychology, 47,* 191–196.

Brodzinsky, D., & Pinderhughes, E. (2002). Parenting and child development in adoptive families. In M. Bornstein (Ed.), *Handbook of parenting* (2nd ed.). Mahwah, NJ: Erlbaum.

Bronfenbrenner, U. (1978). *The ecology of human development.* Cambridge, MA: Harvard University Press.

Bronfenbrenner, U., & Morris, P. (1998). The ecology of developmental processes. In R. M. Lerner (Ed.), *Handbook of child psychology: Vol. 1. Theoretical models of human development.* New York: Wiley.

———. (2006). The ecology of developmental processes. In W. Damon & R. Lerner (Eds.), *Handbook of child psychology,* (6th ed., pp. 793–829). New York: Wiley.

Bronson, M. (1995). *The right stuff for children birth to 8.* Washington, DC: National Association for the Education of Young People.

Bronson, M. B., Pierson, D. E., & Tivnan, T. (1984). The effects of early education on children's competence in elementary school. *Evaluation Review, 8*(5), 615–629.

Brown, B., Dolcini, M., & Leventhal, A. (1997). Transformations in peer relationships at adolescence: Implications for health-related behavior. In J. Schulenberg & J. L. Maggs (Eds.), *Health risks and developmental transitions during adolescence* (pp. 161–189) New York: Cambridge University Press.

Bugental, D. B., & Happaney, K. (2004). Predicting infant maltreatment in low-income families: The interactive effects of maternal attributions and child status at birth. *Developmental Psychology, 40*(2), 234–243.

Buhs, E., & Ladd, G. (2001). Peer rejections as an antecedent of young children's school adjustment: An examination of mediating processes. *Developmental Psychology, 37*(4), 550–560.

Burgess, E. O. (2004). Sexuality in midlife and later life couples. In J. H. Harvey & A. Wetzel (Eds.), *The handbook of sexuality in close relationships.* Mahwah, NJ: Erlbaum.

Burr, J. A., & Mutchler, J. E. (1999). Race and ethnic variation in norms of filial responsibility among older persons. *Journal of Marriage and the Family, 61*(3), 674–687.

Buss, D. (2001). Cognitive biases and emotional wisdom in the evolution of conflict between the sexes. *Current Directions in Psychological Science, 10,* 219–223.

Byrnes, J. P. (2005). The development of regulated decision making. In J. E. Jacobs & P. A. Klaczynski (Eds.), *The development of judgment and decision making in children and adolescents.* Mahwah, NJ: Erlbaum.

C

Cahan, S., Greenbaum, C., Artman, L., Deluya, N., & Gappel-Gilon, Y. (2006). The differential effects of age and first-grade schooling on the development of infralogical and logico-mathematical concrete operations. *Cognitive Development, 23*(2), 258–277.

Cahill, S. (2000). Elderly husbands caring at home for wives diagnosed with Alzheimer's disease: Are male caregivers really different? *Australian Journal of Social Issues, 35,* 53–66.

Cairns, R., & Cairns, B. (2006). The making of developmental psychology. In W. Damon & R. Lerner (Series Eds.) & R. Lerner (Vol. Ed.), *Handbook of child psychology: Vol. 1. Theoretical models of human development.* New York: Wiley.

Campbell, N., & Reece, J. (2005). *Biology.* New York: Pearson/Cummings.

Campos, S., Poulos, G., & Sipple, J. (2005). Prevalence and profiling: Hazing among college students and points of intervention. *American Journal of Health Behavior, 29*(2), 137–149.

Care for Caregivers. (2009). Retrieved from http://www.eldercare.com/modules.php?op=modload&name=CG_Resources&file=article&sid=861

Carel, J. C. (2005). Growth hormone in Turner syndrome: Twenty years after, what can we tell our patients? *Journal of Clinical Endocrinology and Metabolism, 90,* 3793–3794.

Carlson, B. (2004). *Human embryology and developmental biology.* Philadelphia: Mosby.

Carr, D., House, J., Wortman, C., Nesse, R., & Kessler, R. (2001). Psychological adjustment to sudden and anticipated spousal loss among older widowed persons. *Journal of Gerontology, 56B,* S237–S248.

Carstensen, L. L. (1995). Evidence for a lifespan theory of socioemotional selectivity. *Current Directions in Psychological Science, 4*(5), 151–156.

Carstensen, L. L., Edelstein, B. A., & Dornbrand, L. (1996). *The practical handbook of clinical gerontology.* Thousand Oaks, CA: Sage.

Casas, J., & Pytluk, S. (1995). Hispanic identity development: Implications for research and practice. In J. Ponterotto, J. Casas, L. Suzuki, & C. Alexander (Eds.), *Handbook of multicultural counseling.* Thousand Oaks, CA: Sage.

Centers for Disease Control and Prevention (CDC). (2000a). *Sexually transmitted diseases sourcebook.* Atlanta: Author.

———. (2000b). *State-specific prevalence of obesity among adults—United States, 2005. Sept. 2006/55*(36), 985–988.

———. (2001a). *Women and smoking.* Atlanta: Author.

———. (2001b). *Work-related hearing loss.* Retrieved from http://www.cdc.gov/niosh/hpworkrel.html.

———. (2006a). Tobacco use among middle and high school students–United States, 2005. *Morbidity and Mortality Weekly Report.*

———. (2006b). *Suicide in the U.S.: Statistics and prevention.* Retrieved from http://www.cdc.gov/ncipc/wisqars.

———. (2009a). *Provisional cases of infrequently reported notifiable diseases—United States. Morbidity and Mortality Weekly Report, 55*(19), 538.

———. (2009b). Obesity—halting the epidemic by making health easier: At a glance 2009. Retrieved from http://www.cdc.gov/chronicdisease/resouirces/publications/aag/obesity.htm

Centers for Disease Control and Prevention, AARP, American Medical Association. (2009). *Promoting preventive services for adults 50–64: Community and clinical partnerships.* Atlanta: National association of Chronic Disease Directors. Retrieved from http://www.cdc.gov/aging

Center for Disease Control Online Newsroom. (2009). *Life expectancy at all-time high; death rates reach new low, study sasys.* Retrieved from http://www.cdc.gov/media/pressrel/2009/r090819.htm

Centers for Disease Control and Prevention, National Center for Health Statistics. (2000). *CDC growth charts: United States.* Retrieved from http://www.cdc.gov/growthcharts

Chall, J. (1983). *Stages of reading development.* New York: McGraw-Hill.

Chall, J., Jacobs, V., & Baldwin, L. (1990). *The reading crisis: Why poor children fall behind.* Cambridge, MA: Harvard University Press.

Chao, R. (2001). Extending research on the consequences of parenting style for Chinese Americans and European Americans. *Child Development, 72,* 1832–1843.

Chavous, T., Bernat, D., Schmeelk-Cone, K., Caldwell, C., Kohn-Wood, L., & Zimmerman, M. (2003, July/August). Racial identity and academic attainment among African American adolescents. *Child Development, 74*(4), 1076–1090.

Chen, Z., & Kaplan, H. (2003). School failure in early adolescence and status attainment in middle adulthood: A longitudinal study. *Sociology of Education, 76,* 110–118.

Chess, S., & Thomas, A. (1977). Temperamental individuality from childhood to adolescence. *Journal of Child Psychiatry, 16,* 218–226.

———. (1987). *Know your child.* New York: Basic Books.

———. (1999). *Goodness of fit.* Philadelphia: Brunner/Mazel.

Child and Adolescent Mental Health Government Guide. (?) Retrieved from http://www.nih.gov/&CID=16101830/.

Children's Defense Fund. (2009). *Top 12 children's health coverage myths.* Retrieved from http://www.childrensdefense.org/helping-americas-children/childrens-health/health-coverage-for-all-children-campaign/top-12-childrens-health-coverage-myths.html

Children's Foundation (2003). *The 2003 child care center licensing study.* Washington, DC: Children's Foundation.

Chomsky, N. (1957). *Syntactic structure.* The Hague: Mouton.

Chumlea, A. C., Schubert, C. M., Roche, A. F., Kulin, H. F., Lee, P. A., Himes, J. H., et al. (2003). Age at menarche and racial comparisons in U.S. girls. *Pediatrics, 111*(1), 110–113.

Cicchetti, D., & Toth, S. (1998). Perspectives on research and practice in developmental psychopathology. In W. Damon (Series Ed.) & I. Sigel & K. Renningerg (Vol. Eds.), *Handbook of child psychology: Vol. 4. Child psychology in practice.* New York: Wiley.

Clarke, E., Preston, M., Raksin, J., & Bengtson, V. (1999). Types of conflicts and tensions between older parents and adult children. *The Gerontologist, 39*(3), 261–270.

Clarke-Stewart, K., & Allhusen, V. (2005). *What we know about child care.* Cambridge, MA: Harvard University Press.

Cleveland, H., & Wiebe, R. (2003, January/February). The moderation of adolescent-to-peer similarity in tobacco and alcohol use by school levels of substance use. *Child Development, 74*(1), 279–291.

Cohen, S., & Jaskulsky, S. (2001). Prostate cancer: Therapeutic options based on tumor grade, life expectancy, and patient preferences. *Geriatrics, 56,* 39–52.

Cohen-Mansfield, J., & Werner, P. (1998). Predictors of aggressive behaviors: A longitudinal study in senior day care centers. *Journal of Gerontology, 53B*(5), P300–P310.

Colditz, G. A., & Stein, C. (2005). Smoking cessation, weight gain, and lung function (risk of smoking cessation). *The Lancet, 365*(9471), 1600–1602.

Cole, M. (1996). *Cultural psychology.* Cambridge, MA: Harvard University Press.

———. (1999). Culture in development. In M. Bornstein & M. Lamb (Eds.), *Developmental psychology: An advanced textbook.* Mahwah, NJ: Erlbaum.

Cole, P., Bruschi, C., & Tamang, B. (2002). Cultural differences in children's emotional reactions to difficult situations. *Child Development, 73*(3), 983–996.

Collins, W. A., Maccoby, E. E., Steinberg, L., Hetherington, E. M., & Bornstein, M. H. (2001). Toward nature WITH nurture. *American Psychologist, 56,* 171–173.

Compas, B., Benson, M., Boyer, M., Hocks, T., & Konik, B. (2002). Problem-solving and problem-solving therapies. In M. Rutter and E. Taylor (Eds.). *Child and adolescent psychiatry.* London: Blackwell.

Conger, R., & Chao, W. (1996). Adolescent depressed mood. In R. L. Simons (Ed.), *Understanding differences between divorced and intact families: Stress, interaction, and child outcome.* (pp. 157–175). Thousand Oaks, CA: Sage.

Connors, M. (2001). Relationship of sexual abuse to body image and eating problems. In J. K. Thompson & L. Smolak (Eds.), *Body image, eating disorders, and obesity in youth: Assessment, prevention, and treatment* (pp. 149–167). Washington, DC: American Psychological Association.

Crain, W. (2005). *Theories of development.* Upper Saddle River, NJ: Pearson/Prentice Hall.

Crawford, M., & Unger, R. (2000). Introduction to a feminist psychology of women. In M. Crawford and R. Unger (Eds.), *Women and gender: A feminist psychology* (pp. 2–32). Boston: McGraw-Hill.

Csikszentmihalyi, M., & Rathunde, K. (1998). In R. M. Lerner (Ed.), *Handbook of child psychology: Vol. 1. Theoretical models of human development.* New York: Wiley.

Cummings, E., & Henry, W. (1961). Growing old. New York: Basic Books.

Cummings, S. M., Knopf, N. P., & DeWeaver, K. L. (2000). Knowledge of and attitudes toward aging among non-elders: Gender and race differences. *Journal of Women & Aging, 12,* 77–87.

Curran, J. (2006). Deliberate self-harm in the over 60s. *Mental Health Practice, 10*(1), 29–30.

Czaja, S. J., Charness, N., Fisk, A. D., Hertzog, C., Nair, S. N., Rogers, W. A., & Sharit, J. (2006). Factors predicting the use of technology: Findings from the Center for Research and Education on Aging and Technology (CREATE). *Psychology and Aging, 21,* 333–352.

D

Dacey, J. S. (1989a). Discriminating characteristics of the families of highly creative adolescents. *Journal of Creative Behavior, 24*(4), 263–271.

———. (1989b). *Fundamentals of creative thinking.* Lexington, MA: D. C. Heath/Lexington Books.

Dacey, J. S., & Fiore, L. (2000). *Your anxious child.* San Francisco: Jossey-Bass.

Dacey, J. S., & Fiore, L. B. (2006). *The safe child handbook: How to protect your family and cope with anxiety in a threat-filled world.* San Francisco: Jossey-Bass.

Dacey, J. S., Kenny, M., & Margolis, D. (2002). *Adolescent development,* Houston: Thompson.

———. (2008). *Adolescent development.* Belmont, CA: Cengage Learning.

Darwin, C. (1877). Biographical sketch of an infant. *Mind, 2,* 285–294.

Das, A. (2009, April 21). More Wii warriors are playing hurt. *The New York Times.* Retrieved from http://www.nytimes.com/2009/04/21/health/21wii.html

Dating for the over 50 Crowd. (2009). Retrieved from http://www.articlesbase.com/dating-articles/dating-for-the-over-50-crowd-245733.html

Deblinger, E., Mannarino, A. P., Cohen, J. A., & Steer, R. A. (2006). A follow-up study of a multisite, randomized, controlled trial for children with sexual abuse-related PTSD symptoms. *Journal of the American Academy of Child and Adolescent Psychiatry, 45*(12), 1474–1485.

A Definition of Irreversible Coma: Report of the Ad Hoc Committee of the Harvard Medical School to examine the definition of brain death. (1968). *Journal of the American Medical Association; 205,* 337–340.

Dennis, W. (1966). Creative productivity. *Journal of Gerontology, 21,* 1–8.

Diamond, M. (1999). *Magic trees of the mind.* New York: Penguin.

Divorcerate.com. (2009). American divorce rate.

Dixon, R., & Lerner, R. (1999). History and systems in developmental psychology. In M. Bornstein & M. Lamb (Eds.), *Developmental psychology: An advanced textbook.* Mahwah, NJ: Erlbaum.

Dobratz, M. C. (2003). The self-transacting dying: Patterns of social-psychological adaptation in home hospice patients. *Journal of Death & Dying, 46,* 151–163.

Dodge, K., Lansford, J., Burks, V., Bates, J., Pettit, G., Fontaine, R., & Price, J. (2003). Peer rejection and social information-processing factors in the development of aggressive behavior problems in children. *Child Development, 74*(2), 374–393.

Dorn, L. D., Susman, E. J., & Ponirakis, A. (2003). Pubertal timing and adolescent adjustment and behavior: Conclusions vary by rater. *Journal of Youth and Adolescence, 32*(3), 157–167.

Duncan, G., & Brooks-Gunn, J. (2000). Family poverty, welfare reform, & child development. *Child Development, 71*(1), 188–196.

Dunn, K. M., Croft, P. R., & Hackett, G. I. (2000). Satisfaction in the sex life of a general population sample. *Journal of Sex and Marital Therapy, 26,* 141–151.

Dunne, K. (2004). Grief and its manifestations (Bereavement). *Nursing Standard, 18*(45), 45–54.

Dychtwald, K. (2005). Ageless aging: The next era of retirement; "Old age" and "retirement" must be rethought and redefined as the baby boomers surge through the later stages of life, according to a renowned authority on aging. *The Futurist, 39*(4), 16–22.

E

Eagle, M. (2000). Psychoanalytic theory: History of the field. In A. Kazdin (Ed.), *Encyclopedia of psychology.* Washington, DC: American Psychological Association.

Eastman, P. (2000, January). Scientists piecing Alzheimer's puzzle. *AARP Bulletin, 41*(1), 18–19.

Eccles, J., & Roeser, R. (1999). School and community influences on human development. In M. Bornstein & M. Lamb (Eds.), *Developmental psychology: An advanced textbook.* Mahwah, NJ: Erlbaum.

Edwards, C. P., Gandini, L., & Forman, G. E. (Eds.) (1998). *The hundred languages of children: The Reggio Emilia approach—Advanced reflections* (2nd ed.). Greenwich, CT: Ablex.

Eisenberg, N., Fabes, R., & Spinrad, T. (2006). *Prosocial behavior.* In W. Damon & R. Lerner (Series Eds.) & N. Eisenberg (Vol. Ed.), *Handbook of child psychology: Vol. 3. Social, emotional, and personality development.* New York: Wiley.

Eisenberg, N., Martin, C., & Fabes, R. (1996). Gender development and gender effects. In D. Berliner & R. Calfee (Eds.), *Handbook of educational psychology.* New York: Macmillan.

Elder, G., & Shanahan, M. (2006). The life course and human development. In W. Damon & R. Lerner (Series Eds.) & R. Lerner (Vol. Ed.), *Handbook of child psychology: Vol. 1.Theoretical models of human development.* New York: Wiley.

Eliot, L. (2000). *What's going on in there?* New York: Bantam.

Elkind, D. (1978). *The child's reality: Three developmental themes.* Hillsdale, NJ: Erlbaum.

Elkind, D., & Bowen, R. (1979). Imaginary audience behavior in children and adolescents. *Developmental Psychology, 15,* 38–44.

Ellis, B. J., McFadyen-Ketchum, S., Dodge, K. A., Pettit, G. S., & Bates, J. E. (1999). Quality of early family relationships and individual differences in the timing of pubertal maturation in girls: A longitudinal test of an evolutionary model. *Journal of Personality & Social Psychology, 77*(2), 387–401.

Emde, R. (1998). Early emotional development: New modes of thinking for research and intervention. In J. Warhol & S. Shelov (Eds.), *New perspectives in early emotional development*. New York: Johnson & Johnson Pediatric Institute.

Emery, R., & Laumann-Billings, L. (2002). Child abuse. In M. Rutter and E. Taylor (Eds.), *Child and adolescent psychiatry*. London: Blackwell.

Erikson, E. (1958). *Young man Luther: A study in psychoanalysis and history*. New York: Norton.

———. (1959). Growth and crises of the healthy personality. *Psychological Issues, 1,* 40–52.

———. (1963). *Childhood and society* (2nd ed.). New York: Norton.

———. (1968). *Identity: Youth and crisis*. New York: Norton.

———. (1969). *Gandhi's truth: On the origins of militant nonviolence*. New York: Norton.

———. (1978). *Adulthood*. New York: Norton.

Eriksson, P. S., Perfilieva, E., Bjork-Eriksson, T., Alborn, A., Nordborg, C., Peterson, D. A., & Gage, F. H. (1998). Neurogenesis in the adult human hippocampus. *Nature Medicine, 4*(11), 1313–1317.

European Society for Human Reproduction and Embryology. 2009). *Babies born after freeze-thawing embryos do just as well regardless of whether they were created via ICSI or standard IVF*. Retrieved from http://www.eshre.eu/ESHRE/English/Press-Room/Press-Releases/Press-releases-ESHRE-2009/Neri-ICSI-offspring/page.aspx/753

F

Fantz, R. L. (1965). Visual perception from birth as shown by pattern selectivity. In H. E. Whipple (Ed.), *New issues in infant development. Annals of New York Academy of Science, 118,* 793–814.

Febo, M., Numan, M., & Ferris, C. F. (2005). Functional magnetic resonance imaging shows oxytocin activates brain regions associated with mother–pup bonding during suckling. *Journal of Neuroscience, 25*(10), 11637–11644.

Feldman, R., Weller, A., Sirota, L., & Eidelman, A. (2002). Skin-to-skin contact (kangaroo care) promotes self-regulation in premature infants: Sleep-wake cyclicity, arousal modulation, and sustained exploration. *Developmental Psychology, 38*(2), 194–207.

Ferber, R. *Solve your child's sleep problems*. New York: Simon & Schuster.

Ferris, P. (1997). *Dr. Freud: A life*. Washington, DC: Counterpoint.

Field, T. (2002). Violence and touch deprivation in adolescents. *Adolescence, 37,* 735–745.

Finch, C. (2003). Neurons, glia, and plasticity in normal brain aging. *Neurobiology of Aging, 24* (Suppl. 1), S123–S127.

Finch, J., & Robinson, M. (2003). Aging and late-onset disability: Addressing workplace accommodation. *Journal of Rehabilitation, 69*(2), 38–43.

Findling, R., & others. (2001). Psychotic disorders in children and adolescents. *Developmental Clinical Psychology Psychiatry, 44.* Thousand Oaks, CA: Sage.

Fitzpatrick, M. (2003). Women on the treadmill (doctoring the risk society). *The Lancet, 361*(9361), p. 976.

Flavell, J. (1999). Cognitive development: Children's knowledge about the mind. In J. Spence, J. Darley, & D. Foss (Eds.), *Annual Review of Psychology*. Palo Alto, CA: Annual Reviews.

Fraiberg, S. (1959). *The magic years*. New York: Charles Scribner's Sons.

Franco, O. H., de Laet, C., Peeters, A., Jonker, J., Mackenbach, J., & Nusselder, W. (2005). Effects of physical activity on life expectancy with cardiovascular disease. *Archives of Internal Medicine, 165,* 2355–2360.

Frankenberger, K. (2000). Adolescent egocentrism: A comparison among adolescents and adults. *Journal of Adolescence, 23,* 343–354.

Frankl, V. (1967). *Psychotherapy and existentialism*. New York: Simon & Schuster.

Friedan, B. (1963). *The feminine mystique*. New York: Norton.

Friedman, R., & P. Lindsay Chase-Lansdale. (2002). Chronic adversities. In M. Rutter and E. Taylor (Eds.), *Child and adolescent psychiatry*. London: Blackwell.

Fromm, E. (1968 [1956]). *The art of loving*. New York: Harper & Row.

Fung, H., Cartensen, L., & Lang, F. (2001). Age-related patterns in social networks among European Americans and African Americans: Implications for socioemotional selectivity across the life span. *International Journal of Aging & Human Development, 52,* 185–206.

G

Garbarino, J. (1999). *Lost boys: Why our sons turn violent and how we can save them*. New York: Free Press.

Garbarino, J., & Bedard, C. (2001). *Parents under siege*. New York: The Free Press.

Garbarino, J., & Benn, J. (1992). The ecology of childbearing and childrearing. In J. Garbarino (Ed.), *Children and families in the social environment*. New York: Aldine.

Gardner, D., Weissman, A., Howles, C., & Shoham, Z. (2004). *Textbook of assisted reproductive techniques*. Oxford, England: Taylor & Francis.

Gardner, H. (1983). *Frames of mind: The theory of multiple intelligences*. New York: Basic Books.

———. (1997). *Extraordinary minds*. New York: Basic Books.

———. (2003, September 7). *The real head start*. Boston Globe, pp. D1, D2.

Garmezy, N., & Rutter, M. (1983). *Stress, coping, and development*. New York: McGraw-Hill.

———. (1985). Acute reactions to stress. In M. Rutter & E. A. Taylor (Eds.), *Child and adolescent psychiatry*. Oxford, England: Wiley–Blackwell.

Geary, D., & Bjorklund, D. (2000). Evolutionary developmental psychology. *Child Development, 71*(1), 57–65.

Gebhardt, W. A., Kuyper, L., & Dusseldorp, E. (2006). Condom use at first intercourse with a new partner in female adolescents and young adults: The role of cognitive planning and motives for having sex. *Archives of Sexual Behavior, 35*(2), 217–224.

Gelman, R., & Baillargeon, R. (1983). A review of some Piagetian concepts. In P. Mussen (Ed.), *Handbook of child psychology: Vol. 3.* New York: Wiley.

Gendell, M. (2008, January). Older workers: Increasing their labor force participation and hours of work. *Monthly Labor Review,* pp. 41–54.

Gerard, J. M., Landry-Meyer, L., & Roe, J.G. (2006). Grandparents raising grandchildren: The role of social support in coping with caregiving challenges.(Author abstract). *International Journal of Aging & Human Development, 62*(4), 359–384.

Gibbons, R., Dugaiczyk, L. J., Girke, T., Duistermars, B., Zielinski, R., & Dugaiczyk, A. (2004). Distinguishing humans from great apes with AluYb8 repeats. *Journal of Molecular Biology, 339,* 721–729.

Gibson, E., & Walk, R. (1960). The visual cliff. *Scientific American, 202,* 64–71.

Gibson, E., & Pick, A. (2000). *An ecological approach to perceptual learning and development.* New York: Oxford Press.

Gilligan, C. (1982). *In a different voice.* Cambridge, MA: Harvard University Press.

Gilligan, C., Lyons, N., & Hanmer, T. (1990). *Making connections: The relational worlds of adolescent girls at Emma Willard School.* Cambridge, MA: Harvard University Press.

Goldberg, J., Holtz, D., Hyslop, T., & Tolosa, J. (2002). Has the use of routine episiotomy decreased? Examination of episiotomy rates from 1983 to 2000. *Obstetrics and Gynecology, 99*(3), 395–400.

Goldberg, S., & DiVitto, B. (2002). Parenting children born preterm. In M. Bornstein (Ed.), *Handbook of parenting* (2nd ed.). Mahwah, NJ: Erlbaum.

Gomez, C., & Rosen, B. (2001). The leader–member exchange as a link between managerial trust and employee empowerment. *Group and Organization Management, 26*(1), 53–69.

Gopnik, A., Meltzoff, A. N., & Kuhl, P. K. (1999). *The scientist in the crib: Minds, brains, and how children learn.* New York: HarperCollins.

Gottlieb, G. (1997). *Synthesizing nature–nurture.* Mahwah, NJ: Erlbaum.

Gottlieb, G., Wahlsten, D., & Lickliter, R. (2006).The significance of biology for human development: A developmental psychobiological systems View. In W. Damon & R. Lerner (Series Eds.) & R. Lerner (Vol. Ed.), *Handbook of child psychology: Vol. 1. Theoretical models of human development.* New York: Wiley.

Graham, E. I. (2005). Economic, racial, and cultural influences on the growth and maturation of children. *Pediatrics in Review, 26,* 290–294.

Green, J. (2006, May 19). *U.S. has second worst newborn death rate in modern world, report says.* Retrieved from http://www.cnn.com/2006/HEALTH/parenting/05/08/mothers.index/

Greenfield, P., Suzuki. L., & Rothstein-Fisch, C. (2006). Cultural pathways through human development. In W. Damon & R. Lerner (Series Eds.) & K. Ann Renninger & Irving Sigel (Vol. Eds.), *Handbook of child psychology: Vol. 4. Child psychology in practice.* New York: Wiley.

Grodner, M., Long, S., & DeYoung, S. (2004). *Foundations and clinical applications of nutrition.* Philadelphia: Mosby.

Grossman, J., & Kaufman, J. (2002). Evolutionary psychology: Promise and perils. In R. J. Sternberg, & J. C. Kaufman (Eds.), *The evolution of intelligence.* (pp. 9–25). Mahwah, NJ: Erlbaum.

Grotevant, H. (1998). Adolescent development in family contexts. In W. Damon (Series Ed.) & N. Eisenberg (Vol. Ed.), *Handbook of child psychology: Vol. 3. Social, emotional, and personality development.* New York: Wiley.

Guia, D. M. (2003). Caregivers stress syndrome. Letters to the editor. *Townsend Letter for Doctors & Patients.*

Guttmacher Institute. (2008, April 16). Teen pregnancy rates declined to historic low in 2004—Improved contraceptive use a key factor. Retrieved from http://www.guttmacher.org/pubs/fb_ATSRH.html

Guyer, B., Hoyert, D., Martin, J., Ventura, S., MacDorman, M., & Strobino, D. (1999). Annual summary of vital statistics—1998. *Pediatrics, 104*(6), 1229–1246.

H

Haas, F. (2003). Bereavement care: Seeing the body. *Nursing Standards, 17,* 33–37.

Haliburn, J. (2000). Reasons for adolescent suicide attempts. *Journal of the American Academy of Child & Adolescent Psychiatry, 39*(1), 13–14.

Hall, G. S. (1904). *Adolescence.* (2 vols.) New York: Appleton-Century-Crofts.

Hallett, V. (2005). The power of Potter: Can the teenage wizard turn a generation of halfhearted readers into lifelong bookworms? Retrieved from http://www.usnews.com/usnews/culture/articles/050725/25read_6.htm

Handelsman, D. J., & Liu, P. Y. (2006). Klinefelter's syndrome: A microcosm of male reproductive health. *Journal of Clinical Endocrinology and Metabolism, 91,* 1220–1222.

Harlow, H. F., & Suomi, S. J. (1971). Social recovery by isolation-reared monkeys. *Proceedings of the National Academy of Science of the United States of America, 68*(7), 1534–1538.

Harman, W. (2008). CPR on the *Today Show:* In case you missed it. Retrieved from http://redcrosschat.org/2008/10/20/cpr-on-the-today-show-in-case-you-missed-it/

Harrison, L. (2000). Why culture matters. In L. Harrison & S. Huntington (Eds.), *Culture matters.* New York: Basic Books.

Harter, S. (1999). *The construction of the self.* New York: Guilford Press.

————. (2006). The self. In W. Damon & R. Lerner (Series Eds.) & N. Eisenberg (Vol. Ed.), *Handbook of child psychology: Vol. 3. Social, emotional, and personality development.* New York: Wiley.

Hartl, D., & Jones, E. (2005). *Genetics: Analysis of genes and genomes.* Boston: Jones and Bartlett.

Harton, H. C., & Lyons, P. C. (2003). Gender, empathy, and the choice of the psychology major. *Teaching of Psychology, 30*(1), 19–24.

Harvard Men's Health Watch. (2004, January). Medical memo: An update on calcium and prostate cancer. *Harvard Men's Health Watch, 8* (6), 5.

Harvey, E. (1999). Short-term and long-term effects of early parental employment on children of the National Longitudinal Survey of Youth. *Developmental Psychology, 35*(2), 445–459.

Hays, K. (2004). Coping with college series: Tips for successful career planning for all four years of College. Retrieved from Illinois State Website: http://www. counseling.ilstu.edu/DP/cope tips.html.

Heller, S., Larrieu, J., D'Imperio, R., & Boris, N. (1999). Research on resilience to child maltreatment: Empirical considerations. *Child Abuse & Neglect, 23*(4), 321–338.

Heron, M. P., Hoyert, D. L., Murphy, S. L., Xu, J. Q., Kochanek, K. D., & Tejada-Vera, B. (2009). Deaths: Final data for 2006. *National Vital Statistics Reports, 57*(14). Hyattsville, MD: National Center for Health Statistics.

Hess, T., Auman, C., Colcombe, S., Rahhal, & Tamara, A. (2003). The impact of stereotype threat on age differences in memory performance. *Journals of Gerontology Series B – Psychological Sciences and Social Sciences, 58*(1), 3–11.

Hetherington, E. M. (2005). Divorce and the adjustment of children. *Pediatrics in Review, 26,* 163–169.

Hetherington, M., & Stanley-Hagan, M. (1995). Parenting in divorced and remarried families. In M. H. Bornstein (Ed.), *Children and parenting: Vol. 4.* Hillsdale, NJ: Erlbaum.

———. (2002. Parenting in divorced and remarried families. In M. Bornstein (Ed.), *Handbook of parenting* (2nd ed.). Mahwah, NJ: Erlbaum.

Heywood, C. (2001). *A history of childhood.* Malden, MA: Blackwell.

Hill, J. P. (1973). *Some perspectives on adolescence in American society.* Position paper prepared for the Office of Child Development, U.S. Department of Health, Education, and Welfare.

———. (1987). Central changes during adolescence. In W. Damon (Ed.), *New directions in child psychology.* San Francisco: Jossey-Bass.

Hingson, R. W., Heeren, T., Jamanka, A., & Howland, J. (2000). Age of drinking onset and unintentional injury involvement after drinking. *Journal of the American Medical Association, 284*(12), 1527–1533.

Ho, T., Leung, P., Hung, S., Lee, C., & Tang, C. (2000). The mental health of the peers of suicide completers and attempters. *Journal of Child Psychology and Psychiatry, 41,* 301–308.

Hobson, J. A. (2004). Freud returns? Like a bad dream. *Scientific American, 290*(5), 89.

Horn, J. L. (1978). Human ability systems. In P. B. Baltes (Ed.), *Life-span development and behavior: Vol. 1.* New York: Academic Press.

Horowitz, F. D. (2000). Child development and the PITS: Simple questions, complex answers, and developmental theory. *Child Development, 71*(1), 1–10.

Hough, M. S. (2007). Adult age differences in word fluency for common and goal-directed categories. *Advances in Speech Language Pathology, 9*(2), 154–161.

Huang, B., Cornoni-Huntley, J., Hays, J., Huntley, R., Galanos, A., & Blazer, D. (2000). Impact of depressive symptoms on hospitalization risk in community-dwelling older persons. *Journal of American Geriatric Society, 48,* 1279–1284.

Human Development Report. (2009). *Overcoming barriers: Human mobility and development.* Retrieved from http://hdr.undp.org/en/media/HDR_2009_EN_Complete.pdf

Humes, L. E., & Floyd, S. S. (2005). Measures of working memory, sequence learning, and speech recognition in the elderly. *Journal of Speech, Language, and Hearing Research, 48*(1), 224–236.

Humphrey, S., & Kahn, A. (2000). Fraternities, athletic teams and rape: Importance of identification with a risky group. *Journal of Interpersonal Violence, 15*(12), 1313–1322.

Hussey, J. M., Chang, J. J., & Kotch, J. B. (2006). Child maltreatment in the United States: Prevalence, risk factors, and adolescent health consequences. *Pediatrics, 118*(3), 933–943.

J

Jaquish, G. A., & Ripple, R. E. (1981). Cognitive creative abilities and self-esteem across the adult life-span. *Human Development, 24*(2), 110–119.

Jasper, M. (2000). Antepartum fetal assessment. In S. Mattson & J. Smith (Eds.), *Core curriculum for maternal–newborn nursing.* Philadelphia: Saunders.

Jeng, S. F., Yau, K. I. T., Liao, H. F., Chen, L. C., & Chen, P. S. (2000). Prognostic factors for walking attainment in very low-birth weight preterm infants. *Early Human Development, 59*(3), 159–173.

Jenkins, J., & Astington, J. (1996) Cognitive factors and family structure associated with theory of mind development in young children. *Developmental Psychology, 32,* 70–78.

Jimerson, S., Pavelski, R., & Orliss, M. (2002). Helping children with eating disorders: Quintessential research on etiology, prevention, assessment, and treatment. In J. Sandoval (Ed.), *Handbook of crisis counseling, intervention, and prevention in the schools* (2nd ed., pp. 393–415). Mahwah, NJ: Erlbaum.

Jio, S. (2009). *The truth about sex after menopause: Get 10 facts about what will and won't happen to your body.* Retrieved from http://www.womansday.com/Articles/Health/The-Truth-about-Sex-after-Menopause.html

Joensson, P., & Carlsson, I. (2000). Androgyny and creativity: A study of the relationship between a balanced sex-role and creative functioning. *Scandinavian Journal of Psychology, 41,* 269–274.

Johnson, B. (2002). The intentional mentor: Strategies and guidelines for the practice of mentoring. *Professional Psychology: Research & Practice, 33,* 88–96.

Johnson, R. (2002). The puzzle of later male retirement. *Economic Review (Kansas City), 87*(3), 5–28.

Jones, J. (2009). *Who adopts? Characteristics of women and men who have adopted children* (NCHS Data Brief No. 12). Washington, DC: NCHS.

Jones, S. (1996). Imitation or exploration: Young infants' matching of adults' oral gestures. *Child Development, 67,* 1952–1969.

K

Kachru, Y. (2005). Teaching and learning of world englishes. In E. Hinkel (Ed.), *Handbook of research in second language teaching and learning.* Mahwah, NJ: Erlbaum.

Kagan, J. (1998a). Biology and the child. In W. Damon (Series Ed.) & N. Eisenberg (Volume Ed.), *Handbook of child psychology: Vol. 3. Social, emotional, and personality development.* New York: Wiley.

Kagan, J., & Fox, N. (2006). Biology, culture, and temperamental biases. In N. Eisenberg (Ed.), *Handbook of child psychology: Vol. 3. Social, emotional, and personality development.* New York: Wiley.

Kahn, M. (2002). *Basic Freud.* New York: Basic Books.

Kaiser Family Foundation. (2008). *Sexual health of adolescents and young adults in the United States.* Retrieved from http://www.kff.org/womenshealth/upload/3040_04.pdf

Kallman, F., & Jarvik, L. (1959). Individual differences in constitution and genetic background. In J. Birren (Ed.), *Handbook of aging and the individual.* Chicago: University of Chicago Press.

Kashima, Y., Kim, U., Gelfand, M. J., Yamaguchi, S., Sang-Chin, Choi, & Yuki, M. (1995). Culture, gender, and self: A perspective from individualism–collectivism research. *Journal of Personality and Social Psychology, 69*(5), 925–937.

Keel, P., & others. (2001). Vulnerability to eating disorders in childhood and adolescence. In R. E. Ingram & J. M. Price (Eds.), *Vulnerability to psychopathology: Risk across the lifespan.* (pp. 389–411). New York: Guilford Press.

Kellogg, R. (1970). *Analyzing children's art.* Palo Alto, CA: National Press Books.

Killgore, W., & Oki, M. (2001). Sex-specific developmental changes in amygdala responses to affective faces. *Neuroreport: For Rapid Communication of Neuroscience Research, 12,* 427–433.

Kim, U. (1990). Indigenous psychology: Science and applications. In R. Brislin (Ed.), *Applied cross-cultural psychology*. Newbury Park, CA: Sage.

King, K. (2000, February). Common teen suicide myths undermine prevention programs. *American Academy of Pediatrics News*. Elk Grove Village, IL: American Association of Pediatricians.

Knowles, M. (1989). *The adult learner: A neglected species*. Houston: Gulf.

Kohut, A. (2007). Rising environmental concern in 47-nation survey: Global unease with major world powers. *The Pew Global Attitudes Project*. Washington, DC: Pew Research Center. Retrieved from http://pewglobal.org/reports/pdf/256.pdf

Kozol, J. (1991). *Savage inequalities*. New York: Crown.

Kramer, A., & Willis, S. (2004). Enhancing the cognitive vitality of older adults. In J. Lerner & A. Alberts (Eds.), *Current directions in developmental psychology*. New Jersey: Prentice Hall, 160–166.

Krettenauer, T., Ullrich, M., Hofmann, V., & Edelstein, W. (2003). Behavioral problems in childhood and adolescence as predictors of ego-level attainment in early adulthood. *Merrill-Palmer Quarterly, 49*, 125–138.

L

Labouvie-Vief, G. (2006). Emerging structures of adult thought. In J. J. Arnett & J. L. Tanner (Eds), *Emerging adults in America*. Washington, DC: American Psychological Association.

Lamb, M., & Ahnert, L. (2006). Nonparental child care: Context, concepts, correlates, and consequences. In W. Damon & R. Lerner (Series Eds.) & K. Ann Renninger & Irving Sigel (Vol. Eds.), *Handbook of child psychology: Vol. 4. Child psychology in practice*. New York: Wiley.

Lamb, M., Hwang, C., Ketterlinus, R., & Fracasso, M. (1999). Parent–child relationships. In M. Bornstein & M. Lamb (Eds.), *Developmental psychology: An advanced textbook*. Mahwah, NJ: Erlbaum.

Land, K. C., & Yang, Y. (2006). Morbidity, disability, and mortality. In R. H. Binstock & L. K. George (Eds.), *Handbook on aging and the social sciences* (6th ed.). San Diego: Academic Press.

Lang, F. (2001). Regulation of social relationships in later adulthood. *Journal of Gerontology, 56B*, P321–P326.

Lanman, S. (2009, November). *Fed officials cut forecasts for unemployment rate (Update 1)*. Retrieved from http://www.bloomberg.com/apps/news?pid=20601068&sid=aFbDgcAh319I

Lantz, M. (2001). Suicide in late life: Identifying and managing at-risk older patients. *Geriatrics, 56*, 47–48.

Lee, G., DeMaris, A., Bavin, S., & Sullivan, R. (2001). Gender differences in the depressive effect of widowhood in later life. *Journal of Gerontology, 56B*, S56–S61.

Lee, G., Peek, C. W., & Coward, R. T. (1998). Race differences in filial responsibility expectations among older parents. *Journal of Marriage and the Family, 60*(3), 404–412.

Lee, J. M., Appugliese, D., Kaciroti, N., Corwyn, R. F., Bradley, R. H., & Lumeng, J. C. (2007). Weight status in young girls and the onset of puberty. *Pediatrics, 119*(3), 593–595.

Lehman, H. C. (1953). *Age and achievement*. Princeton, NJ: Princeton University Press.

———. (1962). The creative production rates of present versus past generations of scientists. *Journal of Gerontology, 17*, 409–417.

Lehrer, J. (2009, April 26) Inside the baby mind. *The Boston Globe*, p. C1.

Leifer, G. (2003). *Introduction to maternity and pediatric nursing*. St. Louis: Saunders.

Leinonen, E., Korpisammal, L., Pulkkinen, L., & Pukuri, T. (2001). The comparison of burden between caregiving spouses of depressive and demented patients. *International Journal of Geriatric Psychiatry, 16*, 387–393.

Leon, I. (2002). Adoption losses: Naturally occurring or socially constructed? *Child Development, 73*(2), 652–653.

Leonard, D. (2010). The case for $320,000 kindergarten teachers. *New York Times*.

Lerner, J., & Ashman, O. (2006). Culture and lifespan development. In K. Theis & J. Travers (Eds.), *Handbook of human development for health care professionals*. Sudbury, MA: Jones and Bartlett.

Lerner, R. (1991). Changing organism—Context relations as the basic process of development: A developmental contextual perspective. *Developmental Psychology, 27*(1), 27–32.

———. (2002). *Concepts and theories of human development* (3rd ed.). Mahwah, NJ: Erlbaum.

Lerner, R., Fisher, C., & Weinberg, R. (2000). Toward a science for and of the people: Promoting civil society through the application of developmental science. *Child Development, 71*(1), 11–20.

Lerner, R., & Galambos, N. (1998). Adolescent development: Challenges and opportunities for research, programs, and policies. In J. Spence, J. Darley, & D. Foss (Eds.), *Annual Review of Psychology*. Palo Alto, CA: Annual Reviews.

Lerner, R. M. (Ed.). (1998). Theoretical models of human development. *Handbook of child psychology: Vol. 1* (5th ed.). New York: Wiley.

Levin, D., & Kilbourne, J. (2008). *So sexy so soon: The new sexualized childhood and what parents can do to protect their kids*. New York: Random House.

Levinson, D. (1978). *The seasons of a man's life*. New York: Knopf.

———. (1990a). *Seasons of a woman's life*. Presented at the 98th annual convention of the American Psychological Association, Boston.

———. (1990b). A theory of life structure development in adulthood. In C. N. Alexander & E. J. Langer (Eds.), *Higher states of human development*. (pp.35–54). New York: Oxford University Press.

Levy, B. R., & Banaji, M. R. (2002). Implicit ageism. In T. D. Nelson (Ed.), *Ageism: Stereotypes and prejudice against older persons*. (pp. 49–75). Cambridge, MA: MIT Press.

Lewis, M. (1997). *Altering fate: Why the past does not predict the future*. New York: Guilford Press.

———. (2000). The promise of dynamic systems approaches for an integrated account of human development. *Child Development, 71*(1), 36–43.

Lipkins, S., Levy, J. M., & Jerabkova, B. (2009). *Sexting . . . is it all about power?* Retrieved from http://www.realpsychology.com/content/tools-life/sextingis-it-all-about-power

Lips, H. M. (2007). Gender and possible selves. *New Directions for Adult and Continuing Education, 114*, 51–59.

Ljungquist, B., Berg, S., Lanke, J., McClearn, G. E., & Pedersen, N. L. (1998). The effect of genetic factors for longevity: A comparison of identical and fraternal twins in the Swedish Twin Registry. *Journals of Gerontology Series A – Biological Sciences and Medical Sciences, 53A*, 441–446.

Lloyd, M. (2009). *Supercharged retirement: Ditch the rocking chair, trash the remote, and do what you love.* University Place, Washington: Hankfritz Press.

Lorenz, K. Z. (1965). *Evolution and the modification of behavior.* Chicago: University of Chicago Press.

M

Maccoby, E. E., & Martin, J. A. (1983). Socialization in the context of the family. In E. M. Hetherington (Ed.), *Handbook of child psychology: Vol. 4. Socialization, personality, and social development.* New York: Wiley.

Macera, M. H., & Cohen, S. H. (2006). Psychology as a profession: An effective career exploration and orientation course for undergraduate psychology majors. *Career Development Quarterly, 54*(4), 367–371.

Malloy, L. C., Lyon, T. D., & Quas, J. A. (2007). Filial dependency and recantation of child sexual abuse allegations. *Journal of the American Academy of Child and Adolescent Psychiatry, 46*(2), 162–171.

Malloy, M., & Freeman, D. (2000). *Birth weight and gestational age.* Mahwah, NJ: Erlbaum.

Mann, T. (1939, June 21). *The New York Times.*

Marcus, L. (2002). *Ways of telling: Conversations on the art of the picture.* New York: Dutton Books.

Margolis, D. (2005). Gender. In K. Thies & J. Travers (Eds.). *Handbook of human development for health care professionals.* Sudbury, MA: Jones and Bartlett.

Marlier, L., & Schaal, B. (2005). Hujman newborns prefer human milk: Conspecific milk odor is attractive without postnatal exposure. *Child Development, 76,* 155–168.

Marrs, R., Bloch, L., & Silverman, K. (1997). *Dr. Richard Marrs' fertility book.* New York: Delacorte.

Marshall, P. (2002). *Cultural diversity in our schools.* Belmont, CA: Wadsworth.

Martin, J. A., Hamilton, B. E., Sutton, P. D., Ventura, S. J., Menacker, F., Kirmeyer, S., & Mathews, T. J. (2009). Births: Final data for 2006. *National Vital Statistics Reports, 57*(7).

Maslow, A. (1987). *Motivation and personality.* (Revised by R. Frager, J. Fadiman, C. McReynolds, & R. Cox.) New York: Harper & Row.

McCarthy, M. (2002). U.S. government releases nursing home report cards. *The Lancet, 360*(9346), 1670.

McCool, J. P., Cameron, L. D., & Petrie, K. J. (2001). Adolescent perceptions of smoking imagery in film. *Social Science and Medicine, 52*(10), 1577–1587.

McCrae, R., & Costa, P. T., Jr. (1990). *Personality in adulthood.* New York: Guilford Press.

———. (2004, February). A contemplated revision of the NEO Five-Factor Inventory. *Personality and Individual Differences, 36*(3), 587–596.

McCrae, R., Costa, P. T., Ostendorf, F., Angleitner, A., Hrebíckovú, M., & Avia, M. D., et al. (2000). Nature over nurture: Temperament, personality, and lifespan development. *Journal of Personality and Social Psychology, 78*(1), 173–186.

McEvoy, G. M., & Cascio, W. F. (1989). Cumulative evidence of the relationship between employee age and job performance. *Journal of Applied Psychology, 74,* 11–17.

Meschke, L., & others. (2000). Demographic, biological, psychological, and social predictors of the timing of first intercourse. *Journal of Research on Adolescence, 10,* 315–338.

Meshefedjian, G., McCusker, J., Bellavance, F., & Baumgarten, M. (1998). Factors associated with symptoms of depression among informal caregivers of demented elders in the community. *The Gerontologist, 38*(2), 247–253.

Miller, B. C., Benson, B., & Galbraith, K. A. (2001). Family relationships and adolescent pregnancy risk: A research synthesis. *Developmental Review, 21*(1), 1–38.

Miller, J., Rosenbloom, A., & Silverstein, J. (2004). Childhood obesity. *Journal of Clinical Endocrinology & Metabolism, 89*(9), 4211–4218.

Miller, K. E., Barnes, G. M., Melnick, M., Sabo, D. F., & Farrell, M. P. (2002). Gender and racial/ethnic differences in predicting adolescent sexual risk: Athletic participation versus exercise. *Journal of Health and Social Behavior, 43,* 436–450.

Miniño, A. M., Heron, M., Smith, B. L., & Kochanek, K. D. (2006). Deaths: Final data for 2004. *Health E-Stats.*

Moore, K., & Persaud, T. (2003). *Before we are born: Essentials of embryology and birth defects.* Philadelphia: Saunders.

Moran, B. (2000). Maternal infections. In S. Mattson & J. Smith (Eds.), *Core curriculum for maternal–newborn nursing.* Philadelphia: Saunders.

Morris, K., (2006). Genital mutilation and alternative practices. *The Lancet, 368,* 64–67.

Mosher, C.E., & Danoff-Burg, S. (2004). Effects of gender and employment status on support provided to caregivers. *Sex Roles: A Journal of Research, 51,* 589–596.

Mosher, W. D., Chandra, A., & Jones, J. (2005). Sexual behavior and selected health measures: Men and women 15–44 years of age, United States, 2002. *Advance Data for Vital and Health Statistics, 362,* 1–56.

Muehlenhard, C. L., Friendman, D. E., & Thomas, C. M. (2002). Is date rape justifiable? The effects of dating activity, who initiated, who paid, and men's attitudes toward women. *Psychology of Women Quarterly, 9*(3), 297–310.

Muller, F., Rebiff, M., Taillander, A., Qury, J. F., & Mornet, E. (2000). Parental origin of the extra chromosome in prenatally diagnosed fetal trisomy. *Human Genetics, 106,* 340–344.

Munakata, Y. (2006). Information processing approaches to development. In W. Damon & R. Lerner (Series Eds.) & R. Lerner (Vol. Ed.), *Handbook of child psychology: Vol. 1. Theoretical models of human development.* New York: Wiley.

Murphy, W., & others. (2001). An exploration of factors related to deviant sexual arousal among juvenile sex offenders. *Sexual Abuse: Journal of Research & Treatment, 13,* 91–103.

Muse, D. (Ed.). (1997*). Multicultural resources for young readers.* New York: New Press.

N

National Adolescent Health Information Center, (2006). *Fact sheet on suicide: Adolescents & young adults.* Retrieved from http://www.nahic.ucsf.edu/downloads/Suicide.pdf

National Center for Education Statistics. (2003). *Fast facts.* Retrieved from http://nces.ed.gov/fastfacts/display.asp?id-59

National Center for Health Statistics. (2006a). *Health, United States, 2006: With chartbook on trends in the health of Americans.* Hyattsville, MD: Author.

National Center for Health Statistics. (2006b). *Multiple Causes of Death.* Public Use Data Files, 1990–2004. Hyattsville: U.S. Department of Health and Human Services.

National Household Survey on Drug Abuse (NHSDA) Report. (2002). Retrieved from http://www.oas.samhsa.gov/2k2/ AlcBinge/AlcBinge.htm

National Institute of Mental Health (NIMH). 2009. *Older adults: Depression and suicide facts* (Fact Sheet). Retrieved from http://www.nimh.nih.gov/health/publications/older-adults-depression-and-suicide-facts-fact-sheet/index.shtml

Ngai, S. S., Ngai, N., & Cheung, C. (2006). Environmental influences on risk taking among Hong Kong young dance partygoers. *Adolescence, 41*(164), 739–753.

Nielsen Media Research. (2006). *Nielsen media research reports television's popularity is still growing.* Retrieved from http://www.thinktv.com.au/media/Articles/Nielsen_Media_Reports_TV's_Popularity_Is_Still_Growing.pdf

Nuttall, R., & Nuttall, E. (1980). *Family coping and disasters.* Boulder, CO: National Hazards Research Applications.

O

O'Dea, J. A., & Abraham, S. (1999). Onset of disordered eating attitudes and behaviors in early adolescence: Interplay of pubertal status, gender, weight, and age. *Adolescence, 34*(136), 671–679.

Obeidallah, D. A., Brennan, R. T., Brooks-Gunn, J., Kindlon, D., & Earls, F. (2000). Socioeconomic status, race, and girls' pubertal maturation: Results form the Project on Human Development in Chicago Neighborhoods. *Journal of Research on Adolescence, 10*(4), 443–464.

Office of Head Start. (2007). *FY 2007 funding program instruction.* Retrieved from http://eclkc.ohs.acf.hhs.gov/hslc/Progam-DesignandManagement/HeadStartRequirements/Pls/2007/resour_pri_00112_032707.html

Olds, S., London, M., & Ladewig, P. (1996). *Maternal–newborn nursing.* Reading, MA: Addison-Wesley.

Oregon.gov.Death With Dignity Act (2007). Retrieved from http://Oregon.gov/DHS/ph/pas/oars.html

Ory, M., Hoffman, R. R., Yee, J. L., Tennstedt, S., & Schulz, R. (1999). Prevalence and impact of caregiving: A detailed comparison between dementia and nondementia caregivers. *The Gerontologist, 39*(2), 177–185.

Oswald, D. L., & Russell, B. L. (2006). Perceptions of sexual coercion in heterosexual dating relationships: The role of aggressor gender and tactics. *The Journal of Sex Research, 43*(1), 87–96.

P

Pang, J. W. Y., Heffelfinger, J. D., Huang, G. J., Benedetti, T. J., & Noell, S. (2002). Outcomes of planned home births in Washington State: 1989–1996. *Obstetrics & Gynecology, 100*(2), 253–259.

Papalia, D., & Olds, S. (2004). *Human development.* New York: McGraw-Hill.

Paris, S., & Paris, A. (2006). Assessment of early reading. In W. Damon & R. Lerner (Series Eds.) & K. Renninger & I. Sigel (Vol. Eds.), *Handbook of child psychology: Vol. 4. Child psychology in practice.* New York: Wiley.

Parker-Pope, T. (2009). *Well.* Retrieved from http://well.blogs.nytimes.com/2009/08/19/us-life-expectancy-at-all-time-high/

Parten, M. (1932). Social participation among preschool children. *Journal of Abnormal Psychology, 27* 243–269.

Peake, P., Hebl, M., & Mischel, W. (2002). Strategic attention deployment for delay of gratification in working and waiting situations. *Developmental Psychology, 38*(2), 313–326.

Perry, W. (1968a). *Forms of intellectual and ethical development in the college years.* New York: Holt, Rinehart & Winston.

———. (1968b, April). *Patterns of development in thought and values of students in a liberal arts college: A validation of a scheme.* Washington, DC: U.S. Department of Health, Education, and Welfare, Office of Education, Bureau of Research.

———. (1981). Cognitive and ethical growth. In A. Chickering (Ed.), *The modern American college.* San Francisco: Jossey-Bass.

Petersen, A. (1988). Adolescent development. *Annual Review of Psychology, 39,* 583–607. Palo Alto, CA: Annual Reviews.

Phillips, B. D. (2004). The future small business workforce: Will labor shortages exist? The available evidence is less than perfect. *Business Economics, 39*(4), 19–28.

Piaget, J. (1952a). *The origins of intelligence.* New York; Norton.

———. (1952b). *The origins of intelligence in children.* New York: International Universities Press.

———. (1973). *The child and reality.* New York: Viking.

Piaget, J., & Inhelder, B. (1969). *The psychology of the child.* New York: Basic Books.

Pienta, A. M., Hayward, M. D., & Jenkins, K. R. (2000). Health consequences of marriage for the retirement years. *Journal of Family Issues, 21*(5), 559–586.

Pinker, S. (1994). *The language instinct.* New York: Morrow.

Pitkin, S., & Savage, L. (2004). Age-related vulnerability to diencephalic amnesia produced by thiamine deficiency: The role of time of insult. *Behavioural Brain Research, 148*(1–2), 93–105.

Posner, R. B. (2006). Early menarche: A review of research on trends in timing, racial differences, etiology, and psychosocial consequences. *Sex Roles, 54*(5–6), 315–322.

Pruchno, R. (1999). Raising grandchildren: The experiences of black and white grandmothers. *The Gerontologist, 39*(2), 209–221.

R

Ravitch, D. (2010). *The death and life of the great American school system: How testing and choice are undermining education.* New York: Basic Books.

Reisberg, L. (2000, January 28). Student stress is rising, especially among women. *The Chronicle of Higher Education,* p. A521.

Rogoff, B. (1991). *Apprenticeship in thinking: Cognitive development in social context.* New York: Oxford University Press.

———. (2003). *The cultural nature of human development.* New York: Oxford University Press.

Rose, S. (2005). *The future of the brain.* New York: Oxford University Press.

Rosser, S. V. (2004). Using POWRE to ADVANCE: Institutional barriers identified by women scientists and engineers. *NWSA Journal, 16*(1), 50–79.

Rubin, K., Bukowski, W., & Parker, J. (2006). Peer interactions, relationships, and groups. In W. Damon & R. Lerner (Series Eds.) & N. Eisenberg (Vol. Ed.), *Handbook of child psychology: Vol. 3. Social, emotional, and personality development.* New York: John Wiley

Rubin, R. (1984). *Maternal identity and maternal experience.* New York: Springer.

Ruble, D., & Martin, C. (1998). Gender development. In W. Damon (Series Ed.) & N. Eisenberg (Vol. Ed.), *Handbook of child psychology: Vol. 3. Child psychology in practice.* New York: Wiley.

Ruble, D., Martin, C., & Berenbaum, S. (2006). Gender development. In W. Damon & R. Lerner (Series Eds.) & N. Eisenberg (Vol. Ed.), *Handbook of child psychology: Vol. 3. Social, emotional, and personality development.* New York: Wiley.

Russell, R. B., Petrini, J. R., Damus, K., Mattison, D. R., & Schwarz, R. H. (2003). The changing epidemiology of multiple births in the United States. *Obstetrics and Gynecology, 1001,* 129–135.

Russell, S. T. (2006). Substance use and abuse and mental health among sexual-minority youths: Evidence from add health. In A. M. Omoto & H. S. Kurtzman (Eds.), *Sexual orientation and mental health: Examining identity and development in lesbian, gay, and bisexual people* (pp. 13–35). Washington, DC: American Psychological Association.

Rutter, M. (1983). School effects on pupil progress: Research findings and policy implications. *Child Development, 54*(1), 1–29.

———. (2002a). Development and psychopathology. In M. Rutter and E. Taylor (Eds.). *Child and adolescent psychiatry.* London: Blackwell.

———. (2002b). Nature, nurture and development: From evangelism through science toward policy and practice. *Child Development, 73*(1), 1–21.

———. (2006*). Genes and behavior.* Oxford, England: Blackwell.

Rutter, M., & Nikapota, A. (2006). Culture, ethnicity, society, and psychopathology. In M. Rutter and E. Taylor (Eds.), *Child and adolescent psychiatry.* London: Blackwell.

Rutter, M., & Rutter, M. (1993). *Developing minds.* New York: Basic Books

Rutter, M., & Taylor, E. (Eds.). (2002). *Child and adolescent psychiatry.* London: Blackwell.

S

Salter, D., McMillan, D., Richards, M., Talbot, T. Hodges, J., Bentovim, A., Hastings, R., Stevenson, J., & Skuse, D. (2003). *The Lancet, 361*(9356), 471.

Salthouse, T. A. (2001). Structural models of the relations between age and measures of cognitive functioning. *Intelligence, 29,* 93–115.

SAMHSA, Office of Applied Studies. (2008). *National Survey on Drug Use and Health.* Retrieved from http://www.oas.samhsa.gov/NSDUH/2K8NSDUH/tabs/Sect2peTabs17to21.pdf

Sanders, C. M. (1989). *Grief: The mourning after: Dealing with adult bereavement.* New York: Wiley.

Savage, M. P., & Holcomb, D. R. (1999). Adolescent female athletes' sexual risk-taking behaviors. *Journal of Youth and Adolescence, 28,* 595–602.

Schaie, K. W. (1994). The course of adult intellectual development. *American Psychologist, 49*(4), 304 313.

———. (2005). *Developmental influences on adult intellectual development: The Seattle Longitudinal Study.* New York: Oxford University Press.

Schaie, K. W., & Elder, G. (2005). *Historical influences on lives and aging.* New York: Springer.

Scheinfeld, D. R., Haigh, K. M., & Scheinfeld, S. J. P. (2008). *We are all explorers: Learning and teaching with Reggio principles in urban settings.* New York: Teachers College Press.

Schmader, T., Johns, M., & Barquissau, M. (2004). The cost of accepting gender differences: The role of stereotype endorsement in women's experience in the math domain. *Sex Roles, 50*(11–12) 835–850.

Schwartz, I. (2002). Sexual activity prior to coital interaction: A comparison between males and females. *Archives of Sexual Behavior, 28,* 63–69.

Selfhout, M. H. W., Delsing, M. J. M. H., ter Bogt, T. F. M., & Meeus, W. H. J. (2008). Heavy metal and hip-hop style preferences and externalizing problem behaviors: A two-wave longitudinal study. *Youth and Society, 39*(4), 435–452.

Seligman, M. E. P., & Csikszentmihalyi, M. (2000). Positive psychology: An introduction. *American Psychologist, 55*(1), 5–14.

Seppa, N. (1996, August). Rwanda starts its long healing process. *APA Monitor,* p. 14.

Shaffer, D., & Pfeffer, C. (2001). Practice parameter for assessment and treatment of children and adolescents with suicidal behavior. *Journal of the American Academy of Child and Adolescent Psychiatry, 40,* S24–S51.

Shankaran, S., Laptook, A. R., Ehrenkranz, R. A., Tyson, J. E., McDonald, S. A. & Donovan, E. F. (2005). Whole-body hypothermia for neonates with hypoxic-ischemic encephalopathy. *New England Journal of Medicine, 353,* 1574–1584.

Sharples, T. (2008). Study: Most child abuse goes unreported. *Time.* Retrieved from http://www.time.com/time/health/article/0,8599,1863650,00.html

Sheldon, K., & Kasser, T. (2001). Getting older, getting better? Personal striving and psychological maturity across the life span. *Developmental Psychology, 37,* 491–501.

Shenk, J. W. (2009). What makes us happy? *The Atlantic, 3003*(5), 36–53.

Shonkoff, J. P., & Phillips, D. A. (Eds.). (200). *From neurons to neighborhoods: The science of early childhood development.* Washington, DC: National Academy Press.

Shreeve, J. (2005). *The genome war: How Craig Venter tried to capture the code of life and save the world.* New York: Ballantine Books.

Siegel, D. J. (1999). *The developing mind: How relationships and the brain interact to shape who we are.* New York: Guilford Press.

Siegel, L. S. (2003). Learning disabilities. In I. B. Weiner (Ed.), *Handbook of psychology* (Vol. VI). New York: Wiley.

Siegler, R. (1996). *Emerging minds: The process of change in children's thinking.* New York: Oxford University Press.

Siegler, R., & Alibali, M. (2005). *Children's thinking.* Upper Saddle River, NJ: Prentice Hall.

Siegler, R. S. (1996). *Emerging minds: The process of change in children's thinking.* New York: Oxford University Press.

Siegler, R. S., DeLoache, J., & Eisenberg, N. (2006). *How children develop* (2nd ed.). New York: Worth.

Silliman, R. A., & Baeke, P. (1998). Breast cancer in the older woman. In L. Balducci, W. B. Ersher, & G. H. Lyman (Eds.), Comprehensive geriatric oncology. Amsterdam: Harwood.

Simon, Harvey B. (2007, May). *Harvard Men's Health Watch, 11*(10), 8.

Simons, D. J. (2007). Inattentional blindness *Scholarpedia, 2,* 3244. Retrieved from http://www.scholarpedia.org/article/Inattentional_blindness

Singleton, J. (2000, Summer). Women caring for elderly family members: Shaping non-traditional work and family initiatives. *Journal of Comparative Family Studies, 31*(3), 367–375.

Sleek, S. (1997). Weisel emphasizes need to thank elderly. *APA Monitor, 28*(10), 23.

Smith, K. (2000). Normal childbirth. In S. Mattson & J. Smith (Eds.), *Core curriculum for maternal–newborn nursing.* Philadelphia: Saunders.

Söderlund, H., Nyberg, L., Adolfsson, R., Nilsson, L., & Launer, L. J. (2003). High prevalence of white matter hyperintensities in normal aging: Relation to blood pressure and cognition. *Cortex, 39*(4–5), 1093–1105.

Solm, M. (2004). Freud returns. *Scientific American, 290*(5), 82–89.

Squire, L., & Kandel, E. (2000). *Memory: From mind to molecule.* New York: Scientific American Press.

Sternberg, R. (1990). *Metaphors of mind: Conceptions of the nature of intelligence.* New York: Cambridge University Press.

———. (2000). What's your love story? *Psychology Today, 32*(4), 52–59.

———. (2003). *Cognitive psychology.* Belmont, CA: Wadsworth/Thompson.

Sterns, H. L., & Miklos, S. M. (1995). The aging worker in a changing environment: Organizational and individual issues. *Journal of Vocational Behavior, 47*(2), 248–268.

Stice, E., Presenell, K., & Bearman, S. (2001). Relation of early menarche to depression, eating disorders, substance abuse, and comorbid psychopathology among adolescent girls. *Developmental Psychology, 37,* 608–619.

Storey, A. E., Walsh, C. J., Quinton, R. L., & Wynne-Edwards, K. E. (2000). Hormonal correlates of paternal responsiveness in new and expectant fathers. *Evolution and Human Behavior, 21,* 79–95.

Straus, M. A., & Paschall, M. J. (2009). Corporal punishment by mothers and development of children's cognitive ability: A longitudinal study of two nationally representative age cohorts. *Journal of Aggression, Maltreatment, & Trauma, 18*(5), 459–483.

Studelska, J. V. (2006, Spring). At home in birth. *Midwifery Today,* pp. 332–33.

Substance Abuse and Mental Health Services Administration (AMHSA). (2008). *Results from the 2008 National Survey on Drug Use and Health: National Findings.* Rockville, MD: Department of Health and Human Services.

Sudnow, D. (1967). *Passing on.* Englewood Cliffs, NJ: Prentice Hall.

Sugarman, L. (1986). *Lifespan development: Concepts, theories and interventions.* New York: Methuen.

Sullivan, J., Seem, D. L., & Chabalewski, F. (1999). Determining brain death. *Critical Care Nurse, 19*(2), 37–46.

Surjan, L., Devald, J., & Palfalvi, L. (1973). Epidemiology of hearing loss. *Audiology, 12,* pp. 396–410.

T

Taylor, S. E., Kelin, L. C., Lewis, B. P., Guenewald, T. L., Gurung, R. A., & Updegraff, J. A. (2000). Biobehavioral responses to stress in females: Tend-and-befriend, not fight-or-flight. *Psychological Review, 107,* 411–429.

Thompson, J. A., & Bunderson, J. S. (2001). Work–nonwork conflict and the phenomenology of time. *Work and Occupations, 28*(1), 17–39.

Thompson, L., & Kelly-Vance, L. (2001). The impact of mentoring on academic achievement of at-risk youth. *Children & Youth Services Review, 23,* 227–242.

Thompson, R. (1999). The individual child: Temperament, emotion, self, and personality. In M. Bornstein & M. Lamb (Eds.), *Developmental psychology: An advanced textbook.* Mahwah, NJ: Erlbaum.

Toussaint, L., & Webb, J. R. (2005). Gender differences in the relationship between empathy and forgiveness. *The Journal of Social Psychology, 145*(6), 673–686.

Toussaint, O. (2003). Normal brain aging: A commentary. *Neurobiology of Aging, 24* (Suppl. 1), S129–S130.

Tremblay, K., Piskosz, M., & Souza, P. (2003). Effects of age and age-related hearing loss on the neural representation of speech cues. *Clinical Neurophysiology, 114*(7), 1332–1343.

Twigg, J., & Atkin, K. (1994). *Careers perceived: Policy and practice in informal care.* Buckingham, England: Open University Press.

U

Unger, R., & Crawford, M. (2000). *Women and gender: A feminist psychology* (3rd ed.). New York: McGraw-Hill.

U.S. Census Bureau. (2005). *People.* Washington, DC: U.S. Government Printing Office.

U.S. Census Bureau, Population Division. (2004). *Annual estimates of the population by sex and five-year age groups for the United States: April 1, 2000 to July 1, 2003* (NC-EST2003-01). Retrieved from http://www.census.gov/popest/national/asrh/NC-EST2003/NC-EST2003-Q1.pdf

U.S. Department of Health, Education, and Welfare. (1992). *Vital Statistics of the United States, 1999–Mortality.* Vol. II (part A). Hyattsville, MD: Author.

V

Valliant, G. (2002). *Aging well.* Boston: Little, Brown.

Vaillant, G., & Mukamal, K. (2001, June). Successful aging. *American Journal of Psychiatry, 158*(6), 839–847.

Van der Heide, A., Deliens, L., Faisst, K., Nilstun, T., Norup, M., & Paci, E., et al. (2003). End-of-life decision-making in six European countries: Descriptive study. *The Lancet, 362*(9381), 345–350.

Vartanian, L., & Powlishta, K. (2001). Demand characteristics and self-report measures of imaginary audience sensitivity: Implications for interpreting age differences in adolescent egocentrism. *Journal of Genetic Psychology, 162,* 187–200.

Ventura, S. J. (2009). *Changing patterns of nonmarital childbearing in the United States* (NCHS Data Brief No. 18). Hyattsville, MD: National Center for Health Statistics.

Volling, B., McElwain, N., & Miller, A. (2002). Emotion regulation in context: The jealousy complex between young siblings and its relations with child and family characteristics. *Child Development, 73*(2), 581–600.

Von Eye, A., & Schuster, C. (2000). The odds of resilience. *Child Development, 71*(3), 563–566.

von Gunten, C., Ferris, F., & Emanuel, L. (2000). Ensuring competency in end-of-life care: Communication and relational skills. *Journal of the American Medical Association, 284,* 3051–3057.

Vygotsky, L. S. (1962). *Thought and language.* Cambridge, MA: MIT Press.

———. (1978). *Mind in society.* Cambridge, MA: Harvard University Press.

W

Wagster, M. V. (Interviewee). (2006). *Aging: Preventive maintenance for the brain* [Interview transcript]. Retrieved from Washington Post website: http://www.washingtonpost.com/wp-dyn/content/discussion/2006/02/17/D12006021701615.html

Walker-Barnes, C. J., & Mason, C. A. (2004). Delinquency and substance use among gang-involved youth: The moderating role of parenting practices. *American Journal of Community Psychology, 34*(3–4), 235–251.

Wallerstein, J., Lewis, J., & Blakeslee, S. (2002). *The unexpected legacy of divorce.* New York: Hyperion.

Watson, J. (2003). *DNA: The secret of life.* New York: Knopf.

Weeks, L. (2010, June 9). *In your Facebook: Social sites are everywhere.* Retrieved from http://www.npr.org/templates/story/story.php?storyId=127527648

Werner, E. (1995). Resilience in development. *Currents Directions in Psychological Science, 4,* 81–85.

Werner, E., & Smith, R. (1992). *Overcoming the odds: High-risk children from birth to adulthood.* Ithaca, NY: Cornell University Press.

———. (2001). *Journeys from childhood to midlife: Risk, resilience, and recovery.* New York: Cornell University Press.

Wertheimer, M. (1962). Psychomotor coordination of auditory-visual space at birth. *Science, 134,* 213–216.

Westerhof, G., & others. (2001, November). Beyond life satisfaction: Lay conceptions of well-being among middle-aged and elderly adults. *Social Indicators Research, 56*(2), 179–203.

Westin, D. Psychoanalytic theories. (2000). In A. Kazdin (Ed.), *Encyclopedia of psychology.* Washington, DC: American Psychological Association.

Whitbeck, L., & others. (2001). Deviant behavior and victimization among homeless and runaway adolescents. *Journal of Interpersonal Violence, 16,* 1175–1204.

Whitehead, B. D., & Popenoe, D. (2006). *The state of our unions: The social health of marriage in America.* New Brunswick, NJ: Rutgers University.

Whitehurst, G., & Lonigan, C. (1998). Child development and emergent literacy. *Child Development, 69,* 848–872.

Willat, J. (2005). *Making sense of children's drawings.* Mahwah, NJ: Erlbaum.

Wong, S. (2006). *Dialogic approaches to TESOL.* Mahwah, NJ: Erlbaum.

Wong, T. Y. (2001). Effect of increasing age on cataract surgery outcomes in very elderly patients. *British Medical Journal, 322*(7294), 1104.

Woodward, A., & Markman, E. (1998). Early word learning. In D. Kuhn & R. Siegler (Eds.), *Handbook of child psychology: Vol. 2.* New York: Wiley.

Woodward, L. (2001). Life course outcomes of young people with anxiety disorders in adolescence. *Journal of the American Academy of Child & Adolescent Psychiatry, 40,* 1086–1093.

Wright, D. R., & Fitzpatrick, K. M. (2006). Violence and minority youth: The effects of risk and asset factors on fighting among African American children and adolescents. *Adolescence, 41*(162), 251–263.

Wright, P. J. (2006). PDE5 inhibitors compared. *Journal of Men's Health and Gender, 3*(4), 410.

Wright, V. (1999). Sleeping in adult beds risky for kids under 2. *AAP News, 15*(11), 32.

———. (2000, February). Knowledge, counseling can help prevent job injuries among teens. Elk Grove Village, IL.: American Association of Pediatrics News.

Wyckoff, A. (1999). Physicians should not shy away from confronting parents: Consider religious, ethnic customs when diagnosing child abuse. *AAP News, 13*(5), 18–19.

Y

Yoder, K., & others. (2002). Event history analysis of antecedents to running away from home and being on the street. *American Behavioral Scientist. Special Issue: Advancing the Research Agenda on Homelessness: Politics and Realities, 45,* 51–65.

Yurgelun, Todd D. (1998, November/December). Brain abnormalities in chronic schizophrenia. *Psychology Today,* pp. 56–59.

Z

Zigler, E., & Finn-Stevenson, M. (1999). Applied developmental psychology. In M. Bornstein & M. Lamb (Eds.), *Developmental psychology: An advanced textbook.* Mahwah, NJ: Erlbaum.

Photo Credits

Chapter 1

Opener: Corbis; **4:** (top) © The Star-Ledger / John O'Boyle / The Image Works; (bottom) Front cover of "Choose Your Own Adventure", Book ® "Journey Under the Sea". © Chooseco, LLC.; **5:** (left) © Josef Polleross / The Image Works; (right) Courtesy of Lisa Fiore; **6:** Larry Downing / Reuters / Corbis; **8:** (left, top to bottom) Brand X Pictures / Punchstock; Laurence Mouton / Photoalto / Picturequest; Getty Images / SW Productions; Brornwyn Kidd / Getty Images; Digital Vision; Bananastock / AGE Fotostock; Blue Moon Stock / Alamy Images; Ryan McVay / Getty Images; **10:** Kimberley French © 2009 Summit Entertainment, LLC. All rights reserved; **12:** (left) iStockphoto.com / Oleg Kulakov; (middle) © Image Club; (right) Getty Images; **14:** Geoff Manasse / Getty Images; Getty Images / Digital Vision; © Ariel Skelley / BlendImages / Getty Images; Ryan McVay / Getty Images; © Punchstock / Brand X Pictures; BananaStock / JupiterImages; © BananaStock / SuperStock; Comstock Images; Doug Menuez / Getty Images; © Flying Colours Ltd / Getty Images; © Amos Morgan / Getty Images; **15:** Danita Delimont / Getty Images; **17:** Getty Images; **18:** Mark Garfinkel / Boston Herald / Polaris; **19:** Olivier Voisin / Photo Researchers, Inc.; **20:** © ITV / courtesy Everett Collection.

Chapter 2

Opener: David Sutherland / Getty Images; **28:** Golden Pixels LLC / Alamy; **29:** Bettmann / Corbis; **30:** © Lebrecht / The Image Works; **30:** HBO / courtesy Everett Collection; **32:** Ted Streshinsky / TIME & LIFE Images / Getty Images; **33:** Nigel Parry / Hallmark / The Kobal Collection; **34:** (top) Bill Anderson / Photo Researchers, Inc.; (bottom) Dirk Anschutz / Getty Images; **35:** Carol Guzy / The Washington Post via Getty Images; **36:** Courtesy of James Wertsch; **37:** Wolfgang Kaehler / Corbis; **38:** Creatas / PictureQuest; © iStockphoto.com / Geopaul; **39:** Getty Images; **40:** Nina Leen / Time & Life Pictures / Getty Images; Jon Brenneis / Time & Life Pictures / Getty Images; **41:** (top) Peter Dazeley / Getty Images; (bottom) Courtesy of Albert Bandura; **42:** Courtesy of Cornell University; **46:** Juan Carlos Ulate / Reuters / Corbis; **46:** (clockwise) © iStockphoto.com / Grzegorz Lepiarz; Brand X Pictures/Punchstock; © Digital Vision; Brand X Pictures; © Brooke Fasani / Corbis; © Digital Vision; (bottom of page) Juan Carlos Ulate / Reuters / Corbis.

Chapter 3

Opener: Gareth Brown / Corbis; **54:** (top left) © Anatomical Travelogue / Photo Researchers, Inc.; (top right) Custom Medical Stock Photo; Custom Medical Stock Photo; **55:** Hulton Archive / Getty Images; **58:** Markus Moellenberg / Corbis; **59:** (left) © iStockphoto.com / Jaroslaw Wojcik; (right) iStockphoto.com / Zirafek; **60:** (top) Eye of Science / Photo Researchers, Inc.; **61:** © Peter Arnold, Inc / Alamy; **62:** (top) Robin Layton/file/ AP Images; (bottom) Photo Researchers, Inc.; **64:** Noah K. Murray / Star Ledger / Corbis; **65:** © Andy Walker, Midland Fertility Services / Photo Researchers, Inc.; **66:** © Biophoto Associates / Photo Researchers, Inc.; **67:** © Petit Format / Photo Researchers, Inc.; **68:** © HK / A.B. / Corbis; **69:** (bottom) Stockbyte / Getty Images; (top) Courtesy of Alex Ambrose; **71:** GK Hart / Vikki Hart / Getty Images; **73:** PhotoLink / Getty Images; **74:** (top) Barbara Walton / epa / Corbis; (bottom) Andersen Ross / Getty Images.

Chapter 4

Opener: Karen D'Silva / Getty Images; **80:** David Young-Wolff / Alamy; **81:** Larry Williams / Corbis; **82:** Tom Grill / Getty Images; **83:** (top) © Marjorie Shostak / AnthroPhoto; (bottom) Mark Richards / Photo Edit; **84:** (top) Brand X Pictures / Getty Images; (bottom) The McGraw-Hill Companies, Inc. / Jill Braaten, photographer; **85:** Punchstock / BananaStock; **87:** Courtesy of NATUS; **88:** © David Bacon / The Image Works; **89:** (top) Shaun Best / Reuters / Corbis; (bottom) Louie Psihoyos/ Corbis; **90:** Rasha Madkour / AP Images; **91:** Courtesy of Dr. Tiffany Field from Field, et al., Model and Infant Expression from "Discrimination and Imitation of Facial Expressions by Neonates) in Science, fig.2, Vol.218; **93:** (top left) © Elizabeth Crews / The Image Works; (top middle) © Elizabeth Crews / The Image Works; (top right) DAJ / Getty Images; (bottom left) © Elizabeth Crews / The Image Works; (bottom middle) Jennie Woodcock; Reflections Photolibrary / Corbis; (bottom right) Laura Dwight / Corbis; **94:** altrendo images; **95:** John Sciulli / Getty Images; **96:** © 2010 Fisher Wallace Laboratories, LLC.

Chapter 5

Opener: Gavin Kingcome Photography / Getty Images; **102:** Laura and the watch from the Exhibition "The Hundred Languages of Children", Reggio Emilia Municipal Infant-Toddler Centers and Preschools Archives; **104:** Diane Mcdonald / Getty Images; **107:** (top) YOSHIKAZU TSUNO / AFP / Getty Images; (bottom) © Marc Steinmetz / Visum / The Image Works; **108:** (top, left to right): Barbara Penoyar / Getty Images; Digital Vision / Getty Images; © Image Source / Alamy; Titus / Getty Images; © Digital Vision; Bananastock / PictureQuest; Corbis / PictureQuest; © Brand X Pictures / PunchStock; (bottom) Tom & Dee Ann McCarthy / Corbis; **110:** Courtesy of Alex Ambrose; PNC / Getty Images; Corbis / PictureQuest; **111:** (top) Courtesy of Kiss & Bajs; Courtesy of David Linton; **112:** Mark Richards / PhotoEdit Inc.; **114:** © Ellen B. Senisi / The Image Works; **115:** Simons, D. J., & Chabris, C. F. (1999). Gorillas in our midst: Sustained inattentional blindness for dynamic events. Perception, 28, 1059-1074. Figure provided by Daniel Simons © 1999 Daniel J. Simons. All rights reserved. Image may not be distributed or posted online without written permission; **116:** Photodisc Collection / Getty Images; **117:** © Walt Disney Studios Motion Pictures / courtesy Everett Collection; **119:** Tetra Images / Corbis; **121:** Nina Leen / Time & Life Pictures / Getty Images; Jose Luis Pelaez Inc. / Getty Images; **122:** (top left) Nina Leen / Time & Life Pictures / Getty Images; (top right) Cam Barker / Getty Images; (bottom) Nina Leen / Time & Life Pictures / Getty Images; **124:** Image Source / Getty Images.

Chapter 6

Opener: Smith Collection / Getty Images; **131:** © Ellen B. Senisi / The Image Works; **132:** The McGraw-Hill Companies Inc. / Ken Cavanagh Photographer; **134:** © Jim Pickerell / The Image Works; **135:** © Ellen B. Senisi / The Image Works; **136:** BananaStock / PunchStock; **137:** (top) Mary Altaffer / AP Images; (bottom) © David Young-Wolff / Photo Edit; **138:** (top) © IT Stock Free; (bottom) Photodisc Collection / Getty Images; **139:** (top) Paul Popper / Popperfoto / Getty Images; (bottom) Courtesy of the Reggio Emilia Municipal Infant-Toddler Centers and Preschools Archives; **140:** (top) Najlah Feanny / Corbis; (bottom) Image Source / Getty Images; **142:** Leora Kahn; **143:** Royalty-Free / Corbis; **144:** Purestock / PunchStock; **145:** The Kobal Collection / Walt Disney Pictures; **147:** The McGraw-Hill Companies, Inc. / Ken Karp photographer; **148:** Peter Zander / Getty Images; **150:** Mick Tsikas / Reuters / Corbis; Courtesy of Lisa Fiore.

Chapter 7

Opener: Neil Beckerman / Getty Images; **156**: (left) © Comstock/Alamy; (right) Richard Hutchings/Digital Light Source; **157**: Stockbyte / PunchStock; **158**: (top) © John Birdsall / The Image Works; (bottom) © Bill Bachmann / The Image Works; **159**: (top) Fancy / Veer; (bottom left) PNC/ Corbis; (bottom right) Ryan McVay / Getty Images; (bottom) PNC / Corbis; **160**: © Allan Tannenbaum / The Image Works; **161**: Getty Images / Photodisc; **162**: © Ellen B. Senisi / The Image Works; **163**: © Marty Heitner / The Image Works; **164**: (top, left to right) Alexandra Buxbaum / Retna Ltd. / Corbis; Relativity, 1953, Lithograph by M.C. Escher. ©Topham / The Image Works; Christian Hartmann / Reuters / Corbis; (bottom, clockwise) Laurence Mouton / Getty Images; Barbara Penoyar / Getty Images; Mark Andersen / Getty Images; © Thinkstock / Masterfile; Paul Edmondson / Getty Images; © Corbis; Mel Curtis / Getty Images; Halfdark / Getty Images; **165**: © Bob Daemmrich / The Image Works; **168**: (top) © Cameron / Corbis; (middle) Amos Morgan/Getty Images; (bottom) © iStockphoto.com/Catherine Lane; **169**: Courtesy of Lisa Fiore; **173**: Maya Barnes Johansen / The Image Works; **174**: Eric Charbonneau / Getty Images; **175**: © JGI / Tom Grill / Blend Images / Corbis; **176**: © BananaStock/PunchStock; **177**: IT Stock / PunchStock; **179**: RubberBall Productions; **180**: The Kobal Collection / Celador Films.

Chapter 8

Opener: Digital Vision / Getty Images; **186**: Bryan Bedder / Getty Images; **187**: (left) Image Source / JupiterImages; (right) © Brand X Pictures / PunchStock; **189**: Leonard McLane / Getty Images; **191**: Don Arnold / Getty Images; **193**: © Brand X Pictures / PunchStock; **195**: © PhotoAlto / PunchStock; **196**: (top) © iStockphoto.com / Ju-Lee; (bottom) James A. Finley / AP Images; **198**: © K Doepner / SV-Bilderdienst / The Image Works; **200**: © PhotoAlto / PictureQuest; **201**: Joey Foley / Getty Images; **202**: BananaStock / PunchStock.

Chapter 9

Opener: Roberto Westbrook / Getty Images; **208**: (top) © WWD / Conde Nast / Corbis; (bottom) © iStockphoto.com / Redmal; **209**: (bottom) Richard T. Nowitz / Corbis; (top) Hugh Sitton / Corbis; **210**: (left) RubberBall Productions; (right) RubberBall Productions; **211**: Wally McNamee / Corbis; **212**: Dan Galic / Alamy; **214**: (top) Charles Sykes / AP Images; (bottom) Ed Kashi / Corbis; **215**: © Robb D. Cohen / Retna Ltd. / Corbis; **217**: Mike Coppola / Getty Images; **218**: Natalie Fobes / Corbis; **223**: © BananaStock / PictureQuest; **224**: Corbis / PunchStock.

Chapter 10

Opener: Andersen Ross / Getty Images; **232**: (top) Lee Celano / Getty Images; (bottom left) Chris Pizzello / AP Images; (bottom right) © Qi Heng / XinHua / Xinhua Press / Corbis; **233**: Ryan McVay / Getty Images; **234**: (left) Photoshot / Everett Collection, (UFT_149389_0002); (right) © PhotoAlto / Alix Minde; **235**: (top) © iStockphoto.com / Daniel R. Burch; (bottom) © 2007 Getty Images, Inc.; **236**: © Esbin-Anderson / The Image Works; **237**: © Comstock / Alamy; **241**: (top) Shawn Thew / epa / Corbis; (bottom) John Kelly / Getty Images; **242**: Martha Holmes / Time-Life Pictures / Getty Images; **243**: (top) Getty Images; (bottom) Digital Vision / Getty Images; **244**: © The Star-Ledger / Ben Solomon / The Image Works; **246**: The McGraw-Hill Companies, Inc. / Jill Braaten, photographer; **247**: © iStockphoto.com / Bitter; © iStockphoto.com / Sxasher; **248**: Digital Vision / Getty Images; **250**: ©iStockphoto.com / Anton Seleznev.

Chapter 11

Opener: Ronnie Kaufman / Larry Hirshowitz / Blend Images / Corbis; **256**: Erik S. Lesser / Getty Images; **257**: (left) Ken Usami / Getty Images; (right) © iStockphoto.com / Justin Sneddon; **259**: Alvis Upitis / Getty Images; **260**: © St Petersburg Times / Melissa Lyttle / The Image Works; **261**: (left) Cordelia Molloy / Photo Researchers, Inc.; (right) Jonah Light / Getty Images; **263**: Pasieka / Photo Researchers, Inc.; **265**: (top) Bloomberg via Getty Images; (bottom left) Ariel Skelly / Getty Images; (bottom right) Getty Images; **269**: Columbia / Tri-Star / The Kobal Collection / Marshak, Bob; **272**: TWPhoto / Corbis; **273**: © iStockphoto.com / Lisa F. Young.

Chapter 12

Opener: Lisa Stirling / Getty Images; **281**: (top) ImageSource / Getty Images; (bottom) Lund-Diephuis / Getty Images; **282**: (top) The McGraw-Hill Companies, Inc. / Photo by Chris Hammond; (bottom) Alfred Pasieka / Photo Researchers, Inc. **283**: © Rubberball / Corbis; **284**: (top) Mohammed Abed / AFP / Getty Images; (bottom) © Karen Kasmauski / Science Faction / Corbis; **285**: Peter Foley / Pool / epa / Corbis; **287**: The Kobal Collection / HBO; **288**: © Erin Paul Donovan / Alamy; **289**: © Erin Paul Donovan / Alamy; **290**: Tim Boyles / Getty Images; **294**: Photo by Gary Kramer, USDA Natural Resources Conservation Service.

Chapter 13

Opener: Thomas Northcut / Getty Images; **302**: (bottom) Justin Sullivan / Getty Images; (top) Royalty-Free / Corbis; **303**: Steve Liss / Getty Images; **305**: Rick Friedman / Corbis; **306**: (top) © Darrin Klimek / GettyImages; (middle) © Andersen Ross / Getty Images; (bottom) © Image Source; **307**: © Noah Addis / Star Ledger / Corbis; **309**: Jim West / The Image Works.

Text Credits

Chapter 1

Table 1.1: From *Human Development Across the Lifespan*, 7th edition by John Dacey, John Travers, and Lisa Fiore. Copyright © 2009 The McGraw-Hill Companies, Inc. Reprinted with permission. **Fig. 1.1**: From *Human Development Across the Lifespan*, 7th edition by John Dacey, John Travers, and Lisa Fiore. Copyright © 2009 The McGraw-Hill Companies, Inc. Reprinted with permission. **Fig. 1.2**: From *Life Span Development*, 11th edition by John W. Santrock. Copyright © 2008 The McGraw-Hill Companies, Inc. Reprinted with permission. **Fig. 1.3**: From *SOC*, 1st edition by Jon Witt. Copyright © 2009 The McGraw-Hill Companies, Inc. Reprinted with permission. **Fig. 1.4**: From *Human Development Across the Lifespan*, 7th edition by John Dacey, John Travers, and Lisa Fiore. Copyright © 2009 The McGraw-Hill Companies, Inc. Reprinted with permission.

Chapter 2

Fig. 2.3: From *The Child: Development in the Social Context* by Claire B. Kopp. Copyright © 1982. Printed and electronically reproduced by permission of Pearson Education, Inc., Upper Saddle River, New Jersey. **Table 2.1**: Adapted from *Childhood and Society* by Erik H. Erikson. Copyright © 1950, 1963 by W.W. Norton & Company, Inc., renewed © 1978, 1991 by Erik H. Erikson. Reprinted with permission. **Fig. 2.4**: From "Changing organism – context relations as the basic process of development: A developmental perspective" by Richard M.

Lerner in *Developmental Psychology*, Vol. 27, pp. 27-32. Copyright © 1991 American Psychological Association. **Table 2.4:** From *Human Development Across the Lifespan*, 7th edition by John Dacey, John Travers, and Lisa Fiore. Copyright © 2009 The McGraw-Hill Companies, Inc. Reprinted with permission.

Chapter 3

Fig. 3.2: From *Human Development Across the Lifespan*, 7th edition by John Dacey, John Travers, and Lisa Fiore. Copyright © 2009 The McGraw-Hill Companies, Inc. Reprinted with permission. **Fig. 3.3:** From *Human Development Across the Lifespan*, 7th edition by John Dacey, John Travers, and Lisa Fiore. Copyright © 2009 The McGraw-Hill Companies, Inc. Reprinted with permission. **Fig. 3.4:** From "Corrections to maternal age – specific live birth prevalence of Down's Syndrome" by J. Morris, D. Mutton, and E. Alberman in *Journal of Medical Screening*, 12 (4), 2005, p. 202. Permission granted by the Royal Society of Medicine Press, London. **Fig. 3.5:** Adapted from "Why do humans have so few genes?" by Elizabeth Pennisi in *Science*, Vol. 309, No. 5731, p. 80. July 1, 2005. Copyright © 2005, The American Association for the Advancement of Science. Reprinted with permission. **Fig. 3.6:** From *The Growing Child* by John F. Travers. Published by Scott, Foresman and Company, Glenview, IL, 1982. Reprinted by permission of the author. **Fig. 3.7:** From "Suffer Little Children" in *The Economist*, June 25, 2009. Copyright © The Economist Newspaper Limited, London 2009. Reprinted with permission. **Fig. 3.8:** Teratogens and the Timing of Their Effects on Prenatal Development adapted from K.L. Moore and T.V.N. Persaud from *Before We Are Born*, p. 130. J.B. Saunders, 1992. Copyright © 1993, with permission from Elsevier.

Chapter 4

Fig. 4.4: From "Breaking the Cycle of Poverty: Reducing the Disparities in Children's Achievement Will Require Reaching Beyond the Educational System" by L. Olson in *Education Week, 17*, pp. 20-22, 24, 26-27. As first appeared in *Quality Counts 2007*. Reprinted with permission from Editorial Projects in Education. **Fig. 4.5:** Adapted from "A Proposal for a New Method of Evaluation of a Newborn Infant" by Virginia A. Apgar in *Anesthesia and Analgesia*, Vol. 21, pp. 260-267, 1975. **Fig. 4.6:** From *Child Development*, 10th edition by John W. Santrock. Copyright © 2004 The McGraw-Hill Companies, Inc. Reprinted with permission. **Fig. 4.7:** Figure 1 from "Changing Patterns of Nonmarital Childbearing in the United States" by Stephanie J. Ventura, M.A., Division of Vital Statistics. NCHS Data Brief, No. 18, May 2009, Centers for Disease Control and Prevention.

Chapter 5

Fig. 5.1: From "U.S. Still Struggling with Infant Mortality" by Nicholas Bakalar in *The New York Times*, April 6, 2009. Copyright © The New York Times Company. All rights reserved. Used with permission. **Fig. 5.2:** From *Children*, 9th edition by John W. Santrock. Copyright © 2007 The McGraw-Hill Companies, Inc. Reprinted with permission. **Fig. 5.3:** From *Human Development Across the Lifespan*, 7th edition by John Dacey, John Travers, and Lisa Fiore. Copyright © 2009 The McGraw-Hill Companies, Inc. Reprinted with permission. **Fig. 5.5:** From "The Denver Development Screening Test" by W.K. Frankenburg and J.B. Dodds in *Journal of Pediatrics*, 71, August 1967, pp. 181-191. Copyright © 1967, Elsevier. Reprinted with permission. **Fig. 5.6:** From *Child Development*, 11th edition by John W. Santrock. Copyright © 2007 The McGraw-Hill Companies, Inc. Reprinted with permission. **Fig. 5.7:** From *Human Development Across the Lifespan*,

7th edition by John Dacey, John Travers, and Lisa Fiore. Copyright © 2009 The McGraw-Hill Companies, Inc. Reprinted with permission. **Fig. 5.8:** From *Child Development*, 10th edition by John W. Santrock. Copyright © 2004 The McGraw-Hill Companies, Inc. Reprinted with permission.

Chapter 6

Fig. 6.4: From *Human Development*, 7th edition by Diane Papalia and Sally Olds. Copyright © 1998 The McGraw-Hill Companies, Inc. Reprinted with permission. **Fig. 6.6:** From *Educational Psychology: Theory and Practice*, 6th edition by Robert E. Slavin. Copyright © 2000, 1997, 1994, 1991, 1988, 1986 by Allyn & Bacon. **Fig. 6.8:** From "The Effects of Corporal Punishment. Corporal Punishment by Mothers and Development of Children's Cognitive Ability: A Longitudinal Study of Two Nationally Representative Age Cohorts" by Murray A. Straus and Mallie J. Paschall in *Journal of Aggression, Maltreatment & Trauma*, 18:459-483. Copyright © 2009 Taylor & Francis Group LLC. Reprinted by permission of the authors. **Fig. 6.9:** From Chart E, p. 32 in "Perceived Importance of Playful and Creative Activities," *Crisis in the Kindergarten: Why Children Need to Play in School* by Edward Miller and Joan Almon. College Park, MD: Alliance for Childhood, 2009.

Chapter 7

Fig. 7.1: "Breakdown of Uninsured Children by Race, Ethnicity 2006" from *Racial and Ethnic Disparities*. Copyright © 2010 Children's Defense Fund. All rights reserved. **Fig. 7.3:** From *Human Development Across the Lifespan*, 7th edition by John Dacey, John Travers, and Lisa Fiore. Copyright © 2009 The McGraw-Hill Companies, Inc. Reprinted with permission. **p. 161:** Prescription Drug Usage in Children with ADHD or LD, 2004-2006 in "Patterns of Diagnosed ADHD and LD, 1997-2006" by Somnath Pal in *U.S. Pharmacist*, November 18, 2008. Reprinted with permission. **Fig. 7.7:** Reprinted with permission of Greg Kearsley, Theory into Practice. **Fig. 7.8:** From Artful Thinking Project, Project Zero, Harvard Graduate School of Education. Reprinted with permission. **Fig. 7.9:** Reprinted with permission of Hispanic Marketing and Public Relations (HispanicMPR.com). **Fig. 7.10:** From "Ecology of the family as a context for human development: Research perspectives" by Urie Bronfenbrenner in *Developmental Psychology*, 22, (2) pp. 723-742. Copyright © 1986 American Psychological Association. **Fig. 7.11:** From *Life Span Development*, 11th edition by John W. Santrock. Copyright © 2008 The McGraw-Hill Companies, Inc. Reprinted with permission.

Chapter 8

Fig. 8.4: From *Human Development Across the Lifespan*, 7th edition by John Dacey, John Travers, and Lisa Fiore. Copyright © 2009 The McGraw-Hill Companies, Inc. Reprinted with permission. **Fig. 8.5:** Rate of height increase, p. 4.4 in *Introduction to Coaching Theory*, written and edited by Peter J.L. Thompson, Copyright © International Amateur Athletic Federation, 1991. Reprinted with permission. **Fig. 8.6:** From *Life Span Development*, 11th edition by John W. Santrock. Copyright © 2008 The McGraw-Hill Companies, Inc. Reprinted with permission.

Chapter 9

Fig. 9.8: New York Times: http://thenewcivilrightsmovement.com/wp-content/uploads/2009/12/nyt/.jpg. With permission.

Chapter 10

Fig. 10.2: Patterns of Alcohol Use by Sex in Middle-Aged and Elderly Adults in "The Epidemiology of At-Risk and Binge Drinking Among Middle-Aged and Elderly Community Adults: National Survey on Drug Use and Health" by Dan G. Blazer and Li-Tzy Wu, *American Journal of Psychiatry,* October 2009; 166: 1162-1169, Fig. 1, p. 2. Copyright © 2009 American Psychiatric Association. Reprinted with permission. **Fig. 10.4**: Reprinted by permission of Mark Rice/Ranking America (http://rankingamerica.workplace.com.) **Fig. 10.5**: From *Life Span Development*, 11th edition by John W. Santrock. Copyright © 2008 The McGraw-Hill Companies, Inc. Reprinted with permission. **Fig. 10.6**: From *Life Span Development*, 11th edition by John W. Santrock. Copyright © 2008 The McGraw-Hill Companies, Inc. Reprinted with permission. **Fig. 10.7**: From *Human Development Across the Lifespan*, 7th edition by John Dacey, John Travers, and Lisa Fiore. Copyright © 2009 The McGraw-Hill Companies, Inc. Reprinted with permission.

Chapter 11

Fig. 11.2: From *Developmental Physiology and Aging* by Paola S. Timiras. Copyright © 1972. Macmillan. Used with permission. **Fig. 11.3**: From *Human Development Across the Lifespan*, 7th edition by John Dacey, John Travers, and Lisa Fiore. Copyright © 2009 The McGraw-Hill Companies, Inc. Reprinted with permission.

Chapter 12

Fig. 12.2: Drawing by inventor Franz Vester, first published in 1868. **Fig. 12.3**: From *Life Span Development*, 11th edition by John W. Santrock. Copyright © 2008 The McGraw-Hill Companies, Inc. Reprinted with permission. **Fig. 12.4**: Erin N. Perdu, AICP, GISP, Principal, ENP & Associates. Reprinted with permission.

Chapter 13

Fig. 13.1: From *SOC*, 1st edition by Jon Witt. Copyright © 2009 The McGraw-Hill Companies, Inc. Reprinted with permission.

duration of marriages that end in, 247f
emotional, 247
increase in rates of, 222–223
in middle adulthood, 247
rate of, 144, 248
Dixon, R., 44
Dizygotic (fraternal) twins, 61, 259
DNA (deoxyribonucleic acid), 54
    Human Genome Project, 59
    mitosis and, 56
    mutation and, 56
Dobratz, M.C., 291
Doctor of philosophy (PhD), 306
Doctor of psychology (PsyD), 306
Doctors without Borders, 302
Dodge, K., 175
DONA International, 84
Dorn, L.D., 190
Double helix, 54
Doulas, 84
Downsizing, 249
Down syndrome, 57–58, 166
Drake, P., 70, 80
Drawings, children's, 151
Driving, by the elderly, 261
Drug use. see also Substance abuse
    adolescent sexual behavior and, 196–197
    during pregnancy, 73–74
Dual-career family, 225
Dualism, 215
Duncan, G., 177
Dunham, Ann, 6
Dunne, K., 284
Dunn, K.M., 268
Durex Global Sex Survey, 237
Dusseldorp, E., 197
Dychtwald, K., 273

E

Eagle, M., 31
Early adulthood, 207–226
    careers and, 223–226
    characteristics of, 8t
    cognitive development during, 214–216
    cohabitation during, 221–222
    friendship during, 220
    gender roles and, 216–218
    health and, 211–214
    initiation rites, 208–210
    love relationships during, 220–221
    marriage and, 221–222
    physical development during, 210–214
    rape and sexual harassment in, 214
    sexual behavior during, 218
    social development during, 218–221
    suicide and, 292
Early childhood, 130–151
    artwork and, 150–151
    brain development during, 130–131
    characteristics of, 8t, 130
    cognitive development during, 133–138
    development of self during, 141

education, 138–140
    gender development during, 146–147
    information-processing theory on, 136–137
    language development during, 140–141
    motor skill development during, 132
    physical development during, 130–133
    Piaget's preoperational stage, 133–135
    play and, 149–150
    social development during, 141–145
    Vygotsky's theory on, 136
Early childhood education, 138–140
    constructivist approach, 138–139
    Head Start program, 139–140
    Montessori approach, 139
    Reggio Emilia approach, 139
Early Head Start, 68
Early-onset trajectory, 201
Eastman, P., 263
Eating disorders, 190–191
Eating habits, 158, 211. see also Nutrition
Eccles, J., 176
Ecological model of teachers' knowledge and beliefs, 176f
Ectoderm, 65–66
Edelman, Marion Wright, 305
Education. see also Schools
    of children, 303
    early childhood, 138–140
    English language learners and, 171–172
    infant/toddler, 102
    parental expectations and, 178
    sex, 198–199
    socioeconomic status and outcomes in, 177
    for special needs children, 162
Education for All Handicapped Children Act (IDEA) (1990), 162
Edwards, C.P., 139
EEG (electroencephalogram), 105, 282
Efron, Zac, 208
Eggs (reproductive), 61–62
Ego, 30
Egocentric speech, 116, 117
Egocentrism, 112, 134, 192–193
Eisenberg, N., 143, 146
Ejaculation, first, 189
Elaboration, 167
Elder, Glen, 44, 240
Elderly, the. see also Aging; Later adulthood
    driving by, 261
    opinions about, 257
Electroencephalogram (EEG), 105, 282
Electronic book readers, 266
Elementary processes, 36
Eliot, E., 106
Eliot, Lise, 133
Elkind, D., 192, 193
Ellis, B.J., 190
Emanuel, L., 290
Emberley, R., 172
Embryonic period, 65–67

Emde, R., 119
Emergent readers, 170–171
Emerging adulthood, 208
Emery, R., 179
Emotional abuse (of children), 179
Emotional divorce, 247
Emotional expressions, 13, 120–121
Emotions. see also Grief
    defined, 120
    dying process and, 287–288
    in infancy, 119–121
    play and, 149–150
    during pregnancy, 68–69
Employment. See Careers; Work
Empty nest syndrome, 247
Endoderm, 66
English language learners (ELLs)
    culturally sensitive practice and, 172
    number of, 171
    teaching language to, 171–172
    test scores of, 171f
Environmental factors
    genes and, 55
    in infant brain development, 107
    language development and, 119
    operant conditioning theory on, 39
Environment, goodness of fit between temperament and, 123
Epidural blocks, 84
Epigenetic view, 13
Episiotomy, 81
Equilibration, 36, 38t
Erectile dysfunction (ED), 238, 268
Erikson, Erik, 22, 32–33, 141, 173, 194, 219–220, 244, 245, 267
Eriksson, Peter, 265
Erin Brockovich (film), 242
Erling, A., 219
Ethical development, during early adulthood, 215
Ethics of care, 169
Ethnicity. see also Race
    adolescent suicide and, 199
    life expectancy and, 257
    onset of puberty and, 190
Ethology, 121
European Society for Human Reproduction and Embryology, 65
Euthanasia, 288–289
Evening (film), 264
Evolutionary developmental psychology, 44–45
Evolutionary psychology, 216–217
Exceptional children, 162
Excretory system, 66
Executive functioning, 193
Exercise
    in early adulthood, 212
    during pregnancy, 68
Exosystem, 43
Experiential components, 164
Experiments, on attachments, 121–122. see also Research

Trait theorists, 245
Transitivity, 162
Treatment (manipulative experiments), 19
Tremblay, K., 264
Triangular theory of love, 221
Triarchic theory of intelligence, 164–165
Turner syndrome, 58
Twain, Mark, 244
Twigg, J., 270
Twilight (film), 190
Twilight (Meyer), 9–10
Twilight Zone (television series), 268
Twins, 61–62, 259
Two-word sentences, 117

U

Ultrasound, 67
Umbilical cord, 64
Unconscious, the (Freudian theory), 29
Unemployment, 308
Unger, R., 146
UNICEF, 302
Uninsured children, in the U.S., 156f
Uninvolved/neglectful parenting, 142, 143
United Nations Convention on the Rights of the Child, 149
Unmarried women, births to, 96–97, 97f
Unoccupied play, 148
Unresolved grief, 285–286
Up (film), 309
U.S. Bureau of Labor Statistics, 306
U.S. Census Bureau, 222, 257, 271
U.S. Department of Health and Human Services, 122, 270
U.S. Department of Health, Education, and Welfare, 22
U.S. Department of Justice, 214
U.S. Prevention Services Task Force, 233
Uterine contractions, 81

V

Vacuum extractor, 86
Vaillant, George, 11, 20, 245–246, 256
Validation, 221
Van der Heide, A., 290
Variables
  dependent, 19
  independent, 19
  in manipulative experiments, 18–19
Vartanian, L., 192
Vegetarian diet, 158
Viagra, 238, 268
Videatives, 134
Violence
  gang, 201
  spanking and, 41
  television, 178
  youth, 201–202
Virtual fitness, 236

Vision
  in later adulthood, 260–261
  in middle adulthood, 234
  of neonates, 91–92
Vision Quest (initiation rite), 209
Visual literacy, 171
Visual perception, in infancy, 111–112
Vitamin supplements, life expectancy and, 17
Vocabulary, in middle childhood, 169
Volling, B., 120
Von Eye, A., 180
Von Gunten, C., 290
Voter turnout, 308–309, 308f
Vygotsky, Lev, 36–37, 115–116, 136, 138, 149, 192

W

Wagster, Molly, 264
Wahlsten, Douglas, 44
Walkabout (initiation rite), 209
Walker-Barnes, C.J., 201
Walking, in infancy, 109
Walk, R., 111–112
Wallerstein, Judith, 144
Walters, R., 40
War of the Roses (film), 248
War on Poverty, 139
"Water breaking," 80
Waterpipes, 213–214
Watson, John, 39
Webb, J.R., 217
Websites
  on aging process, 13
  on chromosomes, 57
  on humanitarian actions, 302
  on pregnancy, birth, and child rearing, 70
Wedekind, Frank, 186
Weeks, L., 301
Weidner, W., 238
Weight. see also Overweight
  adolescence and, 189
  in early adulthood, 210
  infant, 118t
  of newborn, 103
Weight gain, during pregnancy, 68
Weinberg, R., 44
Werner, E., 90, 179, 180
Werner, Emmy, 4–5
Werner, P., 270
Wernicke's area (brain), 118f
Wertheimer, Michael, 92
Westerhof, 256
Westin, D., 31
When Harry Met Sally (film), 220
Whitbeck, L., 199
Whitehead, B.D., 222
Whitehurst, G., 170
"Why" questions, 4
Widowhood, 269
Wiebe, R., 200
Wiesel, Eli, 272
Wii Fit, 236

Wii, the, 270
Wikis, 177
Wild Strawberries (film), 267
Willat, J., 150
Willis, Sherry, 239
Wilson, E.O., 293–294
Wisdom, 266
Women. see also Females
  childless, 63
  feminist movement and, 215
  in the labor force, 225–226
  menopause in, 237–238
  rape and sexual harassment of, 214
  sexual changes in, 236–237
  thinking of, portrayed in films, 216
Wong, S., 172
Wong, T.Y., 260
Woodward, A., 116
Woodward, L., 199
Woolf, Virginia, 18
Word spurt, 116, 117
WordTwist (online game), 194
Work
  best jobs in America, 2009, 307t
  dual-career family, 225–226
  Family Medical Leave Act (FMLA), 97, 309
  in later adulthood, 272–273
  patterns of work in middle adulthood, 249
  work-family conflict and, 249
World AIDS Orphans Day, 284
World Health Organization, 233
World Resources Institute, 302
Wright, Frank Lloyd, 225
Wright, P.J., 238
Wright, V., 201
Wu, 234
Wyckoff, A., 179
Wynne-Edwards, K., 80

X

X chromosome, 58
XYY syndrome, 58

Y

Yang, Y., 257
Yoder, K., 199
You Can Count on Me (film), 249
Young adulthood, suicide and, 292. see also Early adulthood
Youth Risk Behavior Survey (YRBS), 197
YouTube, 43
Yurgelun, T., 192

Z

Zidovudine (ZDV), 72
Zigler, E., 145
Zone of proximal development (ZPD), 37, 136
Zygote, 54, 56, 64